HEALING WITH POISONS

Healing with Poisons

Potent Medicines in Medieval China

YAN LIU

UNIVERSITY OF WASHINGTON PRESS

Seattle

Healing with Poisons was made possible in part by a grant from the Traditional Chinese Culture and Society Book Fund, established through generous gifts from Patricia Buckley Ebrey and Thomas Ebrey.

Additional support was provided by grants from the Chiang Ching-kuo Foundation for International Scholarly Exchange and the Julian Park Publication Fund of the College of Arts and Sciences at the University at Buffalo.

This book is freely available in an open access edition thanks to TOME (Toward an Open Monograph Ecosystem)—a collaboration of the Association of American Universities, the Association of University Presses, and the Association of Research Libraries—and the generous support of the University at Buffalo Libraries. Learn more at the TOME website, available at: openmonographs.org.

Design by Katrina Noble
Composed in Minion Pro, typeface designed by Robert Slimbach

25 24 23 22 21   5 4 3 2 1

Printed and bound in the United States of America

UNIVERSITY OF WASHINGTON PRESS
uwapress.uw.edu

LIBRARY OF CONGRESS CATALOGING-IN-PUBLICATION DATA
Names: Liu, Yan (Cultural historian) author.
Title: Healing with poisons : potent medicines in medieval China / Yan Liu.
Description: Seattle : University of Washington Press, [2021] | Includes bibliographical references and index.
Identifiers: LCCN 2020052168 (print) | LCCN 2020052169 (ebook) | ISBN 9780295749006 (hardcover) | ISBN 9780295748993 (paperback) | ISBN 9780295749013 (ebook)
Subjects: LCSH: Medicine, Chinese. | Traditional medicine.
Classification: LCC R601 .L583 2021 (print) | LCC R601 (ebook) | DDC 610.951—dc23
LC record available at https://lccn.loc.gov/2020052168
LC ebook record available at https://lccn.loc.gov/2020052169

The paper used in this publication is acid free and meets the minimum requirements of American National Standard for Information Sciences—Permanence of Paper for Printed Library Materials, ANSI Z39.48–1984.∞

To Yige

CONTENTS

ACKNOWLEDGMENTS

During the decade-long making of this book, I was fortunate to have had many people who helped me professionally and personally along the way. In the early stages of this project, I benefited immensely from guidance from Shigehisa Kuriyama for his comparative insight and poetic sensibility, Katharine Park for teaching me the history of European medicine, and James Robson for his expertise in Chinese religions (all at Harvard University). These excellent scholars and kind human beings helped me build a solid foundation for this project.

Other scholars in Chinese history and the history of medicine have played a key role in my intellectual growth and the development of this book. Miranda Brown ignited my interest in the history of Chinese medicine when I was studying at the University of Michigan, and has since been a solid support for my scholarly pursuit. TJ Hinrichs has provided much insight into this project and various opportunities to help develop my career. Marta Hanson has been very generous in offering her time and expertise, especially during the later stages of the project. I am also indebted to Li Jianmin, whose expertise in Chinese medical history yielded invaluable advice.

During my writing and revision of this book, I benefited greatly from many colleagues' help and support. Fan Ka-wai, Chen Hao, and He Bian read the entire manuscript and offered critical suggestions to improve the book. Kristin Stapleton, Gianna Pomata, and Lan Li also read various chapters of the manuscript and gave useful comments. I also received excellent feedback from Michael Stanley-Baker, Chen Yun-ju, and Dolly Yang, the nucleus of a decade-long online reading group that I enjoyed greatly. I also appreciate the conversations and correspondence with many colleagues that in various ways helped me identify new directions and articulate my arguments for the book, and here I especially thank Chen Ming, Hsiao-wen Cheng, Constance Cook, Jeremy Greene, David Herzberg, Sean Hsiang-lin Lei, Liao Yuqun, Liu Xiaomeng, Margaret Wee Siang Ng, Michael Puett, Laurent Sagart, Nathan Sivin, Shao-yun Yang, Yanhua Zhang, and Zheng Jinsheng. I am also grateful to Elaine Leong and Pierce Salguero for offering me the opportunities to share my discoveries with public audiences at the Recipes Project and Asian Medicine Zone, respectively.

In the past years, I have presented sections of the book at various conferences, including the Association for Asian Studies (AAS) Annual Conference, the International Congress of History of Science and Technology (ICHST), the American Academy of Religion (AAR) Annual Meeting, and the International Conference on the History of Science in East Asia (ICHSEA). I am grateful for all the insightful comments from the audiences. In addition, I presented chapters of the book at the University of Rochester, Johns Hopkins University, and Binghamton University, and I thank Sarah Higley, Laura Smoller, Marta Hanson, Tobie Meyer-Fong, and Meg Leja for their kind invitation and hospitality.

Research and writing of this book have been generously supported by a number of institutions and fellowships. A Frederick Sheldon Traveling Fellowship at Harvard University (2012–13) supported my one-year research at the British Library, the Bibliothèque Nationale de France, and Academia Sinica to collect research material and interact with experts in the field. In particular, my thanks go to Vivienne Lo, Catherine Despeux, and Li Jianmin for kindly hosting me at these various institutions. The Andrew W. Mellon Foundation supported a wonderful year of postdoctoral fellowship at the Jackman Humanities Institute of the University of Toronto, where I had vibrant conversations with colleagues that extended my knowledge of material culture studies beyond premodern Chinese history. I thank the entire cohort, including the director Robert Gibbs and my postdoctoral peers Matt Cohn, Chris Dingwall, Peter Jones, Eugenia Kisin, Gabriel Levine, and Rasheed Tazudeen, for the stimulating exchanges and fun time together. Special thanks go to Nicholas Everett and Yiching Wu, who helped me navigate my research at the University of Toronto. Other scholars in the Department of East Asian Studies, including Linda Rui Feng, Yue Meng, and Yurou Zhong, provided intellectual fodder to the development of this project.

I have an excellent academic base in the Department of History at the State University of New York (SUNY) at Buffalo. The department has provided a supportive and congenial environment for junior scholars to flourish. I thank Victoria Wolcott and Erik Seeman for cultivating such an environment, and am particularly grateful for mentorship from Kristin Stapleton, whose generosity and kind heart have made my life in Buffalo enjoyable. Other colleagues in the department and beyond, including David Herzberg, James Bono, Susan Cahn, Ndubueze Mbah, and Walter Hakala, helped me think through the project at its various stages of development. Michael Kicey provided critical help with library resources at Buffalo. A Humanities Institute Faculty Research Fellowship and a College of Arts and Sciences Junior Faculty Research Fellowship at Buffalo offered me a much-needed one-year research leave to complete the manuscript. In addition, the Dr. Nuala McGann Drescher Diversity and Inclusion Leave Program at SUNY gave me a one-semester teaching release to finish the revision of the manuscript on time. The completion of this book would have been much harder without such generous support.

At the University of Washington Press (UWP), Lorri Hagman has offered superb editorship that assured the smooth publication of the book. I appreciate her confidence in this project and her professional help at every step of the process. I thank the two anonymous reviewers who offered constructive feedback to improve the manuscript. I am indebted to Oriana Walker, a fellow historian of medicine, who offered excellent substantive suggestions and editorial help in the final stage of revision. Richard Isaac excellently copyedited the manuscript. Susan Stone professionally prepared the index and Judy Loeven helpfully read through the page proofs to eliminate errors. I also appreciate Margaret Sullivan's support during my proofreading of the manuscript, and the suggestion from Beth Fuget who, in collaboration with Christopher Hollister at Buffalo, steered me through the process of producing the open-access edition of the book. My special thanks go to the University at Buffalo Libraries, which generously funded the subvention for publishing the open-access edition.

In addition, I appreciate that the Library of Congress, the Bibliothèque Nationale de France, the Staatsbibliothek zu Berlin, and Wenwu Press granted permission to use their images in the book. Ben Pease offered crucial help to create the map. The publication of the book was generously supported by grants from the Traditional Chinese Culture and Society Book Fund, the Chiang Ching-kuo Foundation for International Scholarly Exchange, and the Julian Park Publication Fund of the College of Arts and Sciences at Buffalo. I would also like to thank Academia Sinica in Taipei, which opened its wonderful database Scripta Sinica to the public during the COVID-19 pandemic, allowing me to track key sources and finish the book on time. All mistakes in the book, naturally, are mine.

In my pursuit of this project and my intellectual journey in general, I am fortunate to have had many friends along the way who not only helped me in my research but also greatly enriched my life: Margo Boenig-Liptsin, He Bian, Kuang-chi Hung, Natalie Köhle, Philip Zhang, Wen Yu, Xin Wen, Chen Liu, Macabe Keliher, Wayne Tan, Daniel Koss, Victor Seow, Kaijun Chen, Lijing Jiang, Edward Boenig-Liptsin, Megan Formato, Jenna Tonn, Wenzhao Meng, Hu Siyuan, and Priti Joshi, among many others. Back at the University of Michigan, when I decided to shift my path from science to humanities, I received unreserved support from Xuan Wang, David Parker, Jinhee Chang, Ken Cadigan, Eric Engel, and Christian de Pee. Without their encouragement, I cannot imagine that I would have reached this point.

Finally, I want to thank my parents for their unfailing belief in me and for understanding the unconventional path I took. My brother has been a source of support, joy, and alternative perspectives, which have sustained me throughout the journey.

I spent the final months of revising this book in the Pacific Northwest, in the midst of an unprecedented global pandemic. At this surreal moment, and facing many uncertainties ahead, I was extremely fortunate to be with Yige. Although writing is often considered to be a solitary endeavor, I never felt alone. Her intellectual power, unflagging encouragement, and keen sense of humor—let alone her many wonderful suggestions to improve the manuscript—have made the writing of the book both fulfilling and enjoyable. In these trying times, her company is a magic elixir in my life. This book is dedicated to her.

CHRONOLOGY OF DYNASTIES

Shang	ca. 1600–1046 BCE
Zhou	ca. 1046–256 BCE
Western Zhou	ca. 1046–771 BCE
Eastern Zhou	770–256 BCE
Spring and Autumn period	770–476 BCE
Warring States period	476–221 BCE
Qin	221–206 BCE
Han	206 BCE–220 CE
Western Han	206 BCE–9 CE
Xin	9–23
Eastern Han	25–220
Era of Division	220–589
Three Kingdoms	220–280
Wei	220–266
Shu-Han	221–263
Wu	222–280
Jin	266–420
Western Jin	266–316
Eastern Jin	317–420
Sixteen Kingdoms	304–439
Southern Dynasties	420–589
Liu-Song	420–479
Southern Qi	479–502
Liang	502–557
Chen	557–589

Northern Dynasties	386–581
Northern Wei	386–534
Eastern Wei	534–550
Western Wei	535–557
Northern Qi	550–577
Northern Zhou	557–581
Sui	581–618
Tang	618–907
Five Dynasties and Ten Kingdoms	907–960
Liao (Khitan)	907–1125
Song	960–1279
Northern Song	960–1127
Southern Song	1127–1279
Western Xia (Tangut)	1038–1227
Jin (Jurchen)	1115–1234
Yuan (Mongol)	1271–1368
Ming	1368–1644
Qing (Manchu)	1636–1912

HEALING WITH POISONS

Introduction

SOMETIME IN THE EARLY NINTH CENTURY, THE SCHOLAR-OFFICIAL
Liu Yuxi (772–842) became ill while serving in southwestern China. He was
afflicted with scorching pain, a sign of "obstructed flows." Following a
friend's advice, Liu went to see a local doctor, who, upon examining him,
blamed his unhealthy lifestyle. The doctor gave him a prescription but
warned, "The medicine possesses *du* 毒 (toxicity or potency), so you must
stop taking it once you are cured. Taking too much will injure your body. So
take only a small dose." The medicine worked: after ten days, Liu's discomforts all vanished; within a month, he had fully recovered. Delighted, Liu
ignored the doctor's warning and continued to take the medicine, hoping to
further enhance his vigor. But five days later, a numbing sensation spread
throughout his body. Realizing his mistake, Liu rushed back to the doctor,
who, of course, reprimanded him. The doctor then prescribed an antidote, and
he was saved.

Liu recounts this episode in a short essay titled "Inspecting Medicines"
(Jianyao).[1] A figure known for his literary talent, Liu, like many of his fellow
literati during the Tang dynasty (618–907), was also keenly interested in medicine, collecting useful formulas and sharing them with his coterie to spread
the knowledge of healing.[2] In this story, he reveals several key issues of classical Chinese medicine: the experience of sickness, the influence of lifestyle
on health, and the trust between patients and doctors. Yet the most telling
feature of the tale is the doctor's prescription of a toxic medicine to cure Liu's
illness. How could a poison heal? And if poisons healed, what exactly was a
medicine?

"Among the myriad things in the world," the famous seventh-century physician Sun Simiao declared, "there is nothing that cannot be a medicine."[3]
There was, in other words, no essential difference between medicines and

nonmedicines; in the right context, anything could be a drug. And indeed, the Chinese pharmacy was vast, containing not just plants but also minerals, animal-derived materials, and foods. The celebrated sixteenth-century pharmacological treatise *Systematic Materia Medica* (Bencao gangmu), for example, included close to 1,900 entries using substances as wide-ranging as water, dirt, textiles, and even human excrement.[4] Chinese pharmacology was thus at its core an exploration of the entire material world seen through the lens of therapeutics.

In this all-encompassing pharmacy, poisons loomed large. This might seem surprising given that today Chinese herbal remedies are widely imagined to be natural, mild, and safe, especially in comparison with the synthetic drugs of modern biomedicine, which are often perceived as artificial, exceedingly strong, and with therapeutic effects inseparable from dangerous side effects. Another familiar dichotomy contrasts the holistic approach of Chinese healing that seeks to restore the harmony of the body with the reductionist methods of biomedicine that eradicate specific diseases.[5] Neither of these perceptions survives scrutiny: Chinese pharmacy has, over its long history, featured a rich miscellany of medicinal therapies that target diverse disorders. There were certainly mild treatments, such as food therapy, that aimed to balance the body and recover its resonance with the cosmos.[6] Equally important but less examined is the tradition of harnessing toxic drugs that would forcefully destroy or expel pathogenic entities. In fact, Chinese doctors regularly relied on substances that they themselves recognized as possessing *du*. Aconite (*fuzi*), for example, a highly toxic herb grown in southwestern China, was one of the most frequently prescribed drugs in classical Chinese medicine. Conceptually, writers on pharmacy identified *du* as the key index for the classification of medicines. The foundational works of materia medica thus grouped drugs in a three-tiered hierarchy based on their toxicity, and revealingly placed most of the powerful drugs used in curing sickness in the most-toxic tier. Medicinal therapy in China, then, was inconceivable without poisons.

Moreover, classical Chinese pharmacy aimed at more than curing sickness; many substances in the least-toxic tier of the drug hierarchy promised to facilitate the cultivation of long life. Alongside its concern with treating illness, Chinese pharmacology was shaped by the goal of transforming the body into higher states of being and achieving longevity. This program of life enhancement involved a purification of the body that cleared its noxious burdens, leading it to ascend to various levels of sublime existence that correlated to one's life span: the higher one reached, the longer one would live. The highest attainment, as expected, was immortality. Medicine in China thus developed through the interaction of two related but distinct enterprises: the fight *against* sickness and the quest *for* ever-enhanced vitality.

Most of the drugs assigned for this second goal were mild and therefore could be consumed regularly to strengthen the body. Yet this group also included a significant number of toxic substances, especially minerals, such as cinnabar, arsenic, and sulfur. The robustness of these minerals, many believed, could be readily transferred to the body, making it resistant to decay. Yet a dilemma naturally arose: while the ingestion of these powerful drugs was thought to transform the body and prolong life, their toxicity often precipitated the quick demise of many fervent users. Importantly, the violent sensations induced by such drugs elicited diverse interpretations that either justified or contested the consumption of these puissant medicines.

Figure I.1 illustrates these two dimensions of the use of poisons in premodern China. In this diagram, any position inside the cone represents a state of the body. The center of the circle at the bottom of the cone refers to a healthy body. Any deviation from this center refers to a state of sickness, with intelligent

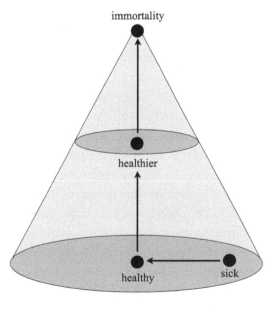

FIGURE I.1. Two dimensions of the use of poisons in classical Chinese medicine.

use of poisons offering the possibility of restoring the body to health. In addition to maintaining a healthy body devoid of illness, classical Chinese medicine strove for a higher goal of elevating the body to a "healthier" state, sometimes aided by toxic minerals. This elevated, "lighter" state of the body was less susceptible to sickness, as indicated by the smaller size of the plane. The ultimate objective was to raise the body to the tip of the cone, where there could be no possibility of becoming ill. This, of course, meant immortality. Poisons in classical Chinese pharmacy acted on a continuum from the elimination of sickness to the enhancement of life, and ultimately the escape from death.

The History of Medicines in China and Beyond

Over recent decades, the study of materiality and material culture has gained momentum in the history of science and beyond. Rather than just adopting a social constructivist approach, scholars have become increasingly sensitive to the material dimensions of the subjects they examine—be it a scientific instrument, a specimen, or an object of daily use. This methodological shift by no means reduces historical inquiries to material determinism; rather, it acknowledges the physical constraints of things and underscores their open-ended potential. Material objects thus offer a unique lens through which one can acquire a sophisticated understanding of the society and culture in which they acted.[7]

This material turn in recent scholarship provides useful insight for the study of the history of Chinese medicine. Early inquiries focused on the theoretical foundations of the healing system and its unique practices, such as acupuncture, interest in which has been influenced by its rising status in contemporary society.[8] Yet the history of Chinese medicine cannot ignore the history of Chinese *medicines*; the rich variety of medicinal substances in Chinese pharmacy constituted a vital part of the healing repertoire. What is striking about these drugs is their fluid materiality; that is, each of them was viewed not as fixed matter with a definite action but as a mutable substance that could undergo manifold transformations and elicit diverse effects.[9] Although *du* is the standard Chinese word for poison today, its core meaning in the past was *potency*—the power not just to harm as a poison but also to cure as a medicine. This duality was central to classical Chinese pharmacy: no material essence marked off poisons from medicines; the effect of any given substance—whether it healed as a medicine, or sickened or killed as a poison, or altered a person in myriad other ways—varied greatly according to the way in which it was prepared and deployed, the bodily sensation it induced, and its assigned value in society. In short, when we ponder what was a medicine, context mattered.

No example illuminates this transformative capacity of medicines better than the regular use of poisons. Yet, despite their importance in Chinese pharmacy, they have largely escaped the attention of medical historians. One notable exception is Frédéric Obringer's *L'aconit et l'orpiment: Drogues et poisons en Chine ancienne et médiévale* (Aconite and orpiment: Drugs and poisons in ancient and medieval China), the most extensive study of the topic to date. The monograph offers a detailed pharmacological analysis of poisons in China from antiquity to the eleventh century, with a focus on the medical understandings of poisons and the pharmaceutical principles underlying their use, but to the exclusion of situating these powerful substances in a broader context.[10] Several other studies have looked beyond the medical realm, exploring poisons in the social, political, and religious culture of premodern China, yet these investigations tend to be brief and episodic, and to focus on the use of poisons for nefarious purposes.[11]

The therapeutic use of poisons was not unique to China. By examining the social history of poisons in colonial India, the historian of medicine David Arnold has demonstrated the complex interplay between European toxicological knowledge and India's "poison culture," which stimulated colonial scholarship and triggered new regulations of these dangerous materials.[12] An important aspect of this culture was the medical use of poisons, which can be traced back to Ayurvedic healing in the premodern era. Although this is not the focus of his study, Arnold muses that "[p]erhaps even among Asian societies, only China, with its ancient use of aconites and orpiment, its Western missionary condemnation of toxic remedies and its recent wholesale descent into industrial pollution, has a comparable tale to tell."[13] The history of poisons in China has yet to be written. By probing the roots of this history in Chinese culture, *Healing with Poisons* seeks to enhance our understanding of the traditional value of poisons in Asia.[14]

There are comparatively more studies of poisons and poisoning in the European context, particularly focusing on their danger and harmful effects.[15] It is useful to recall, however, that the Greek term *pharmakon*, from which the English word "pharmacology" derives, meant both remedy and poison, among other things.[16] This paradoxical sense of drugs in early Western medicine shares much in common with the ancient meaning of *du* in China. Small wonder that the therapeutic use of poisons figured prominently in ancient Greek pharmacy. For example, Dioscorides's *De Materia Medica* (first century), a foundational text in the history of Western pharmacology, contains more than sixty toxic drugs, such as opium poppy, mandrake, and hemlock, that were harnessed to treat diverse illnesses.[17] Analogous to the Chinese case, the use of poisons as curative agents persisted throughout European history.[18] Yet, beginning in the first century, a group of highly toxic substances in Greek pharmacy gradually moved out of the *pharmakon* continuum and were deemed to be absolute poisons without medicinal value. As the historian of medicine Frederick Gibbs has shown, this separation became more pronounced in late medieval Europe when physicians increasingly perceived poisons as ontologically distinct substances from medicines, which paved the way for the rise of toxicology in the early modern period.[19]

The concept of absolute poison, by contrast, never arose in premodern China. The use of toxic substances had constituted the core of Chinese pharmacy since its inception, and it remained so throughout the imperial era.[20] No example better illustrates this divergence than the distinct fates of aconite in Greek and Chinese pharmacies. In *De Materia Medica*, aconite, also called wolfsbane, is described only as a poison to kill wolves, without any curative value. The Greek physician offers treatment for accidental aconite poisoning no less than seventeen times in his text, suggesting that he included the toxic plant simply to warn against its use.[21] But in China, aconite (*fuzi*) was highly valued for its therapeutic power, and even hailed as "the lord of the hundred drugs."[22] This does not mean that there was no knowledge of the danger of poisons in China. Quite the opposite: we find abundant discussion of poison detection and treatment in classical Chinese pharmacy. Yet unlike the study of absolute poisons as substances fundamentally different from medicines in medieval Europe, the understanding of poisons remained an integral part of pharmacological knowledge in premodern China. This striking divergence of European and Chinese pharmacy likely derived from their distinct therapeutic rationales. If European physicians considered toxicity to be the cause of unpleasant side effects, Chinese healers deemed it to be the very source of curative power. In other words, European medicine prescribed poisons in spite of their toxicity; Chinese medicine, because of it.[23]

Medicines in Medieval China

A periodization that has been influential in the existing literature identifies three pivotal turning points in the history of Chinese medicine: the crystallization of medical theories during the Han dynasty (206 BCE–220 CE), the integration of doctrinal learning and empirical knowledge during the Song dynasty (960–1279), and the reinvention of Chinese medicine in the face of modern biomedicine in the nineteenth and twentieth centuries.[24] Accordingly, these crucial moments have been studied in detail. With respect to the premodern period, scholars have extensively investigated the origins of Chinese medicine in the Han dynasty, epitomized by the formation of the foundational theoretical treatise *The Yellow Emperor's Inner Classic* (Huangdi neijing).[25] Other studies have focused on the transformation of medicine during the Song dynasty, examining the emergence of new medical theories, the explosion of medical writings facilitated by printing, the state's effort to establish and disseminate medical canons, and the literati's heightened interest in medicine.[26] But what about the long period between the Han and Song dynasties, which is the focus of this book?

The medieval period in China starts with the collapse of the Han dynasty, followed by three centuries of political disunity, often called the Era of Division (220–589).[27] From the early fourth century, various nomadic peoples from northern and central Asia occupied the north, while a succession of regimes established by the Han people ruled the south.[28] Despite its political turbulence, the period witnessed a flourishing of literature, religion, and medicine. Medical writings were chiefly produced by individual healers and transmitted within powerful clans, reflecting the hereditary nature of medicine at the time.[29] The situation changed in the seventh century, when the unified Sui (581–618) and Tang (618–907) empires, with Chang'an (present-day Xi'an) as their political center, established new institutions, promulgated legal codes, and commissioned authoritative texts to standardize medical knowledge and achieve effective rule. This favorable environment fostered the production of a collection of medical texts that proved influential in Chinese medical history.[30] After the middle of the eighth century, the Tang state was substantially weakened by the devastating An Lushan Rebellion (755–63), which led to the decline of the central authority and the rise of local powers. As a result, the main agency producing medical knowledge shifted from the state to scholar-officials, who became interested in both the practical use of medicine and its allegorical value in political persuasion.

Despite its significance in the history of Chinese medicine, the period stretching from the third to the tenth century has been largely overlooked by medical historians, especially in English-language scholarship.[31] More extensive studies on the medical features of this period have been conducted in Chinese, Japanese, and French scholarship, all of which have informed the writing of this book. In particular, Fan Ka-wai has made a major contribution to our understanding of the medical ideas and practices of this period. In a series of essays, he identifies the changing landscape of medicine from the Era of Division to the Tang dynasty and explores a wide range of issues, situating key medical features in the political, institutional, and literary culture of the time.[32] Other researchers have focused on more specific topics, including the systemization of medical canons, religious healing, women's medicine, and the construction of medical identity.[33] Moreover, scholars have also performed in-depth analysis of a collection of medical manuscripts from Dunhuang and Turfan that offers key insights into the miscellany of healing practice in medieval society and the vibrant exchange of medical knowledge across Eurasia.[34]

What is particularly important about this period in the medical history of China is the growth of pharmacology. Although the roots of drug therapy can be traced back to the Han period, as exemplified by the foundational *The Divine Farmer's Classic of Materia Medica* (Shennong bencao jing) and the excavated medical manuscripts from Mawangdui,[35] its major outlines took shape in the following centuries, which saw the rapid expansion of pharmacy, the spread of pharmaceutical knowledge through society, and, especially relevant to this study, the enhanced understanding of toxic medicines. Two watershed moments warrant our attention as transformative for the therapeutic use of poisons.[36] The first is the fifth century. Building on ancient classics, physicians and pharmacological compilers started to systematize knowledge of drugs by specifying the *du* status of each medicine and providing guidelines on how to prepare and employ drugs. This moment also witnessed increased pharmaceutical specialization, with different groups of actors engaged in harvesting, processing, selling, and prescribing drugs. The second is the seventh century, when the Sui and Tang states played an active role in creating new institutions and producing authoritative texts to regulate the use of poisons and standardize medical knowledge. Sun Simiao, one of the most celebrated physicians in Chinese history, also emerged in this century. Hailed as "the King of Medicines," he integrated state-produced knowledge of drugs into his writings and relied on personal experience to affirm the efficacy of his formulas. By scrutinizing these two crucial moments in the history of Chinese pharmacology, *Healing with Poisons* seeks to unpack the rich culture of drugs in medieval China.

Furthermore, this book situates the study of drugs within the broader context of Chinese political history. A series of social, economic, and intellectual changes took place from the eighth to the twelfth century that profoundly transformed Chinese society. Often called "the Tang-Song transition," these changes include, among others, the rise of meritocracy facilitated by the civil service examination system, the emergence of neo-Confucianism, the development of woodblock printing, and the consciousness of nationalism among literate elites.[37] The transformation of the social order was so significant that some scholars have considered the eleventh century as the start of the modern era in China.[38]

In medical history, what is particularly salient in the new era is the state's active engagement in medicine. The court of the Northern Song (960–1127) took advantage of printing technology to standardize and promulgate medical knowledge to achieve effective governance, an effort seen again only in the twentieth century, when the state reinvented Chinese medicine to cope with the challenge of modern biomedicine.[39] The Song transformation of Chinese medicine is clearly critical, yet the active involvement of the state in medicine is already discernable in the earlier days of the Sui and Tang dynasties. Ending the political division of the preceding three centuries, these unified empires established new policies and legal codes in the seventh and eighth centuries to regulate medical practice and punish poisoners who were accused of witchcraft and menacing the stability of the state. They also sponsored the production of medical texts to standardize and circulate pharmaceutical knowledge. Although state engagement in medicine during the Sui and Tang periods occurred on a smaller scale and via different mechanisms—manuscripts, rather than printed texts, were still the dominant medium of transmitting knowledge—it anticipated the governmental regulation of medicine during the Tang-Song transition that has been extensively examined.[40]

Text and Genre

My emphasis on the materiality of medicines results from a methodological orientation toward a history beyond narratology, discourse analysis, and representations. Yet history is always mediated by texts, and medical history is no exception. What is particularly of note for the period from the Era of Division to the Tang dynasty is that the majority of medical sources in their original form have long been lost; their earliest extant editions were compiled during the Northern Song period (960–1127), driven by the rise of printing and the state's use of the technology to promulgate medical texts. The prestige of the so-called great canonical works of Chinese medicine, such as *The Yellow Emperor's Inner Classic* and *Treatise on Cold Damage and Miscellaneous Disorders* (Shanghan zabing lun) as we know them today, is due in no small part to the systematic effort of the Song state to elevate the status of these works.[41] My study of medieval medical works therefore inevitably relies on these Song compilations and the modern editions based on them.

Before the era of printing, manuscript culture flourished in China.[42] Fortunately, an assortment of pre-Song medical manuscripts from a large collection found in Dunhuang and Turfan and dating from the third to the eleventh century has been discovered. Located on the strategic sites of the Silk Road in the far west, Dunhuang (in present-day Gansu) and Turfan (in present-day Xinjiang) were vibrant frontier towns where, during the Tang period, diverse cultures interacted. The manuscripts, most of which are Buddhist scriptures, contain a sizable collection of medical works that are often lost in printed texts.[43] Although most of these manuscripts are incomplete and lack contextual information, such as the time of compilation and authorship, they are sources without the editorial influences of later periods and are therefore crucial to the study of medical culture in medieval China. Moreover, in contrast to texts produced at the imperial center, these manuscripts carry regional features that reveal the concerns of local actors. They are thus excellent materials for exploring local medical practices.

Among the pre-Song medical sources, two genres are particularly important to my investigation of medicines. The first is the literature of materia medica (*bencao*), which provides detailed entries on drugs, each with its properties, morphology, sources of supply, medical uses, and other categories. The genre originated during the Han dynasty and persisted throughout imperial China.[44] Importantly, the writing of materia medica followed a commentary tradition; that is, later works faithfully preserved the core text formed in the Han period and added, over time, layers of commentaries at the end of each drug entry. This particular structure demonstrates the importance of textual authority in the making of new knowledge of drugs. The second genre is formula books (*fangshu*), which contain a large number of medical formulas usually organized by the types of illness they treat. Compared to the materia medica literature, this genre has neither central text to build on nor commentary tradition to adhere to; it is rather an eclectic assembly of remedies culled from diverse sources. Both genres discuss medicines extensively, but with different epistemic orientations, to borrow a concept developed by the historian of medicine Gianna Pomata.[45] The former manifests the mentality of canon-building and seeks to establish authority and order, whereas the latter speaks more to the production of empirical knowledge that links to medical practice.

Two examples from the seventh century display the difference clearly. The production of the first government-commissioned pharmacological work, *Newly Revised Materia Medica* (Xinxiu bencao, 659), exhibited the state's ambition to standardize pharmaceutical knowledge and exalt the grandeur of the empire, while the personal compilation of Sun Simiao's formula book *Essential Formulas Worth a Thousand in Gold for Emergencies* (Beiji qianjin yaofang, 650s; hereafter *Essential Formulas*) revealed the physician's project of confirming the efficacy of remedies based on his own experience. The two texts thus generated different types of knowledge with specific political and social values. Yet the epistemic distinction between the two genres is by no means absolute: the commentary section of a materia medica text could contain rich empirical information, just as a formula book could be a scholarly project amassing past wisdom and showcasing erudition.[46] Therefore, we must be sensitive to the epistemic variations within a medical genre contingent on the historical condition.

Medicines and the Body

Beyond treating illness, medicines in medieval China also aimed to enhance life. The ultimate goal of the latter pursuit was to evade death altogether (figure I.1), a quest our modern eyes might view as a religious endeavor. Scholars have emphasized the "Daoist" element in classical Chinese pharmacy, since drugs prescribed for nourishing the body also appear in Daoist scriptures.[47]

In particular, a number of toxic minerals were frequently used in Daoist alchemical practices that sought to promote transcendence and escape death. Poisons could be numinous substances that triggered the transformation of the body into higher states of being.

How do we make sense of the "religious" elements in classical Chinese medicine? Rather than treating "medicine" and "religion" as universal categories, it is important to recognize their historical roots in post-Enlightenment Europe and acknowledge their limitations when applied to other times and places.[48] If we refrain from an anachronistic approach, it is hard to separate "medicine" from "religion" at the conceptual, textual, or sociological level in premodern societies. Previous scholarship has amply demonstrated that in medieval and early modern Europe, scientific knowledge was interwoven with religious aspirations in the domains of astrology, alchemy, and medicine.[49] This was also the case in medieval China, where medicine operated in a world suffused with Buddhist, Daoist, and various folk religious activities. At the conceptual level, the effort to combat illness and pursue immortality formed a continuum in classical Chinese pharmacology. At the level of practice, healers in medieval China incorporated a constellation of methods (drug therapy, talismanic healing, meditation, incantation, etc.) that defied the clear boundary between "medicine" and "religion." Like two sides of the same coin, they were inseparable in premodern Chinese culture.[50]

A crucial issue in the study of religious healing in premodern China is how medicines interacted with the body. Scholarship on the history of the body has yielded critical insights into the profound differences in the perception and experience of the body in various medical and religious traditions.[51] Moreover, recent studies of material culture in both Buddhism and Daoism have demonstrated the abundant use of objects in religious practice and the entwined relationship between the spiritual and the material.[52] What has been barely explored, however, is the interaction between the body and things, especially the effect of a given medicine on the body and how such an effect shaped the understanding of the medicine and of the illness it treated.[53] Since toxic substances often induced violent sensations, they offer a window through which to examine the intimate relationship between the ingestion of medicines and the transformation of the body, a theme particularly prominent in Daoist alchemy. Although the interpretations of these sensations could be varied and counterintuitive, they expressed the irreducible physicality of the body, a body that endured pain and even death.[54] The tension between physical anguish and spiritual elevation was precisely what was at stake in the case of elixir poisoning in Chinese alchemy. Examination of these experiences and their diverse explanations illuminates the vital link between the sensations of the body and the knowledge of medicines.

Healing with Poisons is divided into three parts. Parts I and II follow a chronological order, focusing on the therapeutic use of poisons. Specifically, part I explores the prominence of poisons in Chinese pharmacy during its foundational period from the Han dynasty to the Era of Division, investigating the paradoxical meaning of *du* and the diverse techniques that transformed poisons into medicines. Part II examines the changing landscape of Chinese pharmacy in the Sui and early Tang dynasties, inspecting the heightened concern about poisoning and witchcraft in political circles, the state patronage of producing and promulgating pharmaceutical knowledge, and physicians' keen interest in applying such knowledge in practice. Part III, spanning the entire period under study, examines poisons in life enhancement. It moves our story of poisons beyond the realm of curing sickness, scrutinizing their extraordinary power to illuminate the mind and prolong life, in the case of Five-Stone Powder, and to transform the body and confer immortality in alchemy.

Finally, a few words on the translation of *du*. No English expression perfectly captures the paradoxical meaning of *du*. A word like "poisomedicine" might do the job, but creating an awkward neologism is hardly a good choice for translation. Just as the identity of a medicine changed with the context of its formulation and usage, the meaning of *du* varied with the specific text in which it appeared. A medicine in classical Chinese pharmacy, then, was something of a mutable character and transformative potential. Because of *du*'s versatile meanings, in what follows I translate it differently depending on the context. I also leave *du* untranslated in materia medica texts to underscore its ambivalent meaning. In cases where the positive sense of healing is evident, I translate it as "potent" or "potency" to connote the therapeutic power of a medicine. In cases where the negative sense of harm is clear, I translate it as "poisonous" or "poisoning." In addition, I often use the word "poisons" as shorthand for medicines that possess *du* in Chinese pharmacy. This particular way of using the word, I must clarify, does not imply the absolute harmfulness of a substance but rather spotlights the inherent tension between poison and medicine, which is precisely what we are now setting out to explore.

PART I

Malleable Medicines

CHAPTER 1

The Paradox of *Du*

For all things under heaven, nothing is more vicious than the poison
of aconite. Yet a good doctor packs and stores it, because it is useful.

—*MASTERS OF HUAINAN* (SECOND CENTURY BCE)

THE HAN TEXT *HISTORICAL RECORDS* (SHIJI, 91 BCE) PRESENTS A
story that revealingly compares words with medicines. After defeating the
Qin army at the capital, Liu Bang (256–195 BCE), who later became the first
emperor of the Han, was tempted to claim the luxurious palace of the routed
Qin as his own home. One of his generals tried to persuade the greedy lord
to abandon the idea, but to no avail. An advisor named Zhang Liang then
stepped up, admonishing Liu for indulging in the pleasures of victory,
which would only continue the depravity of the regime he had just over-
thrown. Zhang urged the lord to heed the general's warning because "honest
words are unpleasant to hear but good for action; potent drugs are bitter to
ingest but good for healing." Liu eventually took his advice. The message of the
story is clear: harsh words, similar to powerful medicines, are hard to take
yet ultimately provide benefit.[1]

The Han advisor's expression has become a household idiom today in
China, although the term for "potent drugs" (*duyao*) has been replaced by
"good drugs" (*liangyao*).[2] This substitution is telling, which indicates the
changing meaning of *du* over history. Today, it is the standard Chinese word
for poison. Like its English counterpart, the word invites associations with
danger, harm, and intrigue. But *du* was not always noxious: it has carried

diverse, even opposite meanings. The word appears in various medical, philosophical, and institutional texts in ancient China. Although the negative sense
of *du* can indeed be found in these earliest texts, there it can also refer to favorable attributes of a leader, an action, or a medicine. This positive sense of *du*
is evident in the story above; the word denotes a power of medicines that is
crucial to their capacity to cure sickness. This notion of potency, the ability not
just to harm as a poison but also to cure as a medicine, lay at the core of drug
therapy in premodern China. Accordingly, Chinese doctors turned to a large
number of substances perceived as possessing *du* and strategically employed
them for healing. To understand classical Chinese pharmacology, we must
grasp the paradox of *du*.

This crucial tradition of the medical use of poisons is rooted in the formative years of Chinese pharmacology from the Han dynasty to the Era of Division, when a wide array of powerful substances of mineral, animal, and
especially herbal origins were incorporated into the medicinal repertoire.
During the Han period, *du* became a benchmark to classify medicines; by
grouping drugs into a three-tiered hierarchy, Han pharmacological works
linked *du*-possessing drugs to the cure of illness, a therapeutic principle that
lasted throughout the imperial era. During the Era of Division, classical Chinese pharmacy expanded substantially, with more elaborate accounts of the
specification, identification, and deployment of potent drugs. By the sixth
century, *du* had been solidly established as a central criterion to define drugs
and guide therapy in China.

The Etymology of *Du*

To appreciate the significance of *du* in classical Chinese pharmacy, it is neces-
sary to trace the meanings of the word in the broader cultural context of early
China. An informative entry point is the Han text *Explaining Simple and
Analyzing Compound Characters* (Shuowen jiezi, 100; hereafter, *Explaining
Characters*), the first comprehensive dictionary in China. Compiled by Xu
Shen (ca. 55–ca. 149), the text manifests the Han scholar's effort to systematize
written language based on the ancient meanings of characters. Although the
dictionary by no means preserves the "original" sense of *du*, it offers useful
glosses that reveal the multivalent interpretation of the word.[3] Fundamentally,
du is defined as "thickness" (*hou*), which in turn is explained as "thickness of

lofty mountains."[4] *Du* and *hou* share similar features: heavy, dense, and abundant. Neither of the words bears a negative connotation.[5]

Explaining Characters offers a second, less innocuous meaning of *du*. *Du* is compared with a harmful grass that grows invasively, everywhere. A sense of "thickness" is still implied here—the poisonous plant is rampant, wanton, and unrestrained. Luxuriant growth insinuates latent danger. To support this idea, the dictionary partitions the character into two parts: the top part *cao* 屮, which means "grass," and the bottom part *ai* 毒, which means "unvirtuous person" (figure 1.1a). Altogether, *du* denotes an undesirable herb that engenders harm.[6]

Du was not one idea, nor was it written with one character. In addition to the foregoing meanings, there was yet another entirely different graph for *du* that dates to the pre-Han era (figure 1.1b). *Explaining Characters* describes it as an ancient form of *du* that consists of two parts: *dao* 刀 in the lower-right corner, which means "knife," along with *fu* 菖, which designates an invasive plant, anticipating the interpretation of *du* as wild and pernicious grass during the Han period.[7] What is the relationship between the knife and the grass? It has been suggested that because the character *fu*, which is phonetically related to *hou* (thickness), intimates a swelling or ulcer on the body, one could use a knife to cut it away.[8] Although *du* is implicated in treating ulcers in ancient sources, there is no evidence that it directly involved surgery. Instead, the composition of the character for *du*, consisting of the component parts "knife" and "grass," can be interpreted literally: *du* is a knife smeared with the juice of a toxic plant, a deadly weapon for use in hunting or warfare. This was probably an important application of poisons in antiquity, if not earlier.[9]

Although *Explaining Characters* is an important source regarding etymology, its interpretations of *du* were conditioned by Xu Shen's intellectual agenda and political ambition.[10] Can we retrieve other meanings of *du* beyond the Han text? A clue comes from an obscure variant of the word preserved in the sixth-century dictionary *Jade Chapters* (Yupian) (figure 1.1c).[11] This character is derived from an oracle bone script written as in figure 1.1d. Intriguingly, these graphs link *du* to animals: the upper part symbolizes a foot and the lower part a snake; the combination of the two indicates a person stepping on a venomous animal. An ancient meaning of *du*, therefore, pointed to threats posed by dangerous creatures in nature.[12]

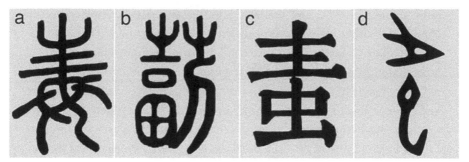

FIGURE 1.1. Variants of *du* in early China. Variants a and b are from *Explaining Characters*. Variant c is from *Jade Chapters*. Variant d is from oracle bones.

In sum, there are at least three different meanings of *du* in ancient China, based on etymological analysis. Before the Han dynasty, the word could refer to a weapon made from poisons or the danger of a pernicious animal. The positive sense of the word is absent in these early graphs. Yet during the Han period, the word acquired the meaning of "thickness," which implies heaviness, intensity, and unconstrained growth. The negative sense of the word still persisted, but this new gloss suggests a changed conception of *du*, whose meaning became more ambivalent. In addition, *du* is explicitly tied to herbs in *Explaining Characters*, indicating the rapid expansion of herbal knowledge at the time. Revealingly, *yao*, the character for drug, also contains the radical for "grass" (*cao* 艸). The meaning of this word, according to the Han dictionary, is "grass that cures illness."[13] As classical Chinese pharmacy by no means contained only herbs, the focus on grass in the definition of *yao* further suggests the growth of herbal medicine during the Han period.

The Meanings of *Du* in Early Chinese Sources

The curious etymological history of *du* offers preliminary insights into its rich meanings. We can bring more focus to the complexity of the word with other types of sources to see how its meanings are expressed in specific contexts. One of the earliest mentions of *du* in Chinese history comes from *The Classic of Changes* (Yijing or I Ching, also known as Zhouyi), a divination text the core of which was formed around the end of the second millennium BCE.[14] The book establishes a spatiotemporal cosmological system manifested by sixty-four hexagrams, each of which is linked to a particular scenario and a prophetic message. In a section called "Gnawing and Chewing" (Shike), the text relates that when one gnaws dry meat and encounters poison (*du*), this causes minor distress but no real troubles.[15] *Du* in this situation carries a negative meaning, much like food poisoning to the modern reader. Poisoning by the corruption of food has been suggested as the original meaning of *du* based on the similarity of the ancient pronunciations of *du* and *shu*, which means "ripe."[16] This type of poisoning is, nonetheless, only perceived as a minor annoyance in the text, not a sign of significant danger.

In another passage, *du* invokes an entirely different meaning. Rather than referring to a vexing matter, it designates a political force: "Remain sturdy at the center to respond to all situations; stay adaptive upon encountering dangers. If a king can rely on these qualities to govern [*du*] the world, people will follow him. Being propitious, how is it possible to cause troubles?"[17] *Du* in this passage can be read as an action performed by a capable ruler. If a leader acts sagaciously, he can rule his people with success. *Du* thus implies the abundance of virtues and the consolidation of capacities. Such virtues and capacities empower the king to achieve effective governance. Here, in one of the earliest books in China, we see two distinct expressions of *du*.[18]

The positive sense of *du* also appears in ancient philosophical texts. For instance, a passage in the foundational Daoist work *Laozi* (ca. fourth century BCE) elucidates the profound importance of the Dao and virtue: "Therefore the Dao creates all things, and virtue raises them—cultivates them and fosters them, rears them and nurtures [*du*] them, nourishes them and protects them."[19] The sentence uses a series of synonymous words, including *du*, to describe the power of virtue (*de*), which facilitates the growth of all things in the world. *Du* embodies the unfolding of the cosmos.

What, then, does *du* mean in the medical context? The key term to examine is *duyao*, which stands for "poison" in modern contexts but had quite different meanings in antiquity. The important text in this respect is *Rites of Zhou* (Zhouli, ca. third century BCE), which presents an idealized structure of the royal bureaucracy in preimperial China.[20] Among the 360-odd offices listed in the book, five are designated for medicine: one for the general supervision of medical affairs and four specialists on preparing foods and treating internal disorders, lesions, and animal maladies. The text defines the duty of the first type of officer, called "master of physicians" (*yishi*), as taking charge of medical policies and orders, as well as collecting substances referred to as *duyao* to supply the practices of physicians.[21] In this early usage, it appears that the word *duyao*, composed of two characters, as are many words in Chinese, referred to two different types of drugs: potent ones (*du*) and mild ones (*yao*). The composite, then, became a term for drugs in general.

This interpretation is supported by another passage in the text that explains the responsibilities of physicians who specialize in treating lesions. They use "five potent drugs [*du*] to attack them, five *qi* to nourish them, five mild drugs [*yao*] to heal them, and five foods to restrain them."[22] Placed in distinct categories, *du* and *yao* are both important for treating lesions. The former, associated with the act of "attack" (*gong*), bears a strong sense of intensity and forcefulness. The latter, associated with the act of "healing" (*liao*), probably refers to drugs of lesser power. In the passage that immediately follows, the text further specifies that these mild drugs are used to nourish (*yang*) different parts of the body, suggesting their tonic value.[23] Among the four types of specialists, only physicians who treat lesions employ *du*, which indicates the emphasis on the topical use of powerful drugs in ancient China.[24] The identity of the exact drugs, however, remains elusive.

The term *duyao* changed its meaning in Han medical sources. Two different usages can be detected in the Han-era *The Yellow Emperor's Inner Classic* (Huangdi neijing), a foundational text in Chinese medical history that served later readers as a crystallization of the basic theories of medicine in antiquity. The first usage there is consistent with the definition in *Rites of Zhou* in the sense that *duyao* refers to both potent and mild drugs. Yet a significant change is that rather than being applied topically, potent drugs were employed, together with mild drugs, to eliminate illness inside the body. Exterior conditions were instead treated by needles and stones.[25] The second usage of the term in *The Yellow Emperor's Inner Classic* is more restrictive, namely, that *duyao* refers only to potent drugs. In a case where the text explains the options for treatment, it lists five in particular, each with a distinct function: "The potent drugs [*duyao*] attack the devious; the five grains provide nourishment; the five fruits provide support; the five livestock provide enrichment; the five vegetables provide replenishment."[26] The verb "attack" resonates with language found in *Rites of Zhou*, indicating the power of the drugs. They contrast with other types of healing that are milder and slower, aiming to nourish the body. This second meaning of *duyao* gradually superseded the first, more inclusive sense of the term in Chinese medical writings from the Han period onward.

Moreover, this second sense of *duyao* has implications beyond the medical context: in the story that opens this chapter, its effects were compared with those of powerful words. The link between *du* and speech is particularly evident in *Discourses Weighed in the Balance* (Lunheng, first century), a collection of essays on history, philosophy, and natural science compiled by the Han scholar Wang Chong. In a chapter titled "Speaking of Poison," Wang associates all potent things with the heat, fire, and *qi* of yang, as perceived in the yin-yang framework.[27] That is, the hot, vehement *qi* in southern regions not only causes the thriving of poisonous plants and animals but also endows local people with a unique capacity to utter especially mighty words. Intriguingly, he uses this theory to explain the shamanistic practices prevalent in the south that often employed incantations to heal or kill. This more expansive interpretation of *du* unified words and things under the scheme of a sultry *qi*, reflecting a southern attitude that was of a piece with the local environment.[28]

Du in the First Chinese Materia Medica

How has the ambivalence of *du* manifested itself in Chinese pharmacy? The question directs us to the first pharmacological treatise in China, *The Divine Farmer's Classic of Materia Medica* (Shennong bencao jing, ca. first century; hereafter, *The Divine Farmer's Classic*). The title of this foundational text merits scrutiny. The term *bencao*, which first appeared during the Han period, refers to knowledge about drugs and the genre producing such knowledge. In the same way that the English word "root" is used metaphorically, *bencao* literally means either "rooted in grass" or "roots and grass," indicating the prominence of herbal medicine in the Han pharmacy.[29] *Bencao* texts in China resemble a type of European pharmacological writing, often called materia medica, that can be traced back to the foundational work *De Materia Medica* by the Greek physician Dioscorides in the first century.[30] Both genres provide a list of drugs, each with an account of the properties, habitats, appearance, and medical uses of the substance. Because of this textual similarity, I translate *bencao* as "materia medica."

But who was "the Divine Farmer" (Shennong)? As the putative author of the book, he was a mythical leader who, at the dawn of civilization, developed agriculture to benefit his people. He was also credited for discovering useful medicines, which won him the reputation as the founder of drug therapy in China. According to an early Han source, the brave man tasted hundreds of herbs to identify suitable medicines for his followers, and encountered seventy potent substances each day. The tale indicates that daily experience and trial-and-error effort played an important role in the accumulation of drug knowledge in early China.[31] The medical identity of the Divine Farmer was firmly established during the Han dynasty; sources at the time considered him, along with several other esteemed figures, such as the Yellow Emperor and Lord Thunder, to be a sage who lived in high antiquity and possessed the true, pristine knowledge of medicine. The attribution of a text to the sage thus suggests the recovery of lost pharmacological wisdom from a glorious past.[32]

The actual author(s) of *The Divine Farmer's Classic*, however, is unknown. It was possibly compiled by a group of Han officials who specialized in drugs. Known as "materia medica specialists awaiting edicts" (*bencao daizhao*), they were summoned by the court when their skills were in demand and dismissed when they were no longer needed. Both knowledgeable and disposable, these specialists are often juxtaposed in Han sources with men of "methods and arts" (*fangshu*), a term that encompasses a wide range of magical and esoteric techniques, such as astrology, geomancy, alchemy, and divination, among others. Possibly, the materia medica specialists exchanged knowledge with these technical adepts, who influenced the former group's understanding of drugs.[33]

The Divine Farmer's Classic, the first systematic writing on drugs in China, was foundational to the theory and practice of Chinese pharmacology. All later materia medica texts adhered to its basic framework of categorizing and defining drugs, and relied on its empirical knowledge to guide medical practice.[34] We know little about the formation of the text and the origins of its sources except that the work was probably a consolidation of drug knowledge accumulated in the preceding centuries. The evidence mainly comes from the medical manuscripts excavated from Han tombs, of which two sets are particularly revealing. The first is an assembly of medical formulas discovered from the tomb of a local lord in Mawangdui (in present-day Hunan, ca. 168 BCE). This collection of silk manuscripts contains close to three hundred formulas that treat fifty-two types of disorders. Based on a conservative estimate, more than two hundred drugs of plant, mineral, and animal origins are deployed, either internally or topically, in this miscellany of remedies. Among them, seventy-odd substances also appear in *The Divine Farmer's Classic*, indicating a process of crystalizing drug knowledge out of formula books during the Han period.[35]

The second set of manuscripts suggests a different route to the formation of the Han pharmacopoeia. Unearthed from a local nobleman's tomb in

Shuanggudui (in present-day Anhui, ca. 165 BCE), this collection of bamboo slips carries a list of more than one hundred drugs, each aiming to treat a medical condition or elicit a magical effect, such as running with high speed and lightening the body, the latter entailing the transformation of the body to higher states of being. Given the term "ten thousand things" (*wanwu*) that appears at the beginning of the slips, the collection offers a type of natural history that seeks to identify the possible uses of all things under heaven.[36] Thus the scope of the work goes beyond healing, describing other uses of things in hunting and fishing, clothes-making, and producing fuels, among others. The slips are just fragments containing miscellaneous information, yet they represent the earliest evidence of a nascent materia medica that embeds drug knowledge within the broader discussion of natural history.[37]

Before investigating the content of *The Divine Farmer's Classic*, it is necessary to position it in the broader Han culture of medical compilation. All medical texts from the Han period have been lost to us; fragments of manuscripts found in excavations, including the two sets mentioned above, are the only sources directly available from the period. Yet *The History of the Han* (Hanshu, first century) preserves an extensive bibliography from the imperial library—the earliest in Chinese history—that lists the titles of close to six hundred families of books organized into distinct categories. The construction of the bibliography was driven by a movement that took place in the last years of the Western Han dynasty, when several imperial scholars systematically collected and organized classic and contemporary works to reestablish textual authority to guide sage governance.[38] Titles on healing are presented at the end of the list, in a section on "methods and techniques" (*fangji*), which is further divided into four subsections: medical classics (*yijing*), classical formulas (*jingfang*), arts of the bedchamber (*fangzhong*), and arts of transcendence (*shenxian*).[39] The second subsection is particularly relevant to pharmaceutical knowledge. Although all eleven titles in this subsection are those of formula books, they relied on the knowledge of individual drugs to offer effective prescriptions. Given that no materia medica titles appear in the bibliography, such drug knowledge was probably still sporadic and unorganized during this period, embedded in formula books and works on natural history, only becoming systematized in the independent genre of *bencao* in the Eastern Han period.

Now let's take a close look at *The Divine Farmer's Classic*.[40] The book contains a short preface that introduces its organization scheme and the basic principles of drug therapy. The main body of the work characterizes a total of 365 drugs corresponding to the number of days in a year, demonstrating the cosmological framework grounding this early pharmacopoeia. Significantly, the book parses these drugs into three categories. The opening of the text defines these categories as follows:

> The higher-level drugs of 120 kinds are the lords. They govern the cultivation of life and correspond to heaven. *They do not possess* du. Taking them in large amounts or for long periods does not harm people. Those who wish to lighten the body and enhance *qi*, prevent aging, and prolong life should rely on the higher-level drugs in [*The Divine Farmer's*] *Classic*.
>
> The middle-level drugs of 120 kinds are the ministers. They govern the cultivation of the human nature and correspond to man. *Some of them do not possess* du; *others do*. One needs to gauge carefully the proper use of them. Those who wish to prevent illnesses and replenish the weak body should rely on the middle-level drugs in [*The Divine Farmer's*] *Classic*.
>
> The lower-level drugs of 125 kinds are the assistants and envoys. They govern the curing of illnesses and correspond to earth. *Most of them possess* du. One may not take them for long periods. Those who wish to eliminate cold, heat, and devious *qi*; to break stagnations; and to cure illnesses should rely on the lower-level drugs in [*The Divine Farmer's*] *Classic*. [Emphases added.][41]

The passage reveals two key features of classical Chinese pharmacology. First, drugs are divided into three groups, and *du* stands out as the defining characteristic for each category. This *du*-centered classification of drugs would remain fundamental to Chinese pharmacy throughout the premodern era. Second, *du* figures not as something to be avoided at all costs but as potency valuable for curing illness. Precisely because of this perceived therapeutic power, drugs in the bottom group, most of which possess *du*, are deployed to treat a variety of disorders. The ambivalence of *du* is manifest in *The Divine Farmer's Classic*: since it could evoke both benefit and danger, one should resort to a potent drug only for short periods, use it with caution, and stop using it once the illness was eliminated. A *du*-possessing drug, the text implies, cures if used properly and harms if it is not.

Although potent drugs are useful therapeutic substances, *The Divine Farmer's Classic* places most of them at the bottom of the hierarchy and regards them as inferior to those in the middle and top groups. Rather than treating illnesses, drugs in the middle category serve to strengthen the body in order to prevent it from falling sick. This goal aligns well with a medical philosophy that was developing during the Han dynasty, captured in an aphorism from *The Yellow Emperor's Inner Classic*: "The sage only treats people who are not yet sick, not people who are already sick."[42] It is always better to prevent maladies from occurring than to treat them after they arise.

Moreover, drugs in the top group, which do not possess *du*, are intended for an even higher goal: to prevent aging and prolong life, an aspiration that resonates with the ideal of "nourishing life" (*yangsheng*) in China. This ancient tradition proposes the regular ingestion of tonic substances, such as mushrooms, resin, and minerals like mica, combined with bodily movement, breathing, and meditation techniques in order to achieve longevity.[43] These methods aim to replenish *qi* and eliminate internal poisons that cause bodily decay. Drugs without *du* thus "lighten the body" and purify it of its toxic burdens. Meanwhile, drugs that possess *du*, with their characteristic "thickness," invigorate the body in order to combat maladies. A potent substance effectively cures sickness but impedes one from achieving a loftier goal: the cultivation of a healthy, long life.[44]

The main body of *The Divine Farmer's Classic* describes 365 drugs in detail, which include minerals, plants, animal substances, and foods. For each drug, it specifies its flavor, its *qi* (degree of heat), the illnesses it treats, the benefits it brings to the body, the place of its harvest, and sometimes its alternative names. The first two, flavor and *qi*, warrant further explanation, as they were the basic categories used to define drug properties in classical Chinese pharmacy. Each drug is characterized by one of the following five flavors (*wei*): pungent, sweet, sour, bitter, or salty. These flavors do not necessarily match the sensations as we experience them today but rather are abstract concepts positioned in the five-phase system that correlates the flavor of a drug to a particular organ in the body: pungent drugs to the Lungs, sweet drugs to the Spleen, sour drugs to the Liver, bitter drugs to the Heart, and salty drugs to the Kidneys. Such correlations played an important role in guiding prescriptions.[45] Furthermore, the degree of heat, or *qi*, refers to the temperature of a drug that could be cooling, warming, or plain, as established in *The Divine Farmer's Classic*. Each of these three properties is often an indicator of the corresponding bodily sensation induced by the drug; a warming drug, for example, generates heat in the body. This definition of *qi*, which speaks to the materiality of drugs, is related to but distinct from the meaning of *qi* as a vital force circulating in the body.

Despite the general outline of the *du*-centered organization in the preface, *The Divine Farmer's Classic* does not specify the *du* status, namely, whether a drug possesses *du* or not, for each of its 365 drugs.[46] In the formative years of Chinese pharmacology, such knowledge may not have been systematically developed. It is not until the end of the fifth century, with the rise of an important commentary to the Han text, that an elaborate account of potent drugs emerged.

Potent Drugs in *Collected Annotations*

Collected Annotations on the Classic of Materia Medica (Bencao jing jizhu, ca. 500; hereafter, *Collected Annotations*) is a pivotal text in the history of Chinese pharmacology. Building on the Han classic, the work substantially expands drug knowledge by doubling the number of entries and adding more information about the appearance, source location, and medical uses of drugs. Importantly, it specifies the *du* status of most of its 730 drugs, and provides rich discussion of some oft-used *du*-possessing drugs in Chinese pharmacy. It also explains a variety of techniques for processing and deploying these substances. The text is thus an indispensable source for studying the conceptualization and uses of potent medicines in China.

Collected Annotations emerged at a time of political disunity in China. From the early fourth century to the late sixth century, various groups of nomadic peoples of Turkic, Mongolian, and Tibetan origin invaded the northern lands and pushed the Han people to the region south of the Yellow River, where the latter established a succession of short-lived dynasties. Despite the political turmoil, medicine thrived thanks to the rise of powerful clans devoted to medical practice and the flourishing of religious healing. Specifically, a number of aristocratic families emerged in the south that produced influential medical works. Unlike the Han period, when medical knowledge was chiefly transmitted between a master and his carefully selected disciples, this new era witnessed the ascendancy of hereditary medicine within prestigious elite clans.[47] Furthermore, the fast development of Buddhism and Daoism during this period substantially enriched the repertory of healing; religious devotees of diverse groups adopted drug therapy, incantations, and meditation techniques to cure patients and achieve self-transformation.

In particular, the rise of Daoist alchemy in the southeast, with its rich material practice of manipulating powerful minerals, informed pharmaceutical writings at the time.[48]

The author of *Collected Annotations* is Tao Hongjing (456–536), who grew up in the southeast, near Jiankang (present-day Nanjing), the capital of the Southern Dynasties. Raised in an aristocratic family, Tao was a polymath who, when still in his twenties, became famous for his accomplishments in literature and calligraphy. He was also versed in medicine, which resulted from both family influence and individual initiative. According to Tao's own account, over many generations his family had devoted themselves to studying and practicing curative arts; Tao's father and grandfather both had advanced knowledge of drugs. They relied on a particular formula book called *The Formulary of Fan* to treat thousands of people.[49] Although there is no evidence that Tao himself practiced medicine, his family's active engagement in healing probably contributed to his medical learning. According to a seventh-century bibliography, Tao compiled eight medical texts, including materia medica, formula books, and alchemical treatises, all pointing to his broad knowledge of medicine.[50]

At an early age, Tao also became interested in Daoist writings. The southeastern area where he lived was fertile ground for new Daoist movements that in the fifth century had great appeal to social elites. In 492, after serving for more than a decade as a minor official at the court of the Southern Qi (479–502), he decided to abandon his political career and retire to Maoshan, a range of mountains not far from the capital, where he dedicated himself to Daoist practices of meditation, alchemy, and the compilation of Daoist works. It was also during these years of seclusion that he completed *Collected Annotations*.

As the title indicates, Tao's work is based on *The Divine Farmer's Classic*, but with significant modifications of both the structure and content of the Han pharmacopoeia. The text starts with a lengthy preface in which Tao not only comments on the short preamble of the Han classic but also explains in detail the methods of drug preparation and enumerates drugs for treating major illnesses and countering different types of poisoning, and various ways they could be combined in formulas to treat particular conditions. The hermit makes his motive for compiling the pharmacological treatise clear at the beginning of the preface, observing that in the centuries following the emergence of *The Divine Farmer's Classic*, a number of medical writers either edited the Han text or produced their own unique pharmaceutical works. These efforts often led to errors and confusions that led physicians astray. To rectify this chaos, Tao compiled his new materia medica based on a comprehensive study of all pharmaceutical works available to him. *Collected Annotations* thus reflects Tao's effort to assemble and synthesize pharmaceutical knowledge that combined ancient wisdom with the new understanding of medicines during his time.[51]

There are altogether 730 drugs in *Collected Annotations*. Half of them (365) are copied from *The Divine Farmer's Classic* and the other half from what Tao calls "supplements from eminent physicians," which refers to new accounts on drugs produced by physicians between the Han period and Tao's time.[52] Each drug entry contains three elements. The first is the text from *The Divine Farmer's Classic*, copied faithfully in large red characters. The second, written in large black characters, is from former writings on the drug by post-Han physicians. Importantly, this element specifies whether the drug possesses *du* or not. Although it is impossible to narrow down in which particular text this specification initially appeared, Tao's work was the first to systematically incorporate this knowledge into writings on materia medica.[53] The third element is Tao's own commentaries, written at the end of each entry in small black characters.

By creating this multipart format, Tao initiated a long tradition of commentary writing in Chinese pharmacology. Instead of modifying the Han classic, he preserved it and added information from other sources as well as his own remarks. To distinguish these three elements, he marked them off using different colors and text sizes. It is unclear what writing material Tao used to produce *Collected Annotations* since this text in its original form has long been lost. Although paper was invented during the Han dynasty (first century), it only became a regular medium for court writings in the fifth century, and its spread to other corners of society was probably even slower.[54] Hence the time when Tao completed *Collected Annotations* (ca. 500) was a transitional moment in the evolution of writing technologies in China as paper was gradually replacing the older materials of bamboo and wooden slips. Tao could have used either medium for his writings.

Although the original *Collected Annotations* no longer exists, there is a small fragment of a paper manuscript of the text dating to the seventh century, which offers us a concrete idea of what Tao's text looked like (figure 1.2). The manuscript, discovered in the early twentieth century in the Turfan area

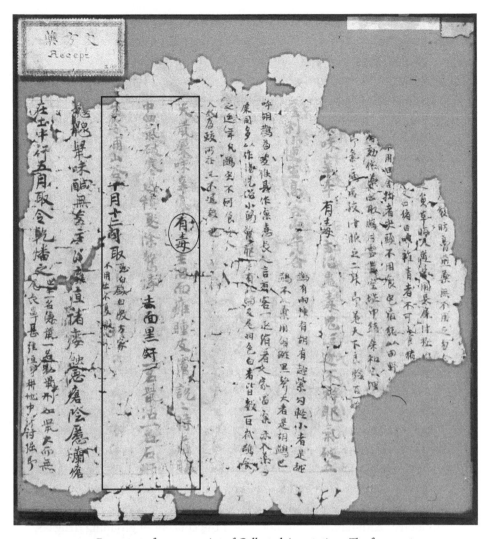

FIGURE 1.2. Fragment of a manuscript of *Collected Annotations*. The fragment contains four animal drug entries. The boxed section shows one of them, bat droppings. The lighter text (red in the manuscript) is from *The Divine Farmer's Classic*, which describes the flavor, degree of heat, medical uses, alternative names, and location of the drug. The darker text (black in the manuscript) is from post-Han medical works that were synthesized by Tao Hongjing, which adds the drug's *du* status, additional medical usage, and time of harvest. The text in small characters at the end is Tao's commentary, pointing out how the drug acts with other substances and how frequently it is used. The circle highlights the black characters *youdu* (possessing *du*), which is Tao's addition. Courtesy of the Deposit of the Berlin-Brandenburg Academy of Sciences and Humanities, State Library of Berlin, Prussian Cultural Heritage, Oriental Department, Turfan Collection Ch. 1036 (back side).

(in present-day Xinjiang), might have been an official copy of the text from the Tang imperial library.[55] It includes the entries for four animal-derived drugs: hog's testicle, swallow droppings, bat droppings, and mole's meat. For each drug entry, excerpts from *The Divine Farmer's Classic* are written in red (shown as light characters in figure 1.2), while the text in black (shown as dark characters in figure 1.2) is Tao's additions (large characters) and commentaries (small characters). Significantly, the information of whether a drug possesses *du* or not is written in black, indicating that this knowledge was later added to the Han work.[56] This particular way of commentary writing persisted in the following centuries; later materia medica texts followed suit by adding new drugs and attaching still more layers of annotation to the existing drug entries. Owing to this format, even though complete works of materia medica from early periods such as *The Divine Farmer's Classic* and *Collected Annotations* are lost to us, their content has been preserved in later sources, allowing for recovery.[57]

In addition to designating the *du* status of each drug, Tao also made one significant change in the organizational scheme of his work. He had based his edition on a version of *The Divine Farmer's Classic* that contained four scrolls, including a short preface and three content scrolls for drugs in the top, middle, and bottom groups, respectively.[58] Tao reorganized the text and created two new versions of his materia medica. The first has three scrolls, with the preface in the first scroll and about half of the 730 drugs in each of the remaining scrolls. The second version, called "the enlarged book" (*dashu*), is divided into seven scrolls: the preface, one scroll on mineral drugs, three on herbal drugs, one on animal-derived drugs, and one on drugs of fruits, vegetables, and grains, as well as drugs that have names but are not used anymore.[59] Although Tao did not invent the concept of grouping drugs by natural category—the idea can be traced back to the Han period—his work was the first in Chinese history to establish this scheme as the basic structure of a text of materia medica.[60]

Besides altering the number of scrolls, *Collected Annotations* also doubles the number of drugs, from 365 to 730. Disregarding those that "have names but are not used anymore," the rest of the drugs (575) are distributed across four natural categories, as shown in table 1.1.

Overall, plants occupy the largest portion in the collection; more than half of the drugs are in this category, indicating the prominence of herbal pharmacology in Tao's days. They are followed by animal-derived products (20%),

TABLE 1.1. Distribution of drugs in *Collected Annotations*

	TOP GROUP	MIDDLE GROUP	BOTTOM GROUP	TOTAL
MINERALS	25	23	23	71
PLANTS	97	91	117	305
ANIMALS	29	39	48	116
FOODS	27	30	26	83
Total	178	183	214	575

Note: The counts are based on Tao, *Bencao jing jizhu*, 2-7.127–516.

foods (14%), and minerals (12%). The drugs are spread across the three-tier hierarchy more or less evenly, with those in the bottom group being slightly more numerous.

How does *du* figure in *Collected Annotations*? Tao inherited the *du*-based organization of drugs from *The Divine Farmer's Classic* and integrated the three-tier hierarchy into each of the four natural categories. Besides defining whether a drug possesses *du* or not, he also created finer distinctions with regard to potency: those possessing "little *du*" (*xiaodu*), those "possessing *du*" (*youdu*), and those possessing "great *du*" (*dadu*), indicating a more nuanced understanding of these substances during his time. The distribution of all the *du*-possessing drugs in *Collected Annotations* is shown in table 1.2.

Overall, about one-fifth (22%) of the 494 drugs in the book are defined as possessing *du*.[61] Consistent with the definition of *du* in *The Divine Farmer's Classic*, the majority of these drugs are in the bottom group (71%); only eight *du*-possessing substances (7%) are in the top group. Moreover, the distribution of the *du*-possessing drugs among the four natural categories is uneven. The plant category contains the largest number (56), meaning more than half of the *du*-possessing drugs are plants. Yet proportionately, the animal category has the highest percentage of potent drugs—almost a third (30%) of the animal-derived medicines possess *du*. These two categories comprise a great majority of the potent drugs (84%). By contrast, the category of foods contains the least number of drugs possessing *du* (8%), which is to be expected, since most of these substances were intended to be consumed regularly.

What are these potent drugs?[62] The group of minerals contains ten *du*-possessing substances, including mercury, sulfur, and four kinds of arsenic compounds.[63] Curiously, most of these drugs are placed in the middle rather than the bottom tier of the hierarchy, which deviates from the *du*-based organizational scheme. It is revealing that besides curing specific illnesses, many

TABLE 1.2. Distribution of *du*-possessing drugs in *Collected Annotations*

	TOP GROUP	MIDDLE GROUP	BOTTOM GROUP	TOTAL
MINERALS	2	5	3	10
PLANTS	4	6	46	56
ANIMALS	1	10	24	35
FOODS	1	2	4	7
Total	8	23	77	108

of these minerals are assigned the power of promoting transcendence, the chief aspiration of Chinese alchemy (see chapter 7). It is probably this lofty promise that enhanced the value of these substances.

The plant group contains a large number of potent drugs, most of which are in the bottom tier. Almost all drugs possessing great *du* are in this tier, among which the most salient example is aconite. Tao lists four kinds of aconite in his book and praises one of them in particular, called "attached offspring" (*fuzi*), as "the lord of the hundred drugs."[64] This is not hyperbole, as aconite was one of the most frequently prescribed drugs in classical Chinese pharmacy.[65] It was also a lethal poison, frequently used in murder in premodern China. Hence proper preparation was the key to harnessing this powerful herb. Other examples of potent plants include "the bean from Ba" (*badou*, croton), the fruit of an evergreen tree growing in the southwest that works as a strong purgative; "the hooking of the throat" (*gouwen*, gelsemium), a poisonous vine from the south that could both kill and heal; "the half summer" (*banxia*, pinellia), the tuber of an herb that is harvested in the summer; and "the seed of derangement" (*langdang zi*, henbane), a hallucinogenic plant that could both induce and cure mania. Tao identifies a variety of uses for these drugs, such as warming the body, breaking stagnation, eliminating swelling, and facilitating movement.[66]

The potent drugs in the animal-derived group are also diverse. Not surprisingly, snakes appear here; their gallbladders are particularly valued for healing.[67] Another important drug in this group is "ox yellow" (*niuhuang*), which refers to bovine bezoars (ox gallstones). Placed in the top tier and defined as possessing little *du*, the drug promises to quell frenzy and pacify the mind. The popularity of the medicine is attested to by its exorbitant price and the proliferation of ersatz products during Tao's time.[68] The most mysterious item in the group is the feathers of a bird called *zhen* (*zhenniao mao*), which were believed to possess great *du*. These special feathers could effectively counter snake poison.[69] They were so poisonous that any alcohol into which they were dipped could kill a person instantly. In fact, alcohol laced with *zhen* feathers was so notorious that the word has become a synonym for poison, as used in the popular idiom "drinking *zhen* to quench thirst" (*yin zhen zhi ke*).[70] The identity of the bird, however, remains murky.[71]

Finally, the group of foods contains several important drugs that possess *du*. One of them is a type of cannabis called "hemp seed" (*mafen*). Placed in the top tier, the drug seeks to treat various kinds of exhaustions and injuries, eliminate cold *qi*, and dissipate pus. Consumed for a long time, it can lighten the body and illuminate the spirit. Yet excessive ingestion of the nutriment makes one "see demons and run crazily"—an indication of a strong disturbance of the mind.[72] Another valuable *du*-possessing drug is alcohol (*jiu*). As a substance of great heating capacity, it is often used as a solvent to release the power of drugs. Similar to cannabis, it could also stir the mind, making one disoriented and confused, an effect that is familiar to many.[73]

Conclusion

One of the defining concepts in classical Chinese pharmacy was *du*. In the formative years of Chinese medicine, the meanings of *du* were more complex than the negative sense of "poison" that is associated with the word today. An important gloss of the word that emerged during the Han period was "thickness," which implied strength, heaviness, and abundance, a characteristic with wide-ranging implications. Early Chinese sources also invoke *du* with a variety of connotations, ranging from effective governance to the nurturing power of virtue, from potent medicines to deadly poisons. *Du* was also used metaphorically to refer to harsh but constructive words. Ultimately, the paradox of *du* lives in its entwined potentials of benefit and harm.

The paradox of *du* is patently expressed in the materia medica of early China. It carries a strong sense of potency that constitutes a medicine's therapeutic power. The three-tier hierarchy established in *The Divine Farmer's Classic* relies on *du* as a principal criterion to categorize drugs. Drugs possessing *du* are valuable for curing illness because of their potency yet could sicken or even kill, also because of their potency. The art of harnessing potent drugs is thus to forcefully eliminate illness without jeopardizing the vitality of life. Later materia medica texts during the Era of Division, exemplified by

Tao Hongjing's *Collected Annotations*, provide more detailed accounts of these powerful substances, which are spread across all the natural categories and are assigned diverse medical uses. By the sixth century, the crucial role of poisons in healing had been firmly established in classical Chinese pharmacy.

What are the possible cultural explanations for the rise of this therapeutic feature in China? The epigraph at the opening of this chapter gives us a clue. The passage, from a second-century BCE philosophical text, stresses the usefulness of aconite, an herb possessing plentiful *du*. This is, of course, medically valid information. Yet the ultimate message of the text is a political one: it uses aconite as a metaphor for emphasizing the value of diverse types of people in the world, which, if recognized by a capable ruler, can greatly benefit the kingdom.[74] Importantly, this all-embracing political vision is aligned with a cosmological view that constitutes the core of the text: the cosmos, originating from the omnipresent Dao, is differentiated into yin and yang complements, the combination of which creates myriad things in the world.[75] As a result, all substances contain both yin and yang forces, which are mutually transformative and in perpetual motion. This cosmology, which finds its roots in ancient philosophical writings such as *Laozi* and *Zhuangzi*, emphasizes the dialectical relationship among all things that defies stable categorization. In this milieu, it is not surprising that poison and medicine, on the pattern of the yin-yang dynamism, are not fixed into distinct, stable categories. They are, in fact, mutually constitutive.

Poisons, with their great healing potential, are, after all, dangerous materials, the misuse of which could result in dire consequences. Physicians in China were fully aware of this, and devised a variety of methods to prepare and deploy them to maximize their benefit and curtail their harm. The central idea underlying the poison-medicine paradox in China is transformation: no fixed distinctions exist; all things are subject to perpetual change. To harness poisons, therefore, one must grasp the techniques of judiciously transforming them into therapeutic agents.

CHAPTER 2

Transforming Poisons

Among herbs there are the long types and the winding types. Ingested separately, they kill people; combined and ingested together, they prolong life.

—*MASTER LÜ'S SPRING AND AUTUMN ANNALS* (THIRD CENTURY BCE)

IN 71 BCE, AT THE CAPITAL OF THE WESTERN HAN, HUO XIAN, THE wife of a powerful general at court, planned to murder Empress Xu so as to seize the position for her daughter. At the time, the empress was frail, as she had just given birth to a child. Huo hired a female physician to prepare a medicine for the empress to help her recover: the physician secretly mixed aconite (*fuzi*) into the medicine and presented it to the empress. On taking some of the "medicine," the empress complained of dizziness and accused the physician of poisoning her, which the latter denied. The empress's condition worsened quickly, leading to her death.[1]

The murder was cunning because of the use of aconite. The herb, a deadly poison, caused the tragic demise of the empress, yet it was also one of the most frequently prescribed medicines in premodern China. In fact, classical Chinese pharmacy rarely used poisons directly; it had developed a variety of pharmaceutical techniques, including dosage control, drug combination, and drug processing, to transform poisons into medicines. Sporadic and terse mentions of these techniques can already be found in ancient medical writings, and more elaborate discussion and dedicated treatises on them arose in the fifth and sixth centuries, which lay the foundation for later pharmaceutical works. The abundant use of potent substances in China thus necessitated the growth of medical technology that tamed these dangerous materials, turning them into useful medicines.

The salience of pharmaceutical techniques in premodern China compels us to rethink the relationship between nature and technology. The increasing appeal of Chinese medicine, and alternative medicine in general today, has much to do with the imagined "naturalness" of herbal remedies in contrast to the artificial quality of Western synthetic drugs. Implicit in this view is a conception of nature that is pure, clean, and safe, a notion derived from the Enlightenment legacy that unambiguously divides nature and culture into separate, mutually exclusive realms.[2] If this legacy propelled a colonial project in the nineteenth and early twentieth century that strove to establish the hegemony of Western medicine over indigenous healing traditions—Chinese medicine included—by discrediting them as "crude" or "unscientific,"[3] the reverse took place in the postcolonial world, when a romanticized view of Chinese medicine made it an attractive alternative to Western biomedicine. Both perspectives are problematic. From the early stages of classical Chinese medicine, technical manipulation of drugs constituted the core of pharmaceutical practice. Potent medicines could be of great value if prepared judiciously. Conversely, a seemingly "natural" substance could seriously injure the body if administered incorrectly. What matters is ultimately not an abstract concept of nature projected by modern minds but the concrete practices of transforming medicines by technical interventions.

Who collected and processed drugs before they reached the hands of physicians? With the expansion of medicinal substances and the increasing sophistication of pharmaceutical techniques from the Han period to the Era of Division, those who prepared and those who sold drugs became gradually separated from those who prescribed them, which, in the eyes of some concerned physicians, affected the quality of ingredients and impeded effective healing. This new situation compelled the latter group to produce treatises that specified the correct techniques of processing and deploying drugs. This significant change marks the heightened attention in medieval China to pharmaceutical preparation so as to guarantee the quality of medicines.

Managing the Dose

In the history of European medicine, the awareness of dosage control in the use of toxic substances can be traced back to antiquity, when Greek physicians noted the danger of prescribing medicines in excess. The importance of dosage control was most explicitly expressed by the Swiss physician Paracelsus (1493–1541), who famously wrote that "all things are poison, and nothing is without poison: the *dosis* alone makes a thing not poison." Throughout Western medical history, careful administration of doses has been key to the therapeutic use of poisons.[4]

Classical Chinese medicine also recognized the significance of dose early on in history. In its preface, the Han pharmacological treatise *The Divine Farmer's Classic* advises, "If one uses a potent drug to cure illness, they should first start with an amount resembling the size of a millet grain, and stop once the illness is eliminated. If not, double the amount. If still not, increase the amount tenfold. Take the measurement according to the elimination of the illness."[5] The amount of a potent medicine, in short, has to be carefully calibrated to the response of the patient.

But this terse statement on dose is still too crude; it sketches a general principle without providing concrete treatment guidelines. Tao Hongjing, in his *Collected Annotations*, further elucidates the passage. He first warns that when using a potent drug on its own, such as croton (*badou*) and euphorbia (*gansui*), one should not recklessly take the maximal dose. He then lays out an elaborate scheme of managing the dose with various combinations of drugs, correlating the amount of a potent drug with the total number of ingredients in a given medicine. The more ingredients with which a potent drug is used, the larger the size of the pill and the greater the number of the pills that Tao recommends.[6] Compared to the discussion of dose in *The Divine Farmer's Classic* that only addresses single-drug therapy, Tao adds more scenarios of compound medicines in his commentary, indicating the rise of such formulas during his time. When suggesting larger doses for multi-ingredient medicines, he probably takes into account the dynamic interaction between these ingredients that curbs the power of the one possessing *du*.

Furthermore, dosage control relies on a stable system of measurement. Elsewhere in the preface, Tao observes that in his time two weight systems coexisted: an ancient system that was coarse, and a more refined one that developed after the Han period. To clear up confusion, he proposes to adhere to the latter system in pharmaceutical preparation to ensure the proper measurement of ingredients.[7] In the case of measuring potent drugs, Tao offers additional advice. For example, he specifies that when using the *du*-possessing fruits of croton (*badou*), an evergreen tree growing in the southwest, one must first remove the pits and skins, and then weigh them using one *fen* to calibrate sixteen pieces of the fruit. This method bypasses the variations introduced by different sizes of fruit, thereby granting a more precise measurement.[8]

Besides these general guidelines on dosage control, Tao also underscores the danger of overdosing in many of his drug entries. Intriguingly, he points out the risk of taking several hallucinogenic drugs. An herb called "the seed of derangement" (*langdang zi*, henbane), for instance, could effectively treat mania. Ingested in excess, however, the drug would cause a person to "run madly." So Tao warns that one must not exceed the suggested doses of the drug. That said, if the drug is taken in small quantities over a long period of time, it could strengthen the body and illuminate the mind. Dose is thus the key factor that could turn the same herb into something curative, harmful, or invigorating.[9] Moreover, Tao particularly emphasizes the problem of consuming certain foods without restraint. Among many cautionary instructions are that immoderate eating of pork could lead to sudden obesity, too much apricot could injure tendons and bones, and eating salt without limit could harm the lungs and induce coughing. Even for these ostensibly benign substances, the price of neglecting proper doses is high.[10]

How should an incident of drug overdose be treated? Tao recommends a list of items that can help to alleviate the symptoms. These include egg yolks, the juice of the indigo plant, mud, water from rinsed rice, and juice from fermented beans, among many others. Notably, most of these substances are ordinary things that could be readily found in a household. Besides treating overdose in general, such commonplace agents could also counter specific types of poisoning, such as spider bites or aconite poisoning. Their easy accessibility probably made them fitting antidotes for handling emergencies.[11]

Combining Drugs

Aside from dosage control, the combination of drugs was another major technique for the safe use of potent medicines, a concept already discernible during the Han dynasty. The rules for combining drugs depended on the structure in *The Divine Farmer's Classic* that has already been discussed. It divides its 365 drugs into three groups, each linked to a specific rank: drugs at the top are the lords; those in the middle are the ministers; those at the bottom are the assistants and envoys. The text then recommends that when combining drugs, one should use one lord, two ministers, and five assistants. One could also use one lord, three ministers, and nine assistants.[12] An effective therapy, like the successful rule of a state, required the cooperation of its constituents.

The correspondence between drug combination and bureaucratic organization is a clear example of the strong influence of political thought on medical writing in early China.[13] In particular, the Han empire established an ideology rooted in the resonance between the cosmos, the state, and the body of the ruler. In this correlative system, a monarch should properly align his body with and model his ways of governance on the patterns of the cosmos. This microcosm-macrocosm resonance promised not just the vitality of the physical body but also the stability of the political body.[14] As a result, medical works during the Han period are replete with political associations. *The Yellow Emperor's Inner Classic*, for instance, assigns an office to each of the twelve organs: the Heart is the office of the lord, the Lungs the office of the minister, the Liver the office of the general, and so forth. When these offices work in harmony, a healthy body is sustained.[15] Drug combination in Han materia medica writings provides another example of this correlative thinking. When the body is in disarray, properly coordinated drugs/officers are dispatched to restore health.

Political alignment, however, was not the only way of perceiving drug relationships during the Han dynasty. Another scheme that stood out was "the seven dispositions" (*qiqing*), which used the analogy of human interaction to define drug relations. *The Divine Farmer's Classic* presents the seven scenarios as follows: drugs that act on their own, ones that need each other, ones that assist each other, ones that fear each other, ones that hate each other, ones that oppose each other, and ones that kill each other.[16] Except for the first type, which refers to single-drug therapy, all the other six dispositions characterize drug combinations with distinct effects, ranging from mutual facilitation to mutual annihilation. The word "disposition" (*qing*) merits our attention. In contrast with political organization discussed above, it points to interpersonal relationships. *Qing* was an important concept in early Chinese thought as disparate definitions emerged out of intellectual debates during the Han period. Some literati understood *qing* to describe the passions or emotions of an individual that required proper control; others took *qing* to be the ways in which one spontaneously responded to specific situations in order to align the self with the natural patterns of the universe.[17] *Qing* in *The Divine Farmer's Classic* meant something still different: rather than referring to sentiments or natural reactions at the individual level, it described the ways people interacted with each other. *Qing* was thus a *relational* concept in the Han pharmacological treatise. That is, a given medicine had no fixed character; its effect would vary greatly depending on the other medicines with which it worked in tandem.

Let us take a closer look at these relationships. In his *Collected Annotations*, Tao Hongjing offers further explanations of them, together with a list of 141 drugs, each with its combinatorial scenarios.[18] The first two dispositions—mutual need (*xiangxu*) and mutual assistance (*xiangshi*)—concern the relationship of two drugs that each enhance the power of the other. In the case of mutual need, the second substance is absolutely required to make a drug work. Tao often identifies these necessary agents as fire, water, or alcohol, indicating the importance of preparing a drug to release its power. In the case of mutual assistance, the second drug could boost the activity of the first one, though it was not essential for efficacy. Sometimes, this involved the use of two potent drugs, such as the combination of gelsemium (*gouwen*) and pinellia (*banxia*). In other cases, ordinary substances were harnessed as "assistants," such as the use of soybeans to activate stellera (*langdu*), an herb possessing great *du*.[19] Tao comments that drugs combined according to mutual need or mutual assistance need not necessarily be of the same type. The combinations resemble cooking, where fish, meat, scallion, and fermented beans are mixed together to bring out the qualities of one another.[20]

The last four types of relationship—mutual fear (*xiangwei*), mutual hatred (*xiangwu*), mutual opposition (*xiangfan*), and mutual killing (*xiangsha*)—seek to constrain a drug's power, with varying degrees of inhibition offered by the second drug. Although *The Divine Farmer's Classic* discourages the use of mutual hatred and mutual opposition in combining drugs because they diminish the power of medicines to the degree that they are not efficacious anymore, Tao does not consider this an absolute rule. If two generals dislike each other, he muses, they can still jointly support the same kingdom. Similarly, although the power of two drugs is reduced, they can still collectively benefit the body.[21] Tao also points out the subtle differences between these two types of combination. For mutual hatred, the inhibition is one-way only—dragon's bone (*longgu*)[22] suppresses bovine bezoar (*niuhuang*), yet the latter enhances the former. Tao explains this using a human analogy: "Although a person hates me, I have no resentment." Mutual opposition, by contrast, is bidirectional—the two "people" are enemies. For example, when orpiment (*cihuang*) and barbarian powder (*hufen*)[23] meet, they become "gloomy and jealous." As a result, barbarian powder blackens, and orpiment also changes color.[24] In the case of potent drugs, the scenario of mutual fear, in which a second drug is required to assuage the potent one without neutralizing its power, is most relevant. For example, whenever using pinellia, Tao stresses that one must add fresh ginger to curb its potency.[25] Without this strategy, the herb is simply too dangerous to ingest.

Finally, the scenario of mutual killing signals the annihilation of the activity of both drugs. This combination, evidently, does not carry therapeutic value. Instead, the goal is to use an antidote to counter a poison. In addition to identifying the medical benefits of poisons, classical Chinese pharmacy recognizes many types of poisoning and offers cures. In fact, Tao provides a list of antidotes in his work to treat cases of poisoning that are derived either from animal attacks (snakebite, beesting, etc.) or from the inept use of powerful medicines.[26] Small wonder that the substances that make potent drugs "fear" overlap with those that "kill" poisons. Examples include licorice, soybean, fresh ginger, ginseng, and the juice of the indigo plant. Dosage is probably the key factor that allows the same substance to work in these two distinct fashions.

Other than dosage control and drug combination, early works of materia medica in China discuss two more factors that condition the use of drugs. First, the method of delivery mattered. According to *The Divine Farmer's Classic*, drugs could be made into pills, powders, decoctions derived from boiling in water or from soaking in alcohol, and pastes formed by pulverizing the ingredients. Each drug could be prepared in one or several of these forms, following strict rules.[27] In general, the liquid forms were thought to deliver the effect of a drug faster than the solid forms, because the former could be easily assimilated into the body. For this reason, drugs possessing *du* were often taken as pills or powders to forestall too vehement a blow to the body. Consistent with this rationale, Tao offered a list of drugs, many of them potent, that he deemed inappropriate for use in decoction.[28]

Second, the effect of a given drug could vary with the state of a particular body. In his *Collected Annotations*, Tao notes that, although a drug's properties were the foundation for its healing power, physicians should also pay attention to the specific condition of a patient's body. For example, they needed to take into account whether a person was deficient, thus requiring replenishment, or replete, thus requiring draining;[29] whether a person was male, female, old, or young; whether a person was sad, happy, vigorous, or exhausted. They should also consider the place where the patient lived and their way of life. All these individual traits could affect the working of drugs. To support this view, Tao offered the example of Chu Cheng, an eminent physician of his time, who treated widows and nuns differently from wives and concubines. In this case, the sexual activity of a woman changed her body to the degree that it required a modified therapy.[30]

Processing Aconite

Many drugs were often subject to various degrees of processing before they were used. A specific term arose in early pharmaceutical sources that designates this set of techniques: *paozhi* (roast and broil).[31] As a result, we find two major types of drugs in Chinese pharmacy: the raw (unprocessed) and the cooked (processed). The latter group included many potent drugs that relied on these techniques to attenuate their power.

How did drug processing in China begin? The etymology of the term *paozhi* offers a clue. Both characters contain the radical for fire, indicating the involvement of heating. According to the Han dictionary *Explaining Characters*, *zhi* means placing meat on fire. The meaning of *pao* is similar but more specific, referring to roasting meat that still has hairs.[32] Evidently, both characters denote ways of cooking. The sense of *pao* as a roasting method can already be found in the first poetry collection in China, *The Book of Odes* (Shijing, ca. 1000 to ca. 600 BCE), in which one poem depicts a host roasting the head of a rabbit to welcome his guests.[33] This early source already considers *pao* and *zhi* to be two distinct cooking techniques: the former refers to the roasting of a newly killed rabbit that still has hairs on its flesh, while the latter designates the broiling of cut rabbit meat that is still soft.[34] Later, *pao* also acquired the meaning of roasting meat coated with a mixture of mud and reed.[35] By the time of the Warring States (476–221 BCE), *pao* had become such a significant method for cooking that it was used interchangeably with its homophone *pao* 庖, which means the person who cooks. The borrowing of this word in labeling drug processing suggests a sharing of culinary and pharmaceutical techniques in early China.[36]

What were the specific techniques and procedures of drug processing? The term *paozhi* implies the use of fire, an essential component in cooking, yet heating constituted only part of the rich repertoire of techniques for drug preparation. For example, *The Divine Farmer's Classic* mentions two ways of drying an herb, under the sun and in the shade, which presumably preserve different levels of moisture in the drug.[37] In his *Collected Annotations*, Tao Hong-jing offers more elaborate explanations of these pharmaceutical techniques, including cutting, pounding, grinding, sifting, rinsing, soaking, boiling, and roasting, among others. He pays keen attention to potent drugs, giving detailed instructions on how to prepare croton, pinellia, and aconite.[38] Skillful preparation was central to taming these poisons for medical use.

Aconite presents an excellent example to illustrate the importance of drug processing. Touted in Tao's text as "the lord of the hundred drugs," it possessed great *du* and hence required careful preparation. The celebrated medicine encompassed a group of herbs of the *Aconitum* genus that Chinese sources refer to by a variety of names (*fuzi, wutou, tianxiong, cezi, wuhui, jin*). It is difficult to precisely identify these plants with species in modern botany given the diverse, sometimes conflicting accounts of them and their shifting referents across disparate sources.[39] In general, these names correspond to different parts of the tubers of the plant collected in different seasons of the year. For example, *wutou*, which literally means "black head," refers to the main tubers of the herb, harvested in the spring when the side tubers have not yet developed, whereas *fuzi*, which literally means "attached offspring," depicts the side tubers that grow in the summer. *Tianxiong*, which literally means "heavenly champion," designates a particular kind of main tuber that never produces side tubers (figure 2.1). Accordingly, these different types of aconite were understood to possess varied levels of potency: *tianxiong*, a plant that consolidated all its medicinal power in its main tubers, was the strongest type, whereas the *fuzi* side tubers were substantially weaker. Classical Chinese pharmacy attributed distinct medicinal uses to each of these varieties of aconite.[40]

More than fifty species of aconite are used in Chinese medicine today, with *Aconitum carmichaelii* from northern Sichuan being the most produced.[41] According to modern pharmacology, the main toxic component in aconite is aconitine-type alkaloid: 0.2 mg of it, taken orally, suffices to poison a person, with symptoms of dizziness, nausea, and numbness of the limbs; 3–5 mg may cause death through cardiovascular and neurological failure.

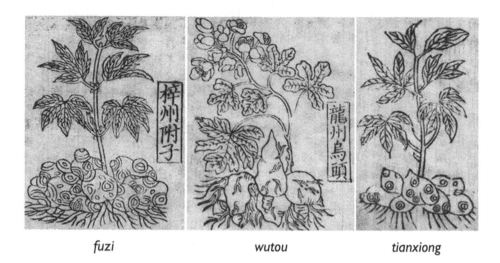

fuzi   wutou   tianxiong

FIGURE 2.1. Three types of aconite. These are depictions from the eleventh-century *Illustrated Materia Medica* (Tujing bencao), the earliest extant pharmacological text that contains drug illustrations. The *fuzi* shown is from Zizhou (northern Sichuan) and the *wutou* shown is from Longzhou (northern Sichuan). These images are preserved in *Revised Zhenghe-Reign Materia Medica Prepared for Usage, Verified and Classified from the Classics and Histories* (Chongxiu Zhenghe jingshi zhenglei beiyong bencao, 1249 Pingyang edition). Courtesy of the Library of Congress.

When administered in smaller doses, however, aconitine and other alkaloids in the herb can relieve pain, reduce inflammation, and strengthen the heart. The use of aconite today, therefore, hinges on the techniques of moderating the herb's toxicity while preserving its therapeutic power.[42]

Evidence for the early medical use of aconite comes from a collection of formulas excavated from Mawangdui in southern China (ca. 168 BCE). Among over two hundred substances that appear in these formulas, aconite, called *wuhui*, is the second most-used drug (twenty-one times), only surpassed by cinnamon (*gui*), another *du*-possessing plant.[43] In most cases, aconite is applied externally, often mixed with other drugs, to treat wounds, abscess, scabies, and itching. When taken internally, it acts as a tonic to replenish *qi*, boost sexual energy, and prolong life. Several formulas also employ aconite to attain the capacity of running with fast speed, evincing its magical power.[44]

Aconite remained popular in the following centuries, with diversified types and altered medical uses. It appears frequently in another set of medical formulas excavated from an unmarked tomb in Wuwei (in present-day

Gansu) dating to the early Eastern Han period (25–220). Prominently, among the one hundred substances included in the thirty-six formulas, aconite stands out as the most often used drug (eighteen times in sixteen formulas). Unlike the Mawangdui formulas, which only employed a strong type of aconite (*wuhui*), the Wuwei formulas primarily used the weaker variety of the plant (*fuzi*), indicating the rising awareness of the drug's power during the Eastern Han period. Subsequently, the herb in the latter collection was often ingested to treat internal disorders such as coughing, "cold damage," and paralysis, whereas its tonic and magical activities receded.[45] That being said, the Wuwei formulas also prescribed *tianxiong*, the most powerful type of aconite, to treat male genital disorders.[46] Consistent with the regular use of aconite in medical manuscripts, *wuhui* and *fuzi* also appear in a list of essential drugs from a first-century BCE primer wordbook for children, indicating that the medicinal use of the herb was common knowledge during the Han period.[47] The drug was fairly affordable at the time, on par with the price of silk products.[48]

Why was aconite so popular in early China? One fundamental guideline of drug therapy in classical Chinese medicine, as established in *The Divine Farmer's Classic*, is the principle of opposites, namely, using warming drugs to treat cold maladies and using cooling drugs to treat hot maladies.[49] Tellingly, aconite is characterized as a substance of great heating power that aims to cure cold conditions such as wind-induced coldness, blood conglomerations, and pain in the joints.[50] The frequent use of the potent herb during the Han dynasty suggests a prevalent concern among healers about the easy loss of the body's vital heat. The warming nature of aconite, therefore, enabled it to powerfully dissipate cold and revive the body.

A potent medicine like aconite could easily turn into a lethal poison. This brings us back to the court murder at the opening of this chapter where the herb figured prominently. Although aconite was a versatile drug, the unprocessed tuber was rarely used due to its extreme toxicity. It is quite possible that the physician introduced some raw aconite into a medicine that was supposed to nourish the empress postpartum but ultimately led to her premature death. An intriguing detail of the story is that the empress complained about feeling dizzy after taking the "medicine," which for us modern readers suggests an alarming sign. Yet medical writings at the time often deemed the strong sensations induced by a potent drug as a marker of its efficacy.[51] This interpretation probably added weight to the words of the physician, who eased the doubts of the empress. The line between medicine and poison is thin; so is that between life and death.[52]

Because of its potency, aconite must be carefully processed prior to medical use. The Mawangdui and Wuwei manuscripts already mention a variety of methods of preparing the plant, including pulverizing (*ye*), soaking in alcohol (*jiuzi*), boiling (*zhu*), decocting (*jian*), roasting (*zhi*), and mincing (*fuju*), although these Han sources offer no technical details.[53] To better understand these pharmaceutical techniques, I now turn to a text that emerged during the Era of Division and offers more detailed accounts. Titled *Treatise on Drug Processing from Lord Thunder* (Leigong paozhi lun; hereafter, *Treatise on Drug Processing*), it is the first book devoted to the discussion of drug preparation in China. The dating of the text is debatable—some scholars have considered it to be a work of the fifth century, while others have argued for later dates, during the Sui or Tang dynasty.[54] The title offers a hint, in that "Lord Thunder" has two possible referents. The name could point to a legendary figure of high antiquity who received the teachings of the Yellow Emperor and became a master in drug processing: this image of Lord Thunder as the founder of Chinese pharmaceutics persisted throughout the imperial era. Alternatively, the name could refer to a historical figure named Lei Xiao, who lived in the fifth century. We know almost nothing about him, except that he was an official in the Liu-Song dynasty established in the south (420–479). He may have written the text based on the teachings of a certain alchemist called Master Yan, as he mentions this name several times in his work.[55] However, particular drugs discussed in the text, such as refined arsenic (*pishuang*), were unlikely to have been available in China during the Era of Division.[56] Most likely, the work took shape over a long period of time, containing a fifth-century core with sections that were added later during the Sui-Tang period.

The treatise contains three scrolls and discusses three hundred drugs altogether.[57] In each entry, the text elucidates the methods of processing the drug, often combined with guidance on how to properly identify the substance in nature. In the case of aconite, the text distinguishes six different types of the plant (*wutou, wuhui, tianxiong, cezi, mubiezi, fuzi*), each with a unique morphology. This is followed by a depiction of two techniques of processing the plant:

> To process ten *liang* [about seven ounces] of aconite, roast it in a gentle fire and
> an intense fire alternately. Eliminate the wrinkles and cracks on the surface of

the tuber. Use a knife to scratch off the hairs at the top and eliminate the fine tip at the bottom. Split the tuber. Dig a pit at the southern ground of *wu* underneath a house, the depth of which could be one *chi* [about one foot].[58] Place the aconite inside overnight. Take it out the next morning. Dry it by baking before use. If one intends to roast aconite, do not use fire generated from impure wood. It is most wonderful to use willow wood. To prepare aconite without heating, eliminate the bottom tip of the tuber. Cut it into thin pieces. Use east-flowing water and black beans to soak the pieces for five days and five nights. Then take them out and drain off the water. Dry them under the sun before use. Whenever one uses aconite, one needs to prepare it without heating. Eliminate the tip of the tuber. For every ten *liang* of aconite, use five *liang* of raw black beans and six *sheng* [about 1.8 liters] of east-flowing water.[59]

Aconite can be prepared in two distinct manners: roasting and soaking. They differ in the time consumed and in the level of technical sophistication. Roasting is faster (one day and one night) but requires delicate manipulation of fire and the use of fine resources (willow wood). It also requires the understanding of a divination system that guides the proper positioning of the tuber for its cooling. Soaking takes longer (five days and five nights) but is easier to execute, given that east-flowing water and black beans were not hard to obtain. The text recommends the latter technique for processing aconite, probably because of its simplicity.

But what is east-flowing water (*dongliu shui*)? Literally, it is water collected from a stream flowing eastward. Such water was deemed to possess the power of purification, an idea that can be traced back to the Han period. According to *The History of the Later Han* (Hou Hanshu, fifth century), each year in the spring, Han officials and common people went to a river that flowed eastward and performed a cleansing ritual to eliminate the filth accumulated over the preceding year.[60] This idea was later adopted by Daoist adepts during the Era of Division, especially those interested in alchemy, who valued the purity of the sites where they compounded elixirs. They often built their alchemical chambers deep in the mountains along a stream flowing eastward, and used its water to ingest the prepared medicines.[61] Certainly easy access to water was important for alchemical exercises, yet we cannot ignore its ritual significance, which aimed to cleanse the site, the alchemical products, and the body of the adept. The water likely served a similar function in the preparation of aconite, that is, to cleanse the herb and eliminate its impurities. It is one of the many examples in *Treatise on Drug Processing* where the text not only discusses material practice in detail but also incorporates ritual thinking prevalent at the time.

Drug Sellers and Medical Markets

Who were the people involved in processing and administering drugs during the formative age of Chinese pharmacology? *The History of the Later Han* recounts a story of a drug seller named Han Kang, who came from a noble family. He harvested drugs in famous mountains and sold them at the market of Chang'an. For more than thirty years, he was unusual in being totally unwilling to negotiate the set price of any of his drugs. This peculiar behavior had made him famous: when he refused to alter the price of a drug that a woman was trying to buy, she immediately recognized who he was.[62] If Han refused to haggle at all, what was his motivation for selling drugs?

The key to this puzzle lies in his prestigious family background, which qualified him for government service. Emperor Huan (132–168) sent envoys with lavish gifts as an invitation to Han to serve at court, but he declined the offer and eventually fled to the mountains to avoid worldly duties altogether. Hence, drug-selling became a façade behind which Han could hide his identity and enjoy his eremitic life. Tellingly, this story appears in a collection of biographies under the category of recluses, people who possessed great talents but had no interest in politics. Besides Han Kang, two other hermits in the section also engaged in harvesting drugs in the mountains to support themselves and escape political burdens.[63] Picking and selling herbs, in other words, was associated with unconventional ways of living.

Other stories from the Han period depict drug sellers as people possessing extraordinary powers. A person named Ji Zixun sold drugs when he was young and after a century, his facial complexion remained unchanged.[64] A healer named Duan Yi offered his disciple an ointment for treating a head injury before the incident occurred, revealing his divinatory power.[65] In another story, an old man hung a gourd in front of his shop when he was selling his drugs at the market. Once the market concluded, he jumped into the gourd. The man later revealed himself to be a master of many kinds of magical arts.[66] Notwithstanding the fantastic aura of these episodes, they disclose an important feature of drug handlers during the Han dynasty:

instead of being devoted specialists, they cultivated multiple skills, often of a magical or occult nature. All these stories appear in a section of *The History of the Later Han* that offers vivid narratives about a group of people generally referred to as *fangshi*, who were technical adepts practicing a variety of magical and esoteric arts, including astrology, divination, exorcism, physiognomy, alchemy, and drug therapy.[67] In comparison to scholars versed in classical learning, these wonder-workers assumed an inferior position in society—standard Han histories treat them as unorthodox and thus less reputable figures, while still depicting their arts with respect. The connection between the preparation of drugs and alchemy was particularly strong, as both activities involved the material practice of transformation.[68] It is possible that certain *fangshi*, such as Han Kang, became hermits and prepared drugs not just to shun politics but also as part of their alchemical practices to prolong their lives. Managing drugs during the Han period was thus linked to a marginalized group of adepts who possessed occult knowledge.

The situation changed during the Era of Division, when we see increasing separation of labor between the different aspects of drug harvesting, selling, and usage. In the preface of his *Collected Annotations*, Tao Hongjing devotes a lengthy section to various methods of preparing drugs. At the beginning of this section, he laments that during his time many drugs were collected from regions south of the Yangzi River instead of from the best sites in the western and northern regions. Due to their inferior quality, these drugs could not effectively cure illness. Tao then remarks:

> Furthermore, the marketmen do not understand the properties of drugs; they only pay attention to their shape and adornment. They no longer sell ginseng from Shangdang,[69] and discard asarum from Huayin like grass.[70] They each follow certain trends, compete with each other, and comply with formulas, accommodating what is needed [in society]. They cannot extensively provide all types of drugs, hence often leave some out. What remains today is about two hundred types. Many physicians do not recognize drugs upon seeing them, so they only listen to the marketmen. Nor are the marketmen able to discriminate among drugs, so they all rely on those who harvest and deliver drugs. Those who harvest and deliver drugs transmit and learn clumsy methods of managing drugs. Thus, it is hard to distinguish the authentic from the fake, the superior from the inferior.[71]

In this passage, Tao identifies three groups of people who act in a chain to handle drugs: those who harvest and deliver drugs (*cai song zhi jia*), the marketmen (*shiren*) who sell drugs, and the physicians who prescribe drugs. We know little about the first group, except that their skills are inferior in Tao's eyes. Besides harvesting drugs, they were probably also involved in processing them, as suggested by the word "manage" (*zhi*), which also appears in *Treatise on Drug Processing*.[72] In his *Collected Annotations*, Tao also uses another term, "drug specialist" (*yaojia*), whose work probably overlapped with that of the first group. Tao holds a critical attitude toward them, claiming that in many cases where a drug proved ineffective, it was due to the incompetence of these drug specialists, not the fault of physicians.[73] Even worse, these suppliers sometimes produced ersatz drugs to make money. Tao writes down a list of ways to produce these counterfeits: whitening stalactite by boiling it in vinegar, straightening the root of asarum by soaking it in water, sweetening astragalus by steaming it in honey, moistening angelica by sprinkling it with alcohol, gluing the eggshells of the mantis to the branches of mulberry trees,[74] and dyeing the legs of centipedes red.[75] What stands out from these examples is Tao's concern about authenticity: the deceptive behavior of the drug suppliers compromised the medical practice of physicians, a situation he tried to rectify by providing reliable pharmaceutical knowledge in his work.

The marketmen, unlike the sagacious, skilled, and somewhat mysterious drug sellers depicted in Han sources, are cast in a negative light in Tao's work, perceived as incompetent and greedy. The competition between these men indicates the booming of the drug market in fifth-century China that drove them to attract consumers by cunning strategies—their attention to the *look* of drugs suggests that the medical uses of these commodities were not necessarily their primary concern. Tao's attitude toward the drug sellers is mixed. On the one hand, he relies on them to obtain pharmaceutical knowledge. In several cases, he points out the obscurity of a drug based on the fact that even the sellers were not able to recognize it.[76] On the other hand, Tao criticizes them for their neglect of drug quality, especially for their selling substitute drugs for profit.[77]

The situation was partly an offshoot of the political turmoil during Tao's days, when the regimes of northern nomadic origin confronted a succession of southern dynasties that Tao was affiliated with. This long-lasting political division impeded the circulation of drugs, leading to the use of ersatz drugs in the south. That being said, markets along the border of the opposing powers allowed a limited exchange of drugs. Previous studies have demonstrated that at least three such markets existed during the fifth century, two in the west—in Liangzhou (present-day Hanzhong in Shaanxi) and Yizhou (present-day Chengdu in Sichuan)—and one on a small island off the east coast, Yuzhou (present-day Lianyungang in Jiangsu). Trade was legal when the two sides were at peace; when political tensions increased, smuggling took the place of open trade.[78] It is conceivable that the marketmen in Tao's account visited similar trading centers and brought valuable drugs from afar back to their local customers.

Sitting at the end of the chain of drug flow, finally, were the physicians. Although Tao himself never practiced medicine, he came from a family that had been involved in healing for generations. By compiling *Collected Annotations*, he hoped to continue his family's engagement in medical enterprise.[79] In this context, Tao's comments on the first two groups of people evince the sentiment of physicians during his days who were concerned about the quality of drugs due to the growth of the market, which distanced them from the source of the medicines they prescribed. By offering elaborate guidelines on the identification and preparation of drugs in his work, Tao sought to clarify the pharmaceutical knowledge that was often opaque to physicians so they would be able to accurately discriminate among drugs and achieve their intended cures.

Tao's observations were echoed by Xu Zhicai (ca. 492–572), an eminent physician and medical officer during his time. Xu came from an aristocratic family that originated from the area of Donghai (in present-day Shandong) and had practiced medicine continuously for eight generations from the fourth to the sixth century. This exceptionally long medical lineage not only brought social prestige to the family but also gained them political capital; several members of the Xu clan served at the courts of both southern and northern dynasties. Xu Zhicai, for his part, was appointed the "director of palace drugs" (*shangyao dianyu*) at the court of the Northern Qi dynasty (550–577), a new position that oversaw the administration of medicines for the imperial house.[80] Among several medical works he compiled, one is titled *Drug Correspondences from Lord Thunder* (Leigong yaodui), a treatise that describes the rules of drug combination. In the preface, Xu notes that in the past, people who were skilled medical practitioners all harvested drugs by themselves. Those healers examined the properties of the drugs and collected them in the right seasons. If a drug was picked too early, its medicinal power would not yet have developed;

if harvested too late, its power would have already diminished. Yet nowadays, he complains, those who practice medicine do not harvest their own drugs. Without knowing in which season a drug should be harvested, they use it indiscriminately. Furthermore, they lack the proper understanding of the cooling and warming properties, administration, and dosage of drugs. As a result, they only desire to cure illness but can never actually obtain the intended results. This is, Xu laments, truly a confusing situation.[81]

Xu attributes his colleagues' insufficient knowledge of drugs partly to their diminished involvement in harvesting, which was likely a result of the separation of labor between collecting, selling, and deploying drugs, as discussed earlier. The distancing of physicians from the sources of their medicines compromised their practice; without knowing the time of a drug's harvest, they missed a crucial piece of information about its power. Yet Xu was not suggesting his readers should go back to the old days. Given the mushrooming of drugs in Xu's time and the sophistication of the techniques of preparation, it had become simply impossible for a physician to know how to do everything. To deal with the new challenge, he established a set of standards for the preparation and administration of drugs to guide physicians' practice. As a court medical officer, he might have produced the text as an institutional response to the chaotic situation of drug usage at the time. Alternatively, considering his family background, it is also possible that he established these pharmaceutical guidelines to assist medical practice in his clan, similar to Tao Hongjing's efforts. Regardless of his motivation, it is evident that fifth- and sixth-century China witnessed increasing concern among physicians about their alienation from the activities of harvesting and preparing drugs and associated therapeutic knowledge. The emergence of the works of Tao and Xu, then, reflects physicians' endeavors to retrieve and standardize that knowledge in order to clear up confusions and improve therapeutic outcomes.

Conclusion

Techniques of preparation and usage were essential in transforming medicines, especially potent ones, from the earliest inception of Chinese pharmacology. Rather than being fixed entities with stable functions, these drugs were malleable substances whose effects varied considerably with the adjustment of dosage, with their interaction with other drugs, and with the methods of processing them. Other factors, such as the form of drugs, the place and time of their harvest, and the constitution of an individual body, mattered too. These diverse techniques were pivotal aspects of drug materiality that constituted a central characteristic of pharmaceutical practice in premodern China: physicians were keenly aware of how the effect of any given medicine changed according to the way in which it was prepared and deployed. Technical interventions were particularly important for the medical use of poisons, such as aconite, as it mitigated their potency yet still preserved their therapeutic efficacy.

This fluid materiality of medicines in classical Chinese pharmacy is in sharp contrast to the concept of "active ingredient" or "active principle" in modern biomedicine, where a specific chemical ingredient isolated from a substance is responsible for its effects. Originating in nineteenth-century Europe, the idea has become the gold standard for drug development in modern pharmacology.[82] In early Chinese pharmaceutical history, however, drugs were not understood to contain such a pure and invariant material core; it was the context of a drug—its interplay with other drugs, its preparation, its mode of acting upon a particular body—that shaped its therapeutic outcome. In this regard, the concept of "drug assemblage" proposed by philosophers Gilles Deleuze and Félix Guattari is relevant. When discussing the function of psychoactive drugs, they challenge the idea of reducing these substances to definitive molecules, and contend that, through dynamic interaction with a fluid body, drugs can produce varied effects that alter a person in myriad ways.[83] Similarly, it is better to consider any given medicine in Chinese pharmacy not as an independent, self-sufficient entity but rather as something working in an assemblage, in which its actions are always *relational*.

These understandings of materiality were put into practice against the backdrop of significant change that took place in the makeup of pharmaceutical practitioners in early China. During the Han period, various aspects of drug management were attended to by *fangshi*, an eclectic group of adepts who possessed occult knowledge and magical power. Although occasionally summoned by the court to offer their expertise, they largely lingered on the margins of the society, living as hermits. In the fifth and sixth centuries, with the expansion of drugs, we see a growing specialization of pharmaceutical activity that separated the collection and selling of drugs from their usage in medical practice. Concurrently, physicians from aristocratic families with strong political connections dominated the production of medical texts, which often reveal their concerns about the new situation. The proliferation of guidelines on how to identify, collect, and prepare drugs during this period manifested their efforts to standardize pharmaceutical knowledge and improve remedies, thereby securing social and political prestige.

The altered landscape of Chinese pharmaceutics in the fifth and sixth centuries was in addition a partial outcome of political conditions, as hostile regimes in the north and south impeded the circulation of medicines. The situation started to change toward the end of the sixth century, when the unified dynasties of the Sui (581–618) and the Tang (618–907) facilitated empire-wide production and dissemination of drug knowledge. Unlike the preceding centuries, when medical works were compiled by capable and concerned individuals, the state became more involved in medicine during the Sui and early Tang periods, resulting in new institutions, legal codes, and pharmacological texts that oversaw the preparation and use of drugs. In this new era, the therapeutic logic of deploying poisons resonated with political rulings, leading to powerful repercussions in society.

PART II

Knowledge, Authority, and Practice

CHAPTER 3

Fighting Poison with Poison

For something that has a shape, one can use a potent medicine to strike it.

—*THE SEQUEL TO RECORDS OF SEARCHING FOR THE SPIRITS*

(FIFTH OR SIXTH CENTURY)

As demons are conjured by humans, killing those conjurers will terminate demons.

—*THE HISTORY OF THE SUI* (SEVENTH CENTURY)

A COLLECTION OF MIRACLE TALES COMPILED BETWEEN THE FIFTH and sixth centuries presents the following story: Xu Yong, an officer in central China, had a brother who had been suffering from pains in the heart and the abdomen for more than a decade. Xu called for a famous doctor named Li Ziyu. The night before the doctor arrived, a demon appeared and whispered to the demon that had been residing in the abdomen of Xu's sick brother, "Why don't you kill him quickly? Otherwise, Li Ziyu will use his red pill to strike you to death." The demon in the abdomen replied, "I am not afraid." The next morning Li showed up. Upon observing the patient, the doctor declared that Xu's brother had contracted a demonic illness. He then took out a medicine called "Red Pill of Eight Poisons" from his drug box and asked Xu's brother to ingest it. In no time, a thundering sound arose from the abdomen of the patient, who then had multiple discharges. After that, he was cured.[1]

The story suggests a crucial link between etiology and therapy. The doctor attributed the illness of Xu's brother to a demon hidden in his body. To eliminate the malign agent, he prescribed a powerful medicine that dealt the demon a lethal blow. The logic of using potent substances to combat illnesses was tied to the ways in which these pathological conditions were understood: etiological ideas justified the use of poisons for healing.

A variety of etiological models existed in medieval China, and demonic sources of illness figured prominently. Originating in antiquity, this family of ideas found new expression in the Daoist movements that flourished during the Era of Division, a time of frequent epidemics. Demonic causes of illness are also discussed extensively in the first treatise on etiology in China, *On the Origins and Symptoms of All Illnesses* (Zhubing yuanhou lun, 610; hereafter *On the Origins and Symptoms*). Among the more than sixty types of disorders discussed in this work sponsored by the Sui court is a set of conditions induced by demons with severe symptoms. The text also elucidates a related but distinct category of illness caused by *gu*, which was a form of poison derived from the manipulation of virulent vermin. A shared characteristic of these illnesses was their source in concrete entities—demons and worms—that could either attack the body from outside or from within. Poisons offered a powerful solution to target and destroy these obstinate but discrete pathological agents.

This rationale was not restricted to medical thinking; it also had significant political ramifications. The demon-induced illnesses were often considered contagious, and responsible for large-scale epidemics that devastated the society. This compelled the state to take swift action to stop these calamities. Moreover, vicious *gu* poisoning, with its elusive nature and dire consequences, posed a serious menace to the political order. During the Sui period (581–618), several new forms of *gu* emerged that generated intense anxiety, even paranoia, at court and beyond. Forceful political responses were triggered to punish the *gu* practitioners, who were mainly women, and push them to the margins of the empire. As we will see, the medical rationale of prescribing poisons would have far-reaching implications for ruling the state.

Demons, Contagion, and Epidemics

The therapeutic principle of utilizing poisons is already visible in *The Divine Farmer's Classic*. In the preface, the Han text recommends the use of different types of drugs to treat different categories of disorders. A warming drug, for example, should be harnessed to counter cold maladies, and vice versa. To treat indigestion, one should take drugs that induce vomiting and draining.

Importantly, the text singles out potent drugs to combat two specific conditions: demonic infestation and *gu* poisoning.[2] What were these disorders? And how do we make sense of the logic of treating them with poisons?

Let's start with demonic infestation (*guizhu*). It is a conspicuous class of illness in *The Divine Farmer's Classic*—more than twenty drugs in the text are recommended to treat the malady. The compound components of the word itself merit explanation. The first component, *gui*, is a multivalent word that in early Chinese sources generally referred to various kinds of spirits, either benevolent or nefarious. *Gui* could refer to the spirit of a dead person, similar to the concept of a ghost, or to a deity offering blessing or protection. It could also designate the spirit of an animal (dog, snake, fox, etc.) or an inanimate thing (mountain, river, tree, etc.).[3] In medical texts, however, the word almost always carries a negative sense, referring to either the disquieted spirit of the deceased haunting the living or demonic entities of diverse origin that assault the body. *Gui*, in short, were believed to be malevolent forces that could trigger devastating illnesses.

If *gui* reveals the cause of sickness, the second component, *zhu*, depicts its dynamics. According to a first-century dictionary, *zhu* means "pouring."[4] Building on this basic sense, a third-century lexicon interprets *zhu* as a condition wherein "when one person dies, another person contracts the illness as the result of *qi* pouring in."[5] This implies that the illness is contagious. Yet unlike the modern conception of contagion, it is only after the afflicted person dies that the illness can be transmitted to others, indicating that the dead body is the source of the pollution.[6] To explain the mechanism, *qi* is the key: a deceased body emanates poisonous *qi*, which pours into a healthy body, leading to its collapse.

Upon investigating its individual components, the meaning of *guizhu* becomes clear: it refers to a set of contagious disorders that are induced by demonic agents. The symptoms of *guizhu* are varied and serious. According to *Formulas for Emergencies to Keep at Hand* (Zhouhou beiji fang), a fourth-century medical work by Ge Hong, demonic infestation expresses itself in sundry symptoms, ranging from thirty-six to ninety-nine different types. The common patterns include alternating chills and fever, dribbling urination, a state of confusion and quietness, not knowing the origin of one's suffering, and pains all over the body. Over time, the patient loses vitality and eventually dies. The illness then spreads to people nearby, sometimes leading to the annihilation of an entire family. When encountering such symptoms, Ge urges, one must take prompt action. Demonic infestation, in brief, signifies a critical situation that demands swift treatment.[7]

Where did the etiology of *guizhu* come from? The notion of illness caused by demonic attack has ancient roots. In the pre-Han era, demons were often held responsible for conditions that were acute, that seemed to occur by chance, and that seemed detached from human culpability. Sometimes, these disorders exhibited contagious symptoms, though the idea of "infestation" (*zhu*) had not arisen.[8] The situation changed in the Eastern Han dynasty (25–220), when demonic maladies became associated with dead bodies that were dangerously contagious. In particular, a new type of funerary writing emerged in the Han tombs that displayed overt concerns about contagion. Called "grave-quelling writs" (*zhenmu wen*), these injunctions aimed to suppress the miasmic influence of a corpse with the help of heavenly deities so as to protect the family of the deceased. Revealingly, the advent of such writings coincided with the occurrence of a series of epidemics in the second and early third centuries that ravaged the country, leading to the development of funeral rituals, possibly mediated by shamans and certain *fangshi*, to manage these devastating events.[9]

With the rise of Daoism at the end of the Han period, the conception of demonic illness changed again. The early Daoist movement known as the Way of the Celestial Masters (Tianshi Dao) that developed in the southwest in the second century used healing as an effective way to recruit followers. In their etiological framework, demons were taken to be the cause of many types of illness.[10] In contrast with earlier views, Daoist practitioners often imagined demonic attack as the unfortunate outcome of the moral failing of the individual. The Celestial Masters, for example, created a ritual space called "the quiet chamber" (*jingshi*) in which patients were to confess their sins and repent before petitions could be sent out to the gods requesting a cure.[11] Illness could also be hereditary: the faults of one's ancestors could affect the body of a descendant, making it susceptible to disasters. In another scenario, the spirits of the dead could file "sepulchral plaints" (*zhongsong*) to the court of the underworld to claim justice, which often entailed punishing the living descendants of the accused with sickness.[12] Therefore, illness in Daoist terms was not just a physiological concept but one entwined with the moral conduct of the individual and its repercussions across generations.

Later Daoist movements followed suit and began blaming demons for epidemics. A Daoist treatise of the fifth century depicts an apocalyptic scene in vivid detail.[13] In an age of moral chaos, swarms of demons plague the human world with myriad illnesses. The Demons of Great Thunder, leading their eighty thousand underlings, spread thirty-six kinds of malady; the innumerable Demons of Youjian are responsible for the sickness of red-swelling; the Demons of Red Eyes induce vomiting and dysentery upon invading the bodies of victims.[14] There is even a kind of demon called "attached offspring" (*fuzi*), which is nine feet tall, with three faces and one eye. The name coincides with that of the potent herb aconite (discussed in chapter 2), revealing the close relationship between powerful drugs and demonic illness.[15] The text conspicuously identifies the names of many demons, as the calling of names was considered an effective way to target and destroy vicious beings in early Daoist rituals. In fact, the entire scripture is devoted to using incantations, often including the invocation of specific names, to annihilate demons.

Medical works from the fifth century on shared the demonic etiology as seen in Daoist healing practices, but with a shifted focus that tied demonic attack to the condition of the body.[16] The issue is elaborated in *On the Origins and Symptoms*, which is the first book devoted to etiology in Chinese history. The text emerged during the Sui dynasty (581–618), the period that marked the end of a three-century-long political division between the northern and southern dynasties. In this new political climate, the court set up medical institutions and sponsored several medical works that paved the way for the governmental regulation of medicine in the centuries to come.

One of these court-commissioned projects was *On the Origins and Symptoms*, produced under the direction of Chao Yuanfang. We know little about Chao, except that he was a head officer in the Imperial Medical Office, a new institution established during the Sui dynasty that aimed to train specialists who would provide medical services for court officials. There were three departments in the office: medicine, therapeutic exercise, and incantation. Although direct evidence is lacking, it is possible that Chao served in the department of therapeutic exercise (*anmo*) given the extensive discussion of the techniques in his work.[17]

On the Origins and Symptoms contains fifty scrolls and sixty-seven categories of illness. For each category, Chao starts with a general discussion of the origin of the illness and its symptoms. This is followed by a series of subsections in which he explains a variety of subtypes of the illness and their respective symptoms. Altogether, he identifies 1,739 symptoms, offering one of the most extensive accounts of etiology and symptomology in premodern China.

The work also recommends remedies for chronic and noncontagious illnesses, chiefly in the form of "guiding and pulling" (*daoyin*), a set of bodily techniques that include stretching, breathing, clacking the teeth, swallowing saliva, and meditation.[18] Drug therapy, by contrast, rarely appears in the book. This is partly due to the immense popularity of *daoyin* at the Sui court, espoused by an avid emperor who promoted it to an unprecedented degree.[19]

How does Chao explain demonic infestation? The condition appears in the category of the illness of infestation, which contains thirty-three subtypes, each with distinct symptoms. In the subtype of demonic infestation, Chao states:

> The reason that infestation means "to reside" is that the illness lingers, stagnates, halts, and resides [in the body]. There are people who initially have no other illness and are suddenly struck by a demon. At that moment, they sometimes feel piercing pains in the heart and the abdomen; sometimes they feel oppressed in the extreme, falling to the ground, resembling the "malignant stroke" type of illness. After one recovers, the residual *qi* does not rest. It halts and resides for a long time, and sometimes agitates and moves. It lingers, stagnates, halts, and resides, eventually leading to death. Upon death, it pours into people nearby. Therefore, it is called demonic infestation.[20]

Two different meanings of *zhu* stand out in this passage. The first is infestation, which echoes the interpretation of the word in the third-century dictionary examined earlier. A second meaning appears for the first time in Chao's text, that is, taking up residence inside the body, indicating that the illness is latent, ever ready to plague the victim again.[21] If the initial attack by demons manifests the sudden and violent aspect of the illness, the lingering *qi* of these vicious entities left in the body poses an ever-present menace to life. In Chao's eyes, demonic infestation is an obstinate condition; early therapeutic success cannot guarantee its thorough eradication.

The symptoms of demonic infestation resemble those of "malignant stroke" (*zhong'e*), a condition in which one is suddenly struck by the *qi* of a demon, which happens when the guarding spirit of the victim is weak. Malignant stroke is an acute condition: the patient falls sick abruptly, with severe symptoms of piercing pain in the heart and the abdomen, and deadly oppression. If the patient survives the initial assault, the residual *qi* of the demon may linger in the body and become the illness of infestation.[22] Although demonic infestation and malignant stroke are similar and related disorders, there is one subtle but important difference: while demons are blamed for the former, the latter is caused by demonic *qi*. In fact, the discourse on *qi* constitutes the most salient feature of Chao's etiological reasoning, yet this *qi*-centered explanation of illness was not invented by the Sui physician—it was already abundantly discussed in the Han medical treatise *The Yellow Emperor's Inner Classic*.[23] What is new in Chao's work is his effort to subsume demonic etiology into this ancient conceptual framework, thereby connecting external insults to the condition of the body. He expresses particular concern about bodies depleted of vitality, which are susceptible to demonic attacks and ensuing total collapse. Departing from the explanations of sickness as a moral failing often seen in early Daoist writings, Chao ascribes the rise of maladies directly to the vulnerability of the body.

Overall, the perception of demonic disorders underwent several transformations in Chao's treatise: a shift in etiological focus from demons to demonic *qi*, the sensitivity of vulnerable bodies, and the tenacity of the illness. The symptoms were acute and severe, often leading to death and causing contagion. How did Chao treat these intractable disorders? Curiously, he offered no remedies. This is likely because he considered therapeutic exercise, the major method of healing in his work, to be particularly effective to treat mild, chronic, and noncontagious illnesses. For acute and life-threatening conditions, however, he may have deemed the method limited.[24]

Other seventh-century physicians, such as Sun Simiao, did propose cures to combat demonic illnesses, primarily through drug remedies. In his *Essential Formulas*, Sun compiled a section with forty-five formulas to treat various types of demonic disorder.[25] These formulas differ considerably in the number of ingredients, ranging from single-drug therapies to compound formulas that contain up to fifty ingredients. A common feature they all share is the regular use of potent drugs. One formula called the Great One's Powder for Emergencies (Taiyi Beiji San), for example, contains nine ingredients, eight of which are potent.[26] As the name implies, the formula is used to treat acute conditions induced by demonic attack. Having ingested the medicine, Sun notes, the patient will have a nosebleed if the illness is located in the head, vomit if it is above the diaphragm, go through draining if it is below the diaphragm, and sweat if it is in the limbs. These therapeutic effects indicate that the medicine powerfully purges the body, expelling poisons in the form of blood, sweat, and bodily waste. In other cases, these toxic matters assume more concrete forms. A large, forty-five-ingredient formula named Powder of Golden Teeth (Jinya San) promises that once the patient takes the potent medicine, worms will be discharged with urine and excrement. Powerful drugs were deployed to drive sinister creatures out of the body.[27]

Finally, there was a strong connection made between demonic infestation and epidemics—contagious illness could inflict large populations with devastating consequences. Epidemics, in fact, constituted a major type of sickness in imperial China, with a history that can be traced back to antiquity.[28] Especially during the tumultuous time of the third century, the collapse of the Han dynasty brought wars, famines, and waves of devastating plagues that decimated the population. The rise of the Daoist movement during this period had much to do with its emphasis on ritual healing that offered attractive antidotes to the gloomy reality.[29] Drug remedies were also utilized to combat epidemics. One story preserved in Sun Simiao's *Essential Formulas* recounts how in 169, an epidemic broke out in Nanyang (in present-day Henan), leading to countless deaths. Witnessing the tragedy, a scholar from Shu offered a pill to the afflicted people, which powerfully expelled demons that caused the suffering. The pill, as revealed by Sun, contained several potent mineral and herbal ingredients. It could not only cure the unfortunate victims who ingested it but also protect anyone from demonic assault who was in a house where the pill had been burned. Potent medicines were mighty weapons to dispel virulent entities.[30]

The sixth century is another moment in Chinese history when epidemics wreaked havoc. Besides the constant wars between the northern and southern powers, another factor that might have contributed to the surge of illnesses was the sudden climate change in the early part of the century, creating a spell of extremely cold weather that ruined crops and caused large-scale famines.[31] Small wonder that during this period, demons proliferated in Daoist writings, which often depicted an apocalyptic scene of the descent of swarms of malign forces spreading illnesses and exterminating large populations. Devotional practices, such as the recitation of scriptures and the invocation of spells, these texts urged, were the only way to obtain salvation.[32] Some of these methods were integrated into the state healing repertoire. Among the three departments established in the Imperial Medical Office of the Sui dynasty, for instance, one relied on incantatory healing, which borrowed both Daoist and Buddhist ritual techniques to fight epidemics.[33] The effort is also seen in the state-sponsored *On the Origins and Symptoms*, which offered substantial discussion of a variety of contagious disorders.³⁴ The institutional responses to epidemics, together with the elaborate conceptualization of such illnesses in medical writings, provided both theoretical reasoning and a practical guide for combatting contagion, which would have repercussions for centuries to come.³⁵

Gu Poison

The other type of illness that potent medicines targeted, encapsulated in *The Divine Farmer's Classic*, was *gu* poison. The meaning of *gu* was complex and changed over time. Its graph, which appeared in oracle bones (second millennium BCE), depicts one or two wormlike creatures sitting in a vessel. It refers to a pathological condition often located at a specific site in the body (bones, teeth, etc.). These early pictographs already imply a connection between *gu* and poison: placing vermin inside a vessel, which may also designate a container for food, could cause serious harm.³⁶

Later sources in antiquity further elucidate the meaning of *gu*. In *Zuo Commentary* (Zuozhuan, ca. fourth century BCE), a work that chronicles the major political events in the ancient state of Lu, we encounter the revealing story of a duke from the state of Jin who summoned a physician to treat his sickness. The physician, named He, claimed that the duke was incurable because he had contracted a *gu*-like illness resulting from sexual indulgence. Later, when a minister approached He and asked him the meaning of *gu*, the physician explained that it was "what excess, indulgence, delusion, and chaos generate." He also considered *gu* to be the way that grains could change into flying vermin. Moreover, he cited *The Classic of Changes* to interpret the word as "women deluding men or the wind blowing down [the trees] in the mountain." Pleased with He's answer, the minister sent him off with lavish gifts.³⁷

Above all, He correlated *gu* with the seductive power of women. The perceptive physician believed that *gu* was induced by intemperance, which spoke to the duke's reproachable and life-limiting sexual indulgence. Earlier in the conversation, he offered a lengthy explanation of this disorder in the framework of "six *qi*" that tied excessive behaviors to the malfunctioning of the body. The sickness of delusion (*huo*), he reasoned, derived from the excess of obscurity, which implied the hours of darkness when intercourse occurs. The sexual excess then generated heat inside the body and turned into *gu* illness.³⁸ To further support the female connection to *gu*, the physician presented evidence from *The Classic of Changes* in which sixty-four hexagrams were used to make predictions. The hexagram for *gu* is ䷑; it consists of the upper trigram ☶, which means "firm" or "mountain," and the lower trigram ☴, which means "supple" or "wind."[39] He thus interpreted the combination as women (a supple force) deluding men (firm beings), or the wind blowing down trees in the mountain, the latter signifying a destructive female power bending and ruining what stands upright, namely, male authority.[40] In addition, the physician also explained *gu* as grains transforming into flying vermin. This possibly refers to the emergence of insects from grains as facilitated by wind, given the close connection between wind and worms in ancient China.[41] More obvious is the idea of transformation associated with *gu*—its potential to morph into myriad things that are hard to predict and elusive to capture. This concept of *gu* became linked to demons in later sources.

Among the diverse meanings of *gu*, the connection to what was referred to as *chong* was the most prominent and enduring. *Chong*, often translated into English as "worm," is impossible to correlate to a single biological entity. The Han dictionary *Explaining Characters* simply defines it as "creatures with feet" and relatedly defines *gu* as "*chong* striking the abdomen," indicating an animal insult on the body.[42] In various contexts, *chong* could refer to animals in general or small, crawling creatures such as reptiles, insects, and worms.[43] As far as *gu* is concerned, it usually designates destructive and sinister agents that either assault the body from the outside or impair it from within. The association of *gu* with animals, large and small, became more conspicuous during the Era of Division. In *Records of Searching for the Spirits* (Soushen ji, fourth century), for example, *gu* was depicted as a demonic agent that could morph into diverse animal forms such as dogs, boars, worms, and snakes. These dangerous creatures would then slyly approach human beings, strike, and kill.[44] In other cases, *gu* referred to malicious human manipulation of vermin. A story in *The Sequel to Records of Searching for the Spirits* (Soushen houji, fifth or sixth century) describes a southeastern family who bred *gu*. Guests who ate their food would spit blood and die. But, the text recounts, when a monk showed up and was offered the poisoned meal, he chanted a spell, which caused two large centipedes to crawl out of the plate. The monk then safely ate his meal uninjured.[45] *Gu* poison here involved the manipulation of dangerous insects to corrupt food. Correspondingly, the removal of them, in this case by a ritual action, neutralized the curse.

The menace of *gu* also drew the attention of medical writers.[46] In his *On the Origins and Symptoms*, Chao Yuanfang dedicates a scroll to the discussion of various illnesses caused by *gu*. It is one of the most elaborate accounts on the deadly poison in medieval China. Chao defines *gu* as follows:

> There are many types of *gu* poison, all of which are *qi* of change and delusion. There are people who deliberately manufacture *gu*. They often catch creatures like worms and snakes, use a vessel to store them, and leave them to freely devour each other. The only thing that remains [in the vessel] is called *gu*. It then can change, and become the source of delusion. Eaten following alcohol and food, it afflicts people with disaster. The affliction of others [in turn] brings fortune to the owner of *gu*. Therefore, untrammeled outlaws store and worship *gu*. There is also flying *gu*, which comes and goes without reason, with the hidden state like demonic *qi*. People who are afflicted by it suddenly contract severe illnesses. Those who are hit by *gu*-induced illnesses often die. Because of its great power of poisoning and harming, it is called *gu* poison.[47]

Chao's formulation clearly links *gu* poison to vermin, but it is not the direct contact of the poisonous creature with the victim's body that causes harm. Instead, illness, misfortune, or death result from the malignant *qi* it emanates, which underscores the elusive and capricious nature of *gu* poison: it can act from a distance, change constantly, and afflict people "without reason." In particular, Chao identifies two basic characteristics of *gu*. The first is its power to change (*bian*). This quality is already visible in some early accounts of *gu*, where it is imagined to assume various animal forms. What is different in Chao's description is his use of amorphous *qi* to replace concrete creatures, a move consistent with the centrality of *qi* as an explanatory framework in his writings. The second is *gu*'s power to delude (*huo*). This sense of *gu* is linked to the seductive danger of women in ancient texts, as discussed before. The association of *gu* with women is not explicit in Chao's account, but what is clear there is that *gu* develops out of the destructive intention of its creators. Because there was always a vicious mind behind each *gu* poisoning, the cure not only concerned the healing of the individual body but also the restoration of social order by eliminating the *gu* poisoners.

According to Chao, illnesses caused by *gu* poison were chiefly of two types, both of which could cause severe symptoms. The first type was chronic, likely the outcome of the deliberate manipulation of *gu* vermin. Chao depicts four kinds of *gu* poison in this category: the *gu* of snakes, the *gu* of lizards, the *gu* of toads, and the *gu* of dung beetles.[48] The maladies caused by this variety of *gu* often lasted for years, and if left untreated would lead to the death of the patient. Tellingly, each of the four kinds of *gu* poison acquired its name from a particular type of vermin. Oftentimes, Chao used these names to delineate the morphology of pathological formations inside the body, which could vigorously devour the viscera. For instance, those who were struck by the *gu* of a dung beetle might spit out something resembling the crawling insect. Since *gu* preparation involved poisonous vermin, they naturally became the source of pathological imagination.

The second type was "flying *gu*," which wandered in nature unattached to a *gu* manipulator. The illnesses it induced were often acute and life-threatening, leading to the rapid collapse of the body. A seventh-century source describes a flying *gu*, invisible but emitting the sound of a bird chirping. If someone was struck by it, they would suffer bloody diarrhea and die within ten days.[49] The acute nature of the condition was obvious. Despite their varied symptoms, both types of *gu* illness were caused by dangerous vermin, which either crushed a victim all of a sudden or slowly ravaged the vital organs of the body.

How could *gu* poisoning be treated? In his *Essential Formulas*, Sun Simiao offered twenty remedies, most of which prescribed potent substances to eliminate vicious vermin. The drugs overlapped substantially with those for expelling demons, such as realgar, croton, aconite, and centipede. Once these powerful medicines were ingested, Sun observed, the patient's body would experience a violent process of purging, leading to the discharge in the form of worms, snakes, and insects. The efficacy of these formulas was thus found in their power to expunge poisons from the body.[50]

There were simpler remedies too. In order to treat two specific types of *gu*, cat-demon *gu* and wild-path *gu*, Sun recommended incinerating a red snake that had happened to die on the fifth day of the fifth month, and eating the ashes with water collected in the morning.[51] The date specified in the remedy is significant, as it was considered a time of extreme yang, when the strength of a poison reached its apex. The vermillion color of the snake also signifies the fiery power of yang. A snake collected on this day, presumably possessing the highest level of poison, could be turned into a potent medicine to counter the similarly poisonous vermin inside the body.[52]

This logic of healing, based on the principle of similarity, was also described in the materia medica literature. A telling example comes from the eighth-century *Supplement to Materia Medica* (Bencao shiyi) compiled by the Tang scholar Chen Cangqi.[53] Among the more than seven hundred drugs in this treatise, one is called "*gu* vermin" (*guchong*), which can be used to treat *gu* poison. Specifically, one collects *gu* vermin expelled out of the body of a victim, dries them, and burns them into black aches. Ingesting these ashes can cure a person with *gu* poisoning. Moreover, the text provides a set of correspondences that act in concert: an illness caused by snake *gu* could be cured by centipede *gu*; an illness caused by centipede *gu* could be cured by toad *gu*; an illness caused by toad *gu* could be cured by snake *gu*. The remedies worked because, the text reasons, "things of the same type can subdue each other." According to this logic, *gu* vermin is *both* a malady and a cure.[54]

Gu Witchcraft

Gu was a medium of poisoning that often involved the manipulation of vermin and the defilement of food, but this was not the only way that *gu* poisoning was imagined and practiced. In many sources from the Han period on, it was also linked to witchcraft. Specifically, the term "shamanistic *gu*" (*wugu*) appeared frequently, referring to various methods of black magic that were deployed to harm the victim.[55] In an often-recounted episode that took place during the Western Han period, a trusted officer of Emperor Wu (reigned 141–87 BCE) accused the prince (and heir apparent) of preparing a type of *gu* witchcraft that operated through a wooden puppet so as to make the emperor sick. Enraged by the accusation, the prince executed the officer, which further aroused the emperor's suspicion. A bloody clash at the court ensued, leading to the death of thousands of courtiers and eventually the suicide of the prince.[56] The event became a watershed in the history of the Han dynasty, resulting in a reshuffling of political power and a sea change in the intellectual culture of the court. Although the accusation was unwarranted, *gu* represented a dangerous menace to the established order, eliciting keen anxieties and harsh actions.[57]

Later sources offer more vivid accounts of *gu* witchcraft. A particular type of *gu*, called "the cat demon" (*maogui*), arose during the Sui dynasty and exerted profound influence on the political culture of the time. Let's first turn to an episode that took place at the end of the sixth century, during the reign of Emperor Wen (reigned 581–604). Dugu Tuo, an official at the court, was interested in "the sinister way."[58] Early on, his mother-in-law worshipped the cat demon and introduced the sorcery into Dugu's household. Later, the empress and the wife of a high-ranking general named Yang Su both fell sick. When physicians were summoned, they all diagnosed it as an illness characteristic of the cat demon. Considering Dugu's special position—he was the half-brother of the empress, and his wife was the half-sister of the general— the emperor questioned him in private, but Dugu denied any involvement. Still suspicious and unhappy with his reluctance to cooperate, the emperor dispatched a group of officers to investigate the case.

Eventually they identified a maid in Dugu's house named Xu Ani, who came from the family of Dugu's mother-in-law. She confessed that she worshipped the cat demon and possessed the power to conjure up the spirit, which could kill a person and secretly transfer the property of the victim to the murderer. She further admitted that early on, Dugu asked her to cast the cat-demon curse on the empress and the general's wife so he could seize their riches. And so she did. After hearing her confession, one officer asked the maid to summon the cat demon back. At midnight, she set up a bowl of fragrant porridge and tapped on it with a spoon. She then called out, "Come, Cat Lady! Don't stay in the palace anymore!" After a while, her face turned completely pale, and she acted as if she were being pulled by someone: she announced that the cat demon had returned. Upon hearing the result of the investigation, the emperor severely punished Dugu and his wife.[59]

This account of the cat demon reveals much about its entanglement with the political life of the Sui court. Let's start with the witchcraft itself. As disclosed by the maid Xu, the practice involved a furtive ritual of conjuring up a demon that inflicted sickness on victims over distance, usurping their wealth. This connection between *gu* and demons in general is not surprising, as we have already seen it in the work of Chao Yuanfang, but what is singular in this episode is the appearance of a demon in the form of a cat. How to make sense of a feline association with *gu*? In his *On the Origins and Symptoms*, the Sui physician explains that the cat demon is the spirit of an old, wild cat (*li*) turned into a demon and attached to human beings.[60] Malicious people store and worship the demon, a typical way of manipulating *gu*, to harm others. The symptoms of cat-demon attack are piercing pains in the heart and the abdomen; the demon would devour the viscera of the victim, leading to death from spitting or discharging blood.[61]

Chao's depiction of the cat demon manifests the ever-changing nature of *gu*, particularly transformations between wild animal and demon. It is important to note that the line between the two was not clear-cut in premodern

China. Early Chinese sources often portray animals as living beings with magical powers they could embody through protean transformations rather than merely biological entities.[62] This is not surprising given the danger posed by animals, especially by ferocious and poisonous animals such as tigers and snakes, to those who ventured into the wilderness. *Gu* was an example par excellence for this type of imagination—the roaming spirits of wild animals, ever ready to morph into malign demons. Vicious people manipulated these demons, turning them into *gu*, which could inflict grievous harm on the targeted victims.

Yet the prominence of the cat in this particular type of *gu* still requires explanation. The portrayal of wild cats in Chinese sources, at least before the tenth century, was mainly negative. Although domesticated cats, since their introduction to China from India during the Era of Division, were valued for practical purposes, especially warding off mice, wild cats were believed to be sly, unpredictable, and inauspicious, often possessing uncanny powers.[63] The fear of cats penetrated the highest echelons of society. In 655, Empress Wu issued an order forbidding cats in the palace because a consort whom the empress had imprisoned vowed a magical revenge against the injustice of her persecution: the empress would turn into a rat and the consort into a cat, ready and able to pounce. Although there is no direct evidence of the practice of the cat demon in this episode, it nonetheless reveals anxiety about devilish feline creatures that could undermine, if not overturn, the political order.[64]

Which brings us back to the story of Dugu. What was the political significance of this dramatic event? Why would Dugu want to poison the empress? The ostensible reason is that he ran short of money, but this is unlikely given his position at the court. Another possibility, suggested by previous studies, is that Dugu devised the sinister plan as a result of family tensions, particularly his jealousy of the empress, who was his half-sister. In earlier days, upon the death of their father, Dugu's family line had enjoyed prominence, since his mother gave birth to six sons. By contrast, his half-sister remained obscure, as she was the only child of her mother. The situation was reversed when the latter became empress in 581, which suddenly raised the status of her family line. This could have elicited Dugu's resentment toward his now-illustrious half-sister. A similar kind of familial resentment may also explain the poisoning of the wife of Yang Su, who was the half-brother of Dugu's wife and a powerful regent at court. Being jealous, Dugu's wife could have deployed the black magic to curse her nemesis.[65]

It is also possible that Dugu and his wife were innocent, and the whole accusation was a conspiracy forged by their political enemies to slander and destroy them. The suspect is Yang Su, who was an ambitious general and a trusted confidant of the crown prince. According to *The History of the Sui* (Suishu, 636), he conspired with the prince to advance a case of witchcraft against one of the latter's brothers, who was rising, threateningly, as a rival, leading to the victim's demotion. The Machiavellian general may even have participated in murdering the emperor to help the impatient prince ascend the throne.[66] Given his record of trickery, it would not be surprising that Yang contrived the whole witchcraft trial to defame and eliminate Dugu.

The mystery of the cat demon scandal remains unresolved, but we know that the state acted swiftly. Initially, the emperor ordered the execution of Dugu and his wife. In response to the pleading of Dugu's brother, he later reduced the penalty to stripping him of his royal position and sending his wife to a convent, a typical punishment for royal women at the time. He also commanded that Dugu's mother-in-law, who was blamed for dispatching the cat demon to kill many people, be banished. Furthermore, the emperor issued an edict in 598 that all families who were accused of practicing cat-demon witchcraft be banished to the remote edges of the empire.[67]

This strong political response to cat-demon witchcraft generated a snowball effect that powerfully shook the country over the next two decades. A seventh-century source provides a sober depiction:

> During the period of Daye of the Sui [605–618], the affair of the cat demon broke out. Some families raised old cats and used them for sorcery, which had quite magical effects. People falsely accused each other [of practicing the sorcery]. Those who were embroiled in the affair and executed in the capital region and in the various prefectures amounted to thousands of families. The Duke of Shu, Yang Xiu, was implicated as well.[68] Once the house of the Sui collapsed, the affair also subsided.[69]

Just like the capricious *gu* that came and went on a whim, cat-demon witchcraft was ephemeral in Chinese history, coinciding with the rise and fall of the short-lived Sui dynasty. Although the widespread persecution of witchcraft may not be the only cause of its collapse, it played an important role in the process, given that these scandals triggered violent court struggles that substantially destabilized the empire.

The state suppression of cat-demon witchcraft and *gu* practices in general continued after the fall of the Sui reign. In the Tang period (618–907) that followed, the court established stringent laws punishing *gu* practitioners. According to *The Tang Code* (Tanglü, 653), those who harbored and dispatched the cat demon and those who taught this black magic would be hanged. If someone practicing sorcery was discovered within a family, all would be exiled to faraway places, even if other members were unaware of her practice. The chief of the precinct in which the accused lived was also banished.[70] Inheriting the Sui model, the Tang state adopted harsh measures to eliminate practitioners of *gu* magic in order to maintain the political order.

Under severe persecution, accused sorcerers were pushed to the peripheral regions of the country. During the Sui-Tang period, this meant primarily the districts south of the Yangzi River. The climate, geography, and local customs of this region were vastly different from the north: it was warm and damp, full of mountains, rivers, and lakes, and associated with the widespread popularity of shamanistic practices. In the eyes of the Sui and Tang rulers, who were of northern origin, the region was uncivilized, mysterious, and dangerous, teeming with poisonous creatures and unruly barbarians.[71]

A connection between poison and heat can be traced back to antiquity, yet it found new expression in the seventh century with the linkages to *gu* in the south. *The History of the Sui*, for example, identifies ten districts where *gu* practices prevailed, all of which were located south of the Yangzi River.[72] This southern proliferation of *gu* practices was partly due to the political expulsion of the practitioners, as just discussed. The mysterious, capricious nature of *gu* and its practices matched up well with the perception of the south as a strange, dangerous environment, abundant with vermin, real and imagined, readily identified as plentiful material for these practices. *Gu* became a perfect embodiment of the south, remote, unfamiliar, and intractable, and the source of serious challenges to state governance.[73]

A salient aspect of the Dugu episode is the involvement of women. Although the central figure of the story is Dugu Tuo, a male official, he was surrounded by a number of women from distinct social backgrounds. These include the wife of Dugu, who—or so we are told—conspired with her husband to devise the sorcery; the two victims, that is, the empress and the wife of Yang Su; Dugu's mother-in-law, who allegedly introduced the cat demon into his household; and last but not the least, the maid Xu Ani, who confessed to having performed the witchcraft. The last figure merits our attention, as all the other women in the story enjoyed lofty social status because of their ties to the imperial house. The maid Xu, by contrast, was merely a servant who was brought into Dugu's house by his mother-in-law. Ani was not a formal name—there is doubt she ever had one—but rather a sort of calling often assigned to servants. Moreover, in the incantation she chanted to call back the cat demon, she referred to the creature as "Cat Lady" (Maonü), a colloquial turn of phrase that betrayed her lowly upbringing.[74] In addition, when the maid claimed that the demon had returned, her face changed color and she lost control of her body as if she were being pulled, indicating that she was possessed by a spirit. All the descriptions suggest that she acted as a shaman (*wu*) who performed a ritual to manipulate the cat demon.

The link between women and shamanism in China can be traced back to the Han period, if not earlier. Having a body that was considered to be more susceptible to external influences and hence easier to be put into a trance, women conducted a variety of shamanistic practices in antiquity. Submitting their bodies to willful spirits through possession, they acted as a crucial medium between numinous powers and human targets. Harnessing techniques such as incantation, spitting, and dancing, they performed rituals that aimed to either obtain benefits, such as healing by calling down deities or the cursing of victims through the manipulation of demons, as evidenced in the case of Dugu. In general, they came from the lower echelons of society and were portrayed as ignorant, incapable, and even dangerous. The energy that elites from the Han to the Tang period spent denigrating them indicates that they were fierce competitors and popular figures. Due to their undistinguished backgrounds—the majority of them were probably illiterate—little is known about these women's lives. Yet occasionally they surface in our sources, such as the vivid depiction of Maid Xu in the examined episode, offering us a rare glimpse of their practices.[75]

Conclusion

A popular saying today aptly summarizes the logic guiding the use of potent drugs in medieval China: use poison to attack poison (*yi du gong du*). Although the expression first appeared in a thirteenth-century text, the idea it conveys has much deeper roots.[76] The first "poison" in the phrase refers to potent medicines; the second designates poisoning, and illness in general. The word "attack" (*gong*) carries two meanings. First, it expresses the violent nature of the remedy. Because the sickness is obstinate, one must apply powerful drugs to eradicate it. Second, the word implies a specific and concrete target that the medicine can latch onto and destroy. The logic of potent treatments was thus linked to a particular way of understanding illness. That is, physicians prescribed poisons as powerful weapons to eliminate tenacious illnesses that often assumed concrete forms, be they demons or *gu* vermin. These malignant entities, which either attacked the body from the outside or ravaged it from within, could induce severe symptoms and trigger deadly epidemics. Poisons were thus used to strike these virulent beings and purge them from the body.[77]

The scholarship on etiological studies provides valuable insights into the understanding of demons and *gu* in Chinese medicine. Previous work on the conceptualization of disease in the history of Western medicine has identified two major models: the ontological, which regards disease as a kind of entity that invades a healthy person, and the physiological, which views disease as a deviation from the normal state of the body.[78] Similar models were proposed within various traditions of Chinese medicine: the ontological approach imagined illness as a concrete agent located at a specific site of the body, while functional orientations saw illness as the aberrant flow of *qi* inside the body and the discordance between the body and the cosmos.[79] The functional model, exemplified by *The Yellow Emperor's Inner Classic*, stresses the importance of harmony and balance in maintaining good health. Since an illness in this model is the result of a body out of kilter, it can be rectified by readjusting the body to the normal state. By contrast, the practice of poisons highlights the ontological model in the imagination of illness during medieval China. In this scenario, illnesses assume concrete forms that are inimical to the body, manifested either as malign agents in nature (demons) or as dangerous creatures prepared by vicious minds (*gu* vermin). They cannot be harmonized or rebalanced; they must be expelled or destroyed.[80]

Furthermore, the medical use of poisons and its underlying etiological rationale had far-reaching political implications in China. Medical writings from the Han period onward conceptualize a system of correspondence that emphasizes the resonance between the individual, the state, and the cosmos. With its focus on harmony and balance, the model presents an ideal body that enjoys physical vigor and social stability. The cases of *gu* witchcraft during the Sui-Tang period, however, present a different scenario. The mysterious and elusive practices elicited great anxiety at court and beyond, and served as justification for strong political action. Similar to physicians' use of potent medicines to eliminate malign forces from the physical body, the state established stringent policies to expel *gu* practitioners themselves, many of whom were women, to sustain a healthy social body. The process continued after the Tang dynasty. As a result, those convicted of practicing *gu* witchcraft were increasingly pushed to the margins of the empire, first to the south, later to the southwest. During the late imperial era, *gu* also became associated with minority peoples, especially the Miao.[81] Despite continuous persecution, *gu* practitioners were never entirely eliminated—we still have ethnographical accounts of their practices today.[82] Hiding in faraway lands, lurking at the edges of empire, they remain a menace to the established order.

The short-lived Sui dynasty was succeeded by the Tang, a powerful and cosmopolitan empire that inherited some of the Sui government's institutional and legal measures on medical regulation but with substantial expansion and changes. In particular, pharmacology flourished in the early Tang period; the court in the seventh century established new institutions, developed a tribute system, and sponsored authoritative texts to collect drugs and standardize the knowledge regarding their use. Such knowledge produced at the political center then quickly spread throughout the empire and underwent fluid transformations in local communities.

CHAPTER 4

Medicines in Circulation

Hence we follow the imperial edict from above and solicit various opinions from below. Promulgating the order under heaven, we seek and pursue medicines.

—*NEWLY REVISED MATERIA MEDICA* (659)

IN 657, A SCHOLAR-OFFICIAL NAMED SU JING PRESENTED A PROposal to Emperor Gaozong, the third monarch of the Tang dynasty. The materia medica compiled by Tao Hongjing a century and a half earlier, he claimed, contained numerous mistakes and hence had to be revised. Convinced, the emperor issued an edict to call together a team of twenty officials tasked with producing a new pharmacological text. In the following two years, the team set out to collect medicines from all corners of the empire, based on which they modified the older drug knowledge, creating updated descriptions and illustrations of these substances. At the beginning of 659, a new pharmacopoeia of fifty-five scrolls was completed and submitted to the emperor, who was pleased and ordered its storage in the imperial library.[1]

The book, titled *Newly Revised Materia Medica* (Xinxiu bencao), is significant in the history of Chinese pharmacology as the first governmentsponsored materia medica in China. The text emerged during the early Tang period (618–755), a period that saw the establishment of a vast empire that enjoyed political stability, economic growth, and cultural flourishing.[2] During this favorable period, the state took an active role in the promotion of medicine, manifested in the building of new institutions, the expansion of a tribute system, and the creation of new and authoritative texts. This state's effort toward new medical regulation was epitomized by *Newly Revised Materia Medica*, which offered the first empire-wide survey of drugs to standardize pharmacological knowledge and guide medical practice.

In this new political environment, potent medicines figured prominently at the intersection of the state and pharmaceutical practice. Given their crucial role in healing, the Tang court collected a set of potent drugs from across the empire through an extensive tribute system, which was an imperial network for the acquisition of natural or manufactured products from local regions. It also tried to standardize the knowledge regarding identifying these drugs and strategies for deploying them in *Newly Revised Materia Medica* in order to forestall the misuse of them in practice, a concern already visible in the fifth and sixth centuries due to the increased specialization of pharmaceutical activity (see chapter 2). Making use of poisons was never a relaxed matter; their potential to kill, either by accident or on purpose, constantly posed a threat to the imperial order. Correspondingly, the state created specific legal codes to regulate the use of poisons and prevent them from falling into the wrong hands.

If the Tang central government developed institutional, legal, and textual measures to standardize drug knowledge and regulate medical activities, what about the situation in local regions? Given the vastness of the Tang empire in the seventh and early eighth centuries, with its territory extending to the far south and to central Asia, there existed considerable variation in pharmaceutical practice that was contingent on climate, geography, the availability of resources, and customs. Pharmacological knowledge produced at the imperial center spread fast to the far ends of the country and beyond, manifesting the majestic power of the state. Yet such knowledge, once it reached remote communities, was subject to rapid transformation shaped by regional conditions and the specific needs of local actors.

Regulation of Medicines by the Tang Court

The institutional supervision of medical practice has a long history in China. The ancient text *Rites of Zhou* (Zhouli, ca. third century BCE) already described specialized departments dedicated to food preparation and treating internal disorders, lesions, and animal maladies as integral elements of the royal bureaucracy. The vision was partly implemented in the Eastern Han period, when the court established offices for the supervision of healing practices and the preparation of drugs for the imperial family and court officials. Furthermore, the Han rulers relied on a system of patronage to recruit capable healers across the country who could provide excellent medical service. Driven by a passion for the practices of immortality, many of these rulers were keen to recruit those who claimed mastery of these occult arts. Upon gaining imperial trust, these adepts often assumed nonmedical positions in the central government. Medicine, therefore, was a means for them to enhance their social prestige and fulfill their political ambitions.[3]

This pattern persisted during the Era of Division. This period saw the rise of hereditary medicine, traditions of medical practices transmitted within aristocratic clans, especially in the south, which produced influential physicians, many of whom enjoyed imperial favor and took up governmental posts. The majority of these appointments, however, were unrelated to medicine, probably because the medical bureaucracy at the time was still limited.[4] The situation changed during the Sui-Tang period, when the state substantially remodeled and expanded medical institutions that systematically selected and trained various types of physicians.

According to *The Six Ministries of the Tang Dynasty* (Tang liudian, 739), a court document that outlined the administrative structure of the central government, three institutions were established during the Tang dynasty. The first was the Imperial Medical Office (Taiyi Shu). This large organization, with 341 personnel, provided medical services for court officials and trained specialists in four departments: general medicine, acupuncture, therapeutic exercise, and incantation. The department of general medicine was the largest and further divided into five subspecialties: internal medicine; treatment of sores and swellings; pediatrics; treatment of ears, eyes, the mouth, and teeth; and cupping. Students in each of these subfields took two to seven years to finish their study. Upon passing an exam, they could start to practice.[5]

The second institution was the Palace Drug Service (Shangyao Ju), which offered medical services to the imperial house. The origins of the institution can be traced back to the end of the fifth century, during the Northern Wei dynasty (386–534), when its major function was the "tasting" of medicines for the emperor to ensure their quality.[6] The Tang court expanded the agency into a multiunit organization that contained eighty-four personnel, including head officers; scribes; specialists in medicine, therapeutic exercise, incantation, and cream-making; and drug preparers.[7] The last group merits our attention, as half of the personnel, forty-two in number, were assigned to this unit, performing tasks including "scraping, trimming, pounding, and sifting." These artisans were supervised by the heads of the service, who directed the combination of drugs based on their characteristics, including their flavors, degrees of heat, and dispositions, following the guidelines in materia medica texts. These carefully prepared drugs were then presented as treatment for the emperor.[8]

A third institution created during the Tang period was the Pharmacy in the Secretariat of the Heir Apparent (Yaozang Ju), which provided medications for the crown prince. The structure of the organization was similar to that of the Palace Drug Service but on a smaller scale, consistent with the hierarchical setup of imperial power.[9]

The administration of drugs for the royal family was a serious matter, with safety being the primary concern. The preparation of medicines was monitored not only by the heads of the Palace Drug Service but also by several officials outside the institution so as to guarantee quality. Once a medicine was ready, all the high-ranking officers in the service would try it first before wrapping it and stamping it with a seal. Together with the seal was a description of the formula, followed by the year, month, and date of the preparation as well as the signatures of all who had overseen its manufacture. On the day it was presented, the medicine was again tasted by the head of the service; his superior, the director of the palace; and then the crown prince before it entered the mouth of the emperor. It is hard to imagine a more stringent system to prevent drug poisoning.[10]

Possibly, some of the medicines presented to the emperor were potent, given the extreme care taken with their preparation and administration. Although this is not explicit in *The Six Ministries of the Tang Dynasty*, there is evidence to be found in a newly discovered legal document that has preserved some eighth-century Tang ordinances on imperial medicine.[11] In particular, a section titled "Ordinances on Curing Illness" (Yiji ling) contains thirty-five regulations on medical education and practice in both central and local governments.[12] One ordinance specifies the presentation of drugs:

> To those in various departments inside the government and those in the ward for the sick, one should present drugs in decoction. If there are also potent drugs, one should present them to the Gates Office as well. One should not present raw drugs.[13]

The passage stipulates the duties of personnel in the Imperial Medical Office who offered medical services to governmental officers. They also took care of the patients in the "ward for the sick" (*huanfang*), a special ward for ailing palace maids.[14] In general, drugs in decoction were prepared, which probably referred to mild substances that were intended to act quickly on the body. But potent drugs were also presented—likely in the form of pills, so they could release their power slowly—which had to be carefully inspected, and possibly tasted, by the Gates Office to guarantee safety.[15] This system of surveillance was simpler than that established for the imperial house, but it was necessary nonetheless, especially when powerful substances were involved. Moreover, raw drugs were forbidden, probably because of their unattenuated strength. The warning also explains the designation of a large number of artisans skilled in drug processing in the Palace Drug Service.

What would happen if one erred in preparing medicines? The punishment was severe. According to *The Tang Code* (Tanglü, 653), the earliest Chinese legal code that is extant in its entirety, negligence in making imperial medicine was a crime of "great disrespect," one of the ten most serious offences at court. Specifically, if a physician failed to follow the formula in preparing a medicine, made mistakes in dosage, or labeled a medicine incorrectly by confusing its warming, cooling, rapid, or slow-acting characteristics, he would be hanged. The punishment also extended to the officers who supervised the preparation; if accessories to a mistake, they would be banished to distant lands. Moreover, if a person failed to correctly prepare each ingredient in a formula by boiling, cutting, rinsing, or soaking, he would be condemned to one year of forced labor.[16] Similar laws also applied to physicians working outside the imperial house, though the punishment was less severe. If a physician inadvertently killed a patient by preparing or labeling a medicine amiss, he would receive a sentence of two and a half years of forced labor.[17] In short, the Tang government established strict laws to regulate medical practice at court and beyond.

Besides creating guidelines for the prevention of medical accidents, the Tang legal system also addressed cases where poisons were used for deliberate killing. Given the ubiquity of potent medicines in Tang medical practice, it would not be surprising to see such crimes occur frequently. In fact, one scholar has identified more than sixty poisonings during the Tang period, suggesting the prevalence of such occurrences at the time.[18] Correspondingly, *The Tang Code* includes an article titled "The Use of Poisons to Poison People":

Those who use poisons to poison people and those who sell these poisons will be hanged. [Note: These substances can kill people. Although they are indeed poisons, they can also cure illness. If the buyer intends to poison a person but the seller does not know this intention, the seller is not punished.] If the transaction is completed but the poison is not used, the buyer and the seller will be banished to places two thousand *li* away.[19]

Revealingly, the law recognized the intention of the sellers: only when they colluded with the buyers would they be punished. This critical specification implies that these sellers could also provide poisons for a legitimate purpose, namely, to cure illness. The ambivalent relationship between medicines and poisons, as we have seen in materia medica writings, was also manifested in the Tang legal code. What defined a poison here was not the substance per se but rather its intended use.

In addition, the commentary on the article specifies four substances commonly deployed for killing: *zhen*-bird poison (*zhendu*), gelsemium (*yege*), and two types of aconite (*wutou* and *fuzi*).[20] All are defined as possessing great *du* and are assigned medical uses in the materia medica literature. But their potential to harm did not escape the state's attention. An ordinance that might have been part of the eighth-century legal document discussed above demands that private families not be allowed to own the first two items. The restriction reveals an effort on the part of the state to control access to dangerous substances and prevent them from falling into the wrong hands.[21]

Imperial Collection of Medicines

The creation of new institutions and legal codes to regulate medical services in the early Tang period relied on a system of drug supply that collected the best ingredients for the court. This goal was achieved by two mechanisms. The first was the cultivation of herbs in the capitals. According to *The Six Ministries of the Tang Dynasty*, the Imperial Medical Office designated land called "the medicinal garden" (*yaoyuan*) to grow medicinal plants, and assigned two masters and eight students to manage the land.[22] "Ordinances on Curing Illness" further elaborates that fertile land of three *qing* (about forty-two acres) was chosen for this purpose at each of the two capitals.[23] The masters taught students who were recruited between the ages of sixteen and twenty. They studied materia medica, which guided them in identifying and cultivating various herbs. If wild forms of these medicinal herbs were available nearby, the office sent people to harvest them. If not, the office ordered those prefectures where the herbs grew naturally to submit the seeds for cultivation. Once successfully transplanted and further assessed, they entered the drug repository for regular use. The students, having completed their study, rose to fill the positions of their masters at the garden.[24]

By cultivating herbs that grew well in the capital regions of northern China, the medicinal gardens provided an assortment of ingredients for the Imperial Medical Office, which in turn processed and deployed them for medical services at court. This strategy of transplantation obviously saved the cost and trouble of transporting medicinal substances over long distances in the vast territory of the empire. As fresh ingredients were preferred in some cases, the presence of a nearby garden was convenient.

But this strategy of growing herbs locally was, after all, limited. Not all plants could adapt to the soil and climate of the capitals. Even if they could, they were found to not necessarily possess the same level of medicinal potency as those growing in their native lands. This is why Chinese materia medica texts specify the location where a drug of the best quality ought to be harvested. Furthermore, the Chinese pharmacopoeia contained not just plants but also minerals and animal-derived materials. These latter two groups were more difficult or even impossible to procure in new environments, and hence had to be collected from their original sites.

This need was met by the second mechanism of drug collection during the Tang period: the tribute system, which was a state network for the procurement of natural or manufactured products from local regions and foreign lands. The idea of such a system can be traced back to antiquity; *The Book of Documents* (Shangshu) envisioned a sage-king convening goods from all corners of his dominion as a "tribute" and symbol of effective governance.[25] The actual practice probably started during the Han dynasty, and had become more elaborate by the time of the Tang. Among the wide-ranging kinds of tribute items, medicines occupied a prominent place. In particular, the Tang court devised two strategies for obtaining local drugs. The first aimed to collect drugs for the Imperial Medical Office, which took care of the health of governmental officials. For this purpose, the court appointed, for each prefecture, a number of "masters of harvesting drugs" (*caiyao shi*) who were responsible for collecting medicinal substances based on the sites specified in the materia medica literature. To facilitate transportation, a donkey was assigned to carry the materials to the capital if their weight exceeded one hundred *jin* (about 68 kg). When necessary, the court also purchased drugs from local markets, though the portion procured in this way was relatively small.[26]

The second strategy had a narrower focus, namely, to collect drugs for the imperial house. It was part of a system called "local tribute" (*tugong*) that not only fulfilled the material needs of the royal family but also symbolized regional submission to central authority. Unlike collection for the Imperial Medical Office, the Tang court designated certain households in a given region, often with hereditary status, to collect or produce local products for tribute. It then appointed a delegate in each prefecture, "the territorial representative" (*chaoji shi*), to purchase these products and present them to the court at the end of each year, where they were prominently and ostentatiously displayed.[27] The amount of these tributes, according to a ninth-century stipulation, should be modest, and their price in a prefecture should not exceed that of fifty rolls of silk, a measure to prevent burdening the community.[28] Based on one modern scholar's calculation, compared to taxes, local tributes constituted only a minuscule portion of state revenue, indicating that their role in the Tang economy was insignificant. That being said, tribute items were not only a symbolic manifestation of imperial power. Many, especially medicines, were practically useful, given their limited supply in the capitals.[29]

A number of Tang sources enumerate these tribute items and their points of origin.[30] Among these, the most elaborate account is found in *Comprehensive Institutions* (Tongdian, 801), a text that surveys political institutions from antiquity to the early Tang period. The book contains an extensive list of tribute items from the mid-eighth century, each with its origin and amount, offering us a concrete picture of the imperial collection of local products.[31] Altogether, 264 items are listed, which include textiles (61); mats and utensils (18); miscellaneous articles such as candles, mirrors, fans, porcelains, silver, and pets (34); foods (28); and above all, medicines (123).[32] The fact that drugs made up nearly half of all tributes suggests their paramount importance for the imperial house. Among the 287 prefectures on the list, 118 from all over the empire presented drugs (map 4.1). Specifically, these prefectures can be divided into eight zones: the capital region (zone A), the Shandong Peninsula in the east (zone B), the Sichuan region in the southwest (zone C), the central region (zone D), the southeastern region (zone E), and three regions at the periphery of the empire: zone F in the far south, zone G in the far north, and zone H in the far west). Among these zones, the southwestern region (zone C) particularly merits our attention, as it contains a concentrated cluster of prefectures, especially those on the eastern edge of the Tibetan Plateau, that submitted a rich variety of medicines to the court. This is probably due to the presence of high mountain ranges and the moist climate characteristic of the region, making it an ideal source of pharmaceutical materials.[33]

Several drugs figure prominently on the tribute list. The one that appears most frequently is musk (*shexiang*)—457 pieces of it were collected from twenty-six prefectures, mainly in the southwest (zone C). The glandular secretion from musk deer, with its strong fragrance, was valued not just as a medicine to treat malaria, counter *gu* poison, and eliminate worms but also as an apotropaic substance that could dispel demons and prevent nightmares. The latter usage likely explains the high demand for the aromatic on the part of the imperial house.[34] Other popular drugs on the list are dendrobium (*shihu*) from eleven prefectures in the central and southern regions (zones D and F), angelica (*danggui*) from six prefectures in the southwest (zone C), and ginseng (*renshen*) from five prefectures in the north and northeast (zones A and G). Intriguingly, all these herbs were believed to possess the power of nourishing the body; their regular ingestion promised to strengthen the viscera, pacify the mind, enhance fertility for women, and prolong life. The benefits of these tonic substances probably made them favorites in the imperial collection.[35]

Besides restoratives, the Tang rulers also gathered potent drugs. Altogether, sixteen such drugs (nine plants, two minerals, and five animal products) appeared on the tribute list, which were presented by twenty prefectures throughout the empire (map 4.1 and table 4.1). Their distribution, however, was uneven. Most of the potent plants came from the central region (zone D), especially the mountainous areas where such herbs grew abundantly. Two potent minerals were collected from distant ends of the empire: mercury from the far south (zone F), where its primary ore, cinnabar (mercury sulfide), was plentiful; and sal ammoniac (*naosha*) from the far west along the Silk Road (zone H). The latter was a foreign drug newly introduced into the Tang pharmacy as a result of the imperial expansion into central Asia.[36] Its inclusion in the tribute list demonstrates not only the imperial interest in trying novel medicines but also the reach of Tang power to the distant edges of its vast territory. Finally, the potent animal products on the list include blister beetles from the capital region (zone A), bovine bezoar from the east (zone B), and most conspicuously, forty pieces of boa gallbladder (*ranshe dan*) collected

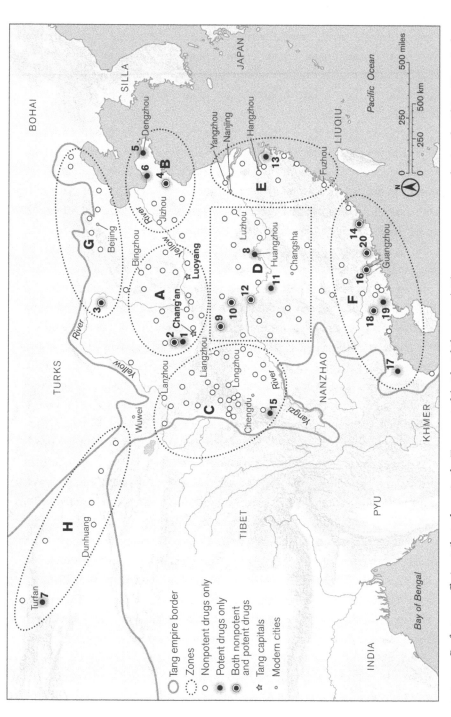

MAP 4.1. Prefectures offering tribute drugs in the Tang period (mid-eighth century). The map was generated using the China Historical GIS and ArcGIS, based on information from *Comprehensive Institutions* (Tongdian, 801).

TABLE 4.1. Potent drugs among Tang local tributes

NO.	SITE	ZONE	ITEMS	TYPE	AMOUNT
1	Binzhou	A	Snake gallbladder (*shedan*)	Animal	10 *jin**
2	Ningzhou	A	Two types of blister beetles (*yuanjing, tingzhang*)	Animal	Unspecified
3	Shengzhou	G	Red peony (*chi shaoyao*)	Plant	10 *jin*
4	Mizhou	B	Bovine bezoar (*niuhuang*)	Animal	1 *jin*
5	Dengzhou	B	Bovine bezoar	Animal	128 pieces
6	Laizhou	B	Bovine bezoar	Animal	122 *liang*
7	Anxi duhufu	H	Sal ammoniac (*naosha*)	Mineral	50 *jin*
8	Huangzhou	D	Horsefly (*mengchong*)	Animal	2 *jin*
9	Jinzhou	D	Dried lacquer (*ganqi*) Omphalia (*leiwan*)	Plant	6 *jin* 5 *liang*
10	Fangzhou	D	Omphalia	Plant	Unspecified
11	Lizhou	D	Dichroa root (*hengshan*) Dichroa leaf (*shuqi*)	Plant	8 *jin* 1 *jin*
12	Xiazhou	D	Dysosma (*guijiu*)	Plant	2 *jin*
13	Mingzhou	E	Aconite (*fuzi*)	Plant	100 pieces
14	Chaozhou	F	Boa gallbladder (*ranshe dan*)	Animal	10 pieces
15	Lizhou	C	Pepper of Sichuan (*shujiao*)	Plant	1 *shi*
16	Guangzhou	F	Boa gallbladder	Animal	5 pieces
17	Annan duhufu	F	Boa gallbladder	Animal	20 pieces
18	Rongzhou	F	Mercury (*shuiyin*)	Mineral	20 *jin*
19	Gaozhou	F	Boa gallbladder	Animal	2 pieces
20	Xunzhou	F	Boa gallbladder	Animal	3 pieces

* During the Tang period, one *jin* was about 661 grams; one *liang*, which was one sixteenth of one *jin*, was about 41 grams; one *shi*, which was equivalent to 120 *jin*, was about 80 kilograms. See Qiu, *Zhongguo lidai duliangheng kao*, 446.

from five prefectures in the far south (zone F). Considered slightly potent, the snake medicine could be either ingested to alleviate pain or applied topically to treat skin disorders. It is unclear why the Tang emperors particularly favored this product since its medical uses were not unique. The drug, though, was extremely hard to acquire, and the Tang materia medica literature advised on how to distinguish the genuine type from the impostors.[37] The rarity of the substance, together with its inconvenient source at the remote south of the empire, may have enhanced its exotic appeal.[38]

The Making of *Newly Revised Materia Medica*

The extensive collection of drugs procured from throughout the empire not only manifested the symbolic authority of the Tang rulers over local domains but also supplied the court with necessary materials for practical needs. What texts did the state rely on to locate and deploy these medicines? As discussed earlier, both the personnel at the medicinal gardens of the capitals and the harvesters in various prefectures relied on materia medica texts to identify herbs and procure drugs. Moreover, according to "Ordinances on Curing Illness," materia medica were among the first texts that the students in the Imperial Medical Office were required to master, allowing them to recognize the morphology of ingredients and understand their medicinal properties.[39] One text in particular, *Newly Revised Materia Medica* (Xinxiu bencao, 659), played a pivotal role in standardizing drug knowledge and guiding medical practice.

As the first state-commissioned materia medica in China, *Newly Revised Materia Medica* was produced under the sponsorship of Emperor Gaozong (reigned 649–683).[40] According to a partial copy of the text preserved in Japan and dating to 731, twenty-two officials were involved in the project. Among them, twelve were medical specialists from the Imperial Medical Office, the Palace Drug Service, and the Pharmacy in the Secretariat of the Heir Apparent. Another seven were nonmedical officers; they either possessed medical knowledge conducive to producing the work or coordinated the effort of medical specialists between different offices. The director of the project, Su Jing, belonged to this group. Although he was not a medical officer, he had advanced knowledge of medicine, with particular skill in treating an illness known as foot *qi* (*jiaoqi*), which brought him great fame.[41] Su's leadership in the project reveals the vital interaction between medical specialists and court officials in the production of standardized drug knowledge. Finally, the last three persons on the list were high officials at court, who were probably only nominally involved in the project to display the support of the state. Taken together, this composite list of authors, consisting of specialists, nonspecialists, and high-ranking statesmen, reveals the agenda of the project that tied the making of pharmacological knowledge to the establishment of political authority.[42]

Newly Revised Materia Medica contains fifty-four scrolls, which include twenty-one scrolls of the main text, twenty-six scrolls of drug illustrations, and seven scrolls mapping source locations of drugs.[43] The latter two parts, which were new additions to the standard materia medica genre, emphasized the importance of the precise identification of drugs. These two sections, however, have been lost. The organization of the main text followed Tao Hong-jing's classification scheme, grouping drugs based on their natural category (minerals, plants, animals, foods), and further divided these groups into finer gradations: the plant group was split into "herbs" and "trees," the animal group into "beasts and birds" and "reptiles and fish," and the food group into "fruits," "vegetables," and "grains."[44]

Altogether, *Newly Revised Materia Medica* lists 850 drugs. Among them, we find 115 new drugs, 193 drugs no longer in use and mentioned only by name, 138 drugs for which the Tang authors endorsed Tao's annotations, and 404 drugs for which they rectified his views.[45] For each drug entry, the compilers copied Tao's writing faithfully, even in the cases where they disagreed with him, and added their own comments at the end marked by "carefully examined" (*jin'an*). Overall, the Tang authors did not challenge the commentary conventions of the materia medica genre initiated by Tao, nor did they alter the basic properties of each drug, which include mention of its potency (*du*). Their comments instead focused on the clarification of the naming, morphology, or source location of each drug for which they considered Tao's knowledge of these to be obsolete or erroneous. The collection of local drugs constituted a vital part of the imperial tribute system, which likely explains the emphasis on accurate drug identification in the Tang commentary.

Before going over each of the entries, *Newly Revised Materia Medica* offers a short preface written by Kong Zhiyue, the director of the Ministry of Rites. The preface starts with an account of the early history of medicine, listing a group of eminent physicians in antiquity who had mastered the art of healing. It then turns to Tao, recognizing his contribution to the writing of materia medica but highlighting the many mistakes he made, necessitating the compilation of the new work. The section that then follows, a sudden change of topic, shifts to extol the grandeur of the Tang empire. The section is omitted in the Song editions but preserved in a manuscript fragment from Dunhuang dating to the late ninth century that has been made open to the public only recently.[46] Written in ornate, rhapsodic style, it proclaims:

> Our great Tang rules under heaven. We have inherited the propitious fortune
> of the Qin and Han.[47] During the devastating time of the Zhou and Sui, we

saved the pivot of Heaven from falling and stabilized the center of Earth to prevent it from toppling.[48] We have recalibrated all kinds of things to continue nourishing human beings. Our magnificent achievements reverberate afar, and orderly rule spreads throughout the world.[49]

Swiftly zooming out from the specific case of Tao Hongjing, the passage depicts a grandiose image of the Tang majestically recovering and sustaining the proper order of the cosmos. After the chaos of the preceding dynasties, the Tang had managed to "recalibrate" (*chonggou*) everything in the world to benefit its people. The standardization of things—medicines included— became a critical approach for the empire to achieve effective governance.

The remainder of the section carries on in the same grand tone, celebrating the unbounded virtue of the Tang rulers and the splendid gifts presented to the court from all parts of the world, a clear reference to the tribute system. After this overtly political passage that glorifies the all-encompassing Tang power, the preface zooms in to the compilation of *Newly Revised Materia Medica*, specifying its authors, principles, and content, and the pivotal role of the state in propelling the project. All in all, weaving medical narrative with political proclamations, the preface reflects a synergistic effort between medical specialists and court officials that sought to standardize pharmaceutical knowledge so as to facilitate the ruling of the empire.

How did *Newly Revised Materia Medica* standardize knowledge of drugs? Significantly, the authors of the Tang work devoted most of their comments to clarifying the morphology and source locations of drugs rather than elucidating their medicinal uses. In their eyes, Tao's text was often erroneous because he had been restricted to the southeast and hence had no firsthand knowledge of medicines from other regions. Moreover, Tao's close association with Daoist practices also tainted his understanding of many drugs. A telling example is gelsemium (*gouwen*), an herb possessing great *du* and deployed mainly for making ointments to treat swellings. It was also a poison frequently used in suicide. The identification of the plant was a thorny issue. In his commentary, Tao depicted the medicine as a type of grass with purple stems and yellow flowers; newly grown, it strikingly resembled another herb called "yellow essence" (*huangjing*, polygonatum).[50] The juxtaposition of the two herbs originally appeared in a late third-century Daoist treatise that discussed the techniques of life cultivation. The text contrasted the yang power of *huangjing*, which nourished life, with the yin power of *gouwen*, which triggered death.

The morphological similarity between the two plants, as described by Tao, fit well with the yin-yang dichotomy articulated in the Daoist writing.[51]

The Tang authors, however, found Tao's view to be mistaken. They instead contended that the two plants were utterly unrelated: *huangjing* grew straight, with two leaves or four to five leaves facing each other, whereas *gouwen* spread on the ground, with leaves resembling those of a willow tree. They also grew in different regions. While the former grew everywhere, the latter was only found in the far south, anywhere south of Guizhou (in present-day Guangxi), a region that Tao probably never visited. The Tang authors asserted that *gouwen* grew "in all the villages and alleys" in that region, with two different names used by local people, suggesting that they obtained direct knowledge of the plant by surveying the area. This is also indicated by another piece of evidence: Tao held that there was a different type of *gouwen* growing in the region of Qin in the northwest, which was far away from where he lived. The Tang authors, however, considered the claim to be nothing but a rumor, as they couldn't find the herb in that region in spite of an exhaustive search. Rectifying Tao's remarks that relied on the accounts of others, the Tang revision offered updated knowledge of the morphology and source locations of drugs based on firsthand observation.[52]

Besides amending the identification of drugs, the Tang authors also strove to standardize their names. Beginning in the period of *The Divine Farmer's Classic*, many medicinal substances had alternative names, including local variations. Over time, the names proliferated, which caused confusion: sometimes two names were thought to refer to two different drugs, but actually these were just variant names for the same plant; other times, the opposite happened. *Newly Revised Materia Medica* tried to clear up these confusions. On the one hand, it verified regional names of drugs by on-site investigation, as seen in the case of *gouwen*. On the other hand, it relied on classical texts to identify the correct pronunciation and meaning of many drug names. Tellingly, the most frequently cited title in the Tang materia medica was not a medical text but an ancient dictionary, *Approaching Correctness* (Erya, ca. third century BCE), suggesting the value of classical knowledge in the naming of medicines.

This scholarly bent is illustrated by the case of aconite. *Newly Revised Materia Medica* presented five names for the potent herb (*wutou, wuhui, tianxiong, fuzi,* and *cezi*), most of which depicted the shape of its tubers. Tao pointed out that *wutou*, which means the head of a black bird, referred to an intact tuber, whereas *wuhui*, the beak of a black bird, specified a tuber that cracks in the middle. The Tang authors, however, did not find such a distinction meaningful. If a cracked tuber of *wutou* justified a different name, they wondered, what would one call a cracked tuber of *tianxiong*, or *fuzi*? Redundant names were bewildering.[53]

Moreover, these authors also challenged Tao's understanding of *cezi*, which literally means "side offspring." They defined *cezi* as the small outgrowth of *wutou*, which is the main tuber of aconite, not the large node of the side tuber *fuzi*, as Tao identified it. In certain regions, they observed, the size of *fuzi*'s nodes was as small as that of a grain of millet, making its use impractical. Moreover, they noticed that the slim *fuzi* used lately in the capital was quite efficacious, but no one took off its nodes for separate use. Empirical knowledge, therefore, informed the proper naming of medicines.[54]

Another name that Tao mentioned is *sanjian*, which referred to three types of aconite (*wutou*, *fuzi*, and *tianxiong*) from the region of Jianping in the southeast. The Tang authors found the name misleading. The best aconite, they declared, grew in Mianzhou and Longzhou in the southwest (in Mianyang in northern Sichuan, see Longzhou on map 4.1); those from the rest of the country possessed only weak powers, while aconite in the southeast was utterly useless. Then where did Tao get the name of *sanjian*? Citing the aforementioned dictionary *Approaching Correctness*, the Tang compilers pointed out that the ancient name for aconite was *jin*, pronounced in a similar way to the place name *jian*. The phonetic resemblance, they reasoned, must have caused Tao's confusion, causing him to mistake the source location of the herb. Classical wisdom was conducive to clarifying dubious names.[55]

Finally, to facilitate standardization, the Tang authors also rectified local drug knowledge, especially that deriving from common people. Given the size of the empire, ordinary people's understanding of drugs differed vastly across regions, often leading to contradictory claims, which compelled the court to establish an authoritative guide to standardize pharmaceutical knowledge and eliminate confusion. The preface of *Newly Revised Materia Medica* pointed out the issue explicitly: there were 404 drugs for which Tao had made wrong annotations. Sometimes he was right about a drug, yet laypeople used it incorrectly; sometimes he was wrong, and laypeople followed his mistaken instructions for how to use the drug.[56] Evidently, the Tang authors were critical of laypeople in general, calling attention to the unreliability of their knowledge of drugs. This ignorance, they indicated, could lead to serious consequences. For instance, in the entry for *duheng* (southern asarum), they observed that laypeople at the time often replaced the herb with *jiji* (chloranthus), a *du*-possessing plant that should only be applied externally to treat ulcers and scabies. The substitution was a dangerous mistake, since ingesting the powerful *jiji* would make a person vomit.[57] Sometimes, the limited availability of drugs compelled lay users to employ inferior substitutes. This was the case for *guijiu* (dysosma), a *du*-possessing herb grown in the deep mountains that was "extremely hard to acquire." Laypeople then used the herb *yegan* (belamcanda), or an unspecified herb from the southeast, both of which the Tang authors deemed inauthentic.[58] The warning reveals a tension between the imperial effort to standardize pharmaceutical knowledge and lay practices that often depended on restricted resources.

Local Adaptations of Drug Knowledge

The making of *Newly Revised Materia Medica* revealed the imperial ambition of standardizing medical knowledge to guide the collection and deployment of drugs. Once the text was created at the imperial center, how did it spread to the rest of the country? What strategies did the Tang court employ to disseminate medical knowledge? Although there is evidence suggesting the use of printing by the court in the early eighth century, the technology was still nascent, with a particular focus on replicating religious texts.[59] Manuscript culture, by contrast, dominated the reproduction of books, including those on healing. In addition, the Tang court put key medical instructions on public display to enhance their accessibility. For example, in 746, Emperor Xuanzong (reigned 713–756) issued an edict requesting that local officials inscribe essential passages from a medical work called *Formulas for Widespread Aid* (Guangji fang) on large slabs and then place them on the main road of each village. Similarly, in 796, Emperor Dezong (reigned 779–805) sponsored the compilation of *Formulas for Widespread Benefit* (Guangli fang) and requested that the work be inscribed and exhibited on the major roads of the empire.[60] In both cases, what was engraved has been lost, but based on the titles of these works, they were probably prescriptions for easy, everyday use. Before the age of print, public display was a vital method of disseminating medical knowledge to the populace.[61]

In the case of *Newly Revised Materia Medica*, the text quickly spread to various regions of the empire, propelled by the government. Before the compilation of the text, the Tang court in 629 had established offices for teaching medicine in the prefectures. In 723, it further appointed an "erudite of medicine" (*yi boshi*) in each prefecture who took charge of medical education, using the materia medica together with an unspecified formula collection as key guidebooks.[62] Yet before the text was fully institutionalized, it had already been diffused to local districts. In the town of Dunhuang in the far west, a manuscript copy of the text has been discovered that dates to as early as 669, that is, merely ten years after the court completed the project.[63] The text also traveled eastward—it reached Japan in the early eighth century, as attested to by an extant copy dating to 731.[64]

The rapid transmission of *Newly Revised Materia Medica* raises the question of how it was used in local communities. The central government had all the resources for procuring the best drugs to serve the top echelons of society, but how did common people harness the text for their own needs? The study of the Dunhuang manuscripts offers clues. Discovered in one of the Buddhist grottoes of Mogao near Dunhuang (in present-day Gansu, see map 4.1) in 1900, the treasure trove contained over forty thousand manuscripts dating from 406 to 1002. The manuscripts were likely the holdings of a local monastic library since most of them are Buddhist scriptures, but there was also a large number of secular documents in the collection, including classics, poems, and governmental edicts.[65]

Among more than one hundred medical manuscripts in the Dunhuang collection are formula books, medical classics, acupuncture guides, and materia medica texts, including five copies of *Newly Revised Materia Medica*, all incomplete.[66] One, dating to the late ninth century, preserves a segment of the preface.[67] One, dating to 669 or later, contains the herbal section of thirty drugs in the bottom group.[68] Another two copies are highly incomplete: one contains nine drugs spread across the sections for fruits, vegetables, and grains, and the other has two drugs from the section for fruits.[69] The three manuscripts that preserve drug entries follow the convention of commentary writing, with the original Han text and both Tao Hongjing's and the Tang authors' commentaries clearly differentiated. The fifth copy (P. 3822), however, is of a different type.[70]

P. 3822 stands out as a unique document (figure 4.1). Above all, its form is intriguing. In contrast to other copies written on standard scrolls, which are often long and bulky, it was written on both sides of a small leaflet made of paper (27 cm long and 8.3 cm wide). It is a self-contained text, because the last

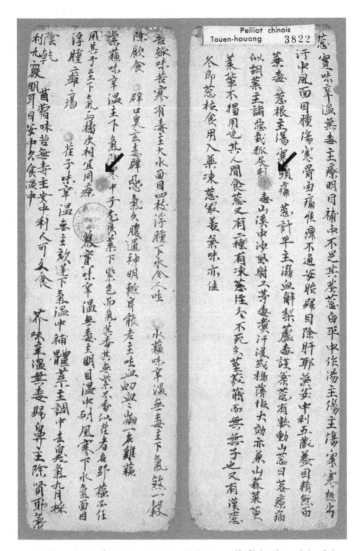

FIGURE 4.1. Dunhuang manuscript P. 3822, (*left*) back and (*right*) front. The arrows point to the hole where multiple leaflets were fastened. Courtesy of Bibliothèque Nationale de France (BnF), Paris.

line was squeezed in on the back to finish a sentence. Revealingly, a small hole is found at the upper center of the leaflet, which would have been the site where multiple such leaflets were bound together. This is characteristic of the so-called *pothi* manuscripts, originally developed in ancient India, where dried palm leaves were used for writing.[71] This form of manuscript had spread to Tibet with Buddhist monks by the Tang period, but with paper replacing leaves as the dominant medium. The Dunhuang collection contains about forty manuscripts of this type, the majority of which are Buddhist scriptures. As Dunhuang was occupied by the Tibetan empire from 786 to 848, it is likely that the *pothi* manuscripts were produced during this period or later. As a primordial form of codex books, these manuscripts were convenient to carry and easy to use by flipping through the fastened leaflets. For an itemized text such as *Newly Revised Materia Medica*, the form would have worked well for a user who wanted to quickly locate a drug entry.[72]

What is written on the leaflet? P. 3822 includes eight drugs from the vegetable section of *Newly Revised Materia Medica* but alters their order from the court-issued version. On the front side is "scallion" (*cong*), a vegetable in the middle group. The back begins with one vegetable from the bottom group, followed by three vegetables from the middle group, and ends with three vegetables from the top group. Moreover, the writing defies the conventional style of materia medica, namely, using red ink for the original *Divine Farmer's Classic*, black ink for the rest, and a smaller font for the commentaries. In P. 3822, every word is written in black, and all characters are the same size. Most significantly, the manuscript does not fully copy each drug entry. On the front side, for example, the content of "scallion" is complete, yet on the back, most of the entries are shortened. Sometimes the omissions are striking—even words from *The Divine Farmer's Classic* are missing, a phenomenon we do not see in any other extant manuscripts of the text.

Obviously, the copying was selective, possibly for practical reasons. The copyist might have chosen the most relevant vegetables from the Tang materia medica and arranged them according to local demands. The elimination of the color and font distinctions suggests a breaking of the textual hierarchy that was strictly followed by the court scribes. Among the eight vegetables, scallion was the most important for the copyist; it occupies the full front side of the leaflet, including the complete original text. This could be due to its diverse medical uses: its seeds brighten the eyes and replenish the body; its stems treat "cold damage," excessive sweating, and a swollen face, as well as annihilate a hundred kinds of drug poisoning; its roots alleviate headache; its juice cures blood in the urine. The plant appears to be a marvelous panacea. Moreover, the Tang compilers' commentary, which was faithfully copied, is particularly useful, because it further identifies three types of scallion for different uses: the mountain scallion, for treating illness; and the frozen scallion and the Han scallion, which are consumed as foods.

The availability of the plants may have been another factor in the selective copying. The text does not specify the location of scallion, suggesting its widespread growth. By contrast, the three plants written on the back of the leaflet only grew along the rivers and lakes of specific regions that were far away from Dunhuang: bitter calabash (*kuhu*) from the land of Jin (in present-day Shanxi), water betony (*shuisu*) from Jiuzhen (in present-day northern Vietnam), and the fruit of knotweed (*liaoshi*) from Leize (in present-day Shandong). It is perhaps not a coincidence that these three entries suffered severe editing, as the information was not as relevant as that for local plants.[73] In comparison, the complete copying of the text for purple betony (*zisu*) immediately after water betony makes sense. The plant probably grew locally, suggested by its unique name—possibly a regional name—chosen by the copyist.[74] To help one recognize the plant, the copyist also included the key information for its identification: the back of its leaves is purple, and it gives off a strong fragrance. It may have been a suitable local substitute for water betony: the plant has the same properties (warming and pungent), with a similar medical usage of precipitating *qi* in the body. Textual modification in P. 3822, therefore, evinces a deliberate effort to adapt imperial knowledge to local needs.[75]

Who might have used the leaflet? Given that the Dunhuang manuscripts were part of the library collection of a Buddhist monastery and that the *pothi* texts were predominantly produced and employed by Buddhist monks, it is likely that local monks utilized the leaflet for their medical practice. As mentioned earlier, the Tang court's management of medicine spread to all corners of the empire in the seventh and early eighth centuries by appointing medical personnel and circulating standardized texts in various prefectures. Dunhuang was no exception: located in Shazhou in the far west, it established an office of medical education with its own "erudite of medicine," appointed by the court. Yet after the Tibetan empire seized the town in the late eighth century, Tang influence declined. As a result, the center of medical service shifted from governmental offices to local monasteries. In fact, scholarship has identified several prominent monks in Dunhuang who practiced medicine and obtained great reputations in the community. The leaflet, with its modified knowledge of drugs for local needs, could have been an important guide for their practice.[76]

Furthermore, the vegetables listed on the leaflet could have been cultivated in local monasteries and consumed for dietary instead of medical purposes. This hypothesis, developed by the historian Iwamoto Atsushi, is reasonable

given the intimate relation between food and medicine in the Tang pharmacy.[77] However, if local monasteries did intend to grow these vegetables as
foods, they probably would have consulted an agricultural manual rather than
a pharmacological text. In addition, the most prominent entry on the leaflet
is scallion, which was one of the five pungent vegetables (*wuxin*) forbidden by
Buddhist doctrines, because its strong flavor was believed to disturb the body
and poison the mind.[78] This prohibition made the consumption of scallion as
a regular food unlikely. On the other hand, the plant could still be used as a
medicine, taken periodically to treat specific illnesses. Alcohol was consumed
in a similar manner in monasteries. Ultimately, it was not the substance itself
but the particular purpose it served that mattered.[79]

   Finally, it merits our notice that not every manuscript stored in Dunhuang
was copied there. Some Buddhist scriptures, especially the esteemed ones,
were copied at the capital, where the court had established copying offices and
employed professional scribes to reproduce texts that were often long and
didactic. These court-sponsored manuscripts were typically written in standard script and subject to multiple rounds of proofreading.[80] P. 3822, however,
was probably not the product of such systematic copying. There is no evidence
that any extant *pothi* manuscript was produced by the Tang government,
considering its characteristic form of Indian-Tibetan origins. Its portable lay-
out made it easy to use but not necessarily an object that manifested imperial
majesty. What is more, the writing on the leaflet was casual and unstylish,
with the frequent use of nonstandard words and more than twenty copying
errors. Clearly, this was a text produced by an untrained hand, not at an official copying center. Although we cannot be entirely certain of its provenance,
given that a significant number of manuscripts in Dunhuang were donated
by pilgrims from other places, it is probably safe to say that the leaflet was
linked to local medical practice, either in Dunhuang or elsewhere.[81]

Conclusion

The seventh and early eighth centuries witnessed the active engagement of
the state in standardizing pharmaceutical knowledge and regulating medical
practice. Institutionally, the Tang court established several offices to train specialists and provide medical services for the imperial house and governmental officials. Legally, it created a series of ordinances to inspect the quality of
drugs and guarantee the safe use of them in practice. Moreover, it cultivated

herbs in the medicinal gardens of the capitals and built an extensive tribute system to collect drugs throughout the empire, which not only manifested the pervasive spread of imperial power but also supplied necessary medicinal substances for the court. Finally, it commissioned the production of medical texts, epitomized by *Newly Revised Materia Medica*, which critically edited, corrected, and updated existing knowledge of drugs, standardizing it as a guide for medical practice both at court and in local regions.

Among these various strategies, poisons figured prominently. Instead of shunning dangerous substances entirely, the Tang court recognized their medicinal value and tried to collect the most useful substances throughout the empire. The imperial effort was aided by *Newly Revised Materia Medica*, whose authors paid keen attention to the appearance, names, and local uses of drugs, and generated new knowledge that combined classical wisdom with empirical observation. The state was fully aware of the danger of poisons, though, as revealed by the elaborate drug-tasting system to protect the emperors, and strict laws to punish those who either misused poisons in their medical practice or manipulated them for nefarious purposes. This is unsurprising given the plentiful incidents of poisoning, murder, and witchcraft at court. Poisons hence presented both opportunities and challenges for sustaining effective rule.

Most of the actions taken by the Tang government to regulate drugs were not entirely new. For instance, the Sui authority had already established the Imperial Medical Office and the Palace Drug Service, which the Tang court inherited in the seventh century and substantially remodeled during the favorable environment of political stability and imperial expansion.[82] After the devastating An Lushan Rebellion in the mid-eighth century, though, the Tang central power waned—no state-sponsored medical projects appeared in the ninth and early tenth centuries. It was not until the Northern Song period (960–1127) that the state resumed enthusiastic engagement in medicine; the historian of medicine TJ Hinrichs has demonstrated how the Northern Song court achieved effective governance by systematically producing and disseminating medical texts, deploying them to suppress unorthodox local customs.[83] Although such efforts seem to resemble those of the early Tang period, there is one key difference: in the earlier period, the state relied heavily on the copying of manuscripts, accompanied by the public display of concise guidelines, to spread medical knowledge, while in the later dynasty, printing played a central role. Utilizing this new technology that could quickly reproduce authoritative texts, the state became more efficient in establishing standards and circulating them throughout the empire.

How was the government-produced medical knowledge received by local communities? Compared to the court, where the most skilled physicians and the finest medicines were available, ordinary people—especially those living in regions far away from the imperial center, such as Dunhuang—faced the challenge of limited medical resources. Consequently, they adopted various methods to overcome these obstacles, such as harnessing herbs available in their area and identifying drug substitutes. The rise of authoritative, standardized medical knowledge thus went hand in hand with its fluid transformations in distant regions. From the tenth century, the development of printing effectively promulgated standardized texts that suppressed local practices. During the Tang period, however, a different picture emerged: the flexible and adaptive character of manuscripts allowed local actors to resourcefully cope with established medical knowledge and modify it for their own needs. When manuscript culture flourished, the power of the textual regime was limited, leading to rich varieties of regional writings that informed diverse practices.[84]

The Dunhuang manuscripts reveal the importance of practice in guiding the production of local medical knowledge. Due to the fragmented nature of these manuscripts, we know little about who the authors were and what might have motivated them to create the texts. Fortunately, for more elaborate discussion of medical practice, we have the writings of Sun Simiao, the subject of the next chapter, an eminent Tang physician who wrote profusely on drug remedies, many of which were based on his own experience.

CHAPTER 5

Medicines in Practice

I realized that the efficacy of spectacular things is not bound by common rules. . . . This is without understanding why it is so—even sages cannot discern the reason.

—SUN SIMIAO, *ESSENTIAL FORMULAS WORTH A THOUSAND IN GOLD FOR EMERGENCIES* (650S)

IN ONE OF HIS FORMULA BOOKS, THE SEVENTH-CENTURY PHYSI-cian Sun Simiao included a prescription named Genkwa Powder (Yuanhua San). This large formula, which uses sixty-four herbs, including eighteen *du*-possessing ones, promised to cure a variety of obdurate disorders. After providing an elaborate account of ways to prepare and employ the formula, Sun mulls over its healing logic; the choice of the included drugs and the methods of their use are, he writes, beyond his understanding, as they do not accord with set principles. Upon trying it, however, he finds the remedy "spectacularly efficacious" (*shenyan*), especially for treating acute conditions. Pondering this, he concludes that certain things in the world do not act according to regular rules, but their efficacy has to be acknowledged nonetheless.[1]

Sun's remarks reveal the key role of practice in his evaluation of the efficacy of the powerful formula. This is not surprising, as empirical knowledge was crucial for physicians when deploying poisons; any misuse of these dangerous substances would lead to dire consequences. More broadly, the Tang physician's reflection on the unusual formula points to a critical issue in the study of medical history in China, namely, the relationship between doctrine and practice. Today, the word *jingyan*, which can be translated as "experience," refers to embodied skills of diagnosis and treatment, such as feeling the pulse, observing the face, and prescribing drugs, all of which are only acquired and improved by continuous practice. Although *jingyan* underlines the empirical nature of the practice of Chinese medicine, scholarship has tended to emphasize the indispensable role of the theoretical apparatus endorsed in medical canons, in guiding practice in both historical and contemporary settings. In other words, embodied knowledge acquired through practice works hand in hand with textual learning.[2]

In the premodern era, however, *jingyan* carried a different sense. Its original meaning was "having been tested," which, rather than referring to the skills of a medical practitioner, designated the quality of a formula that had been tried in practice.[3] Implied in this definition is the efficacy (*yan* or *xiao*) of the remedy. The term *jingyan* only appears once in sources prior to the tenth century; from the Song period on, it proliferated in medical texts, primarily associated with tested formulas.[4] Related terms, though, emerged earlier in the Sui and Tang bibliographical records, such as "personally tested formulas" (*shenyan fang*), "collected tested formulas" (*jiyan fang*), and "efficacious formulas" (*xiaoyan fang*). Such expressions evince the keen attention to efficacy in medical writings.[5]

One medical work in which many "efficacious" remedies appear is Sun Simiao's *Essential Formulas Worth a Thousand in Gold for Emergencies* (Beiji qianjin yaofang, 650s). The text belongs to the genre of formula books (*fangshu*), which collect prescriptions, organize them by types of illness, and offer instructions on the preparation and use of each of these remedies. Compared to theoretical treatises confined by intellectual frameworks, these formula collections are more miscellaneous and idiosyncratic, and offer insights into medical practice. Although the genre appeared in antiquity, it flourished in Tang China, as attested to by the emergence of a number of influential works compiled by the state, physicians, or scholars. What is particularly significant is Sun's incorporation of twenty-five medical cases into his *Essential Formulas*, a new feature in the writing of formula books. Scholars have examined the evolution of the genre of medical case literature (*yi'an*), which blossomed from the sixteenth century on.[6] Although Sun's text is not devoted to medical cases, his integration of them into the presentation of his formulas reveals a heightened attention to the value of personal experience in the treatment of patients. The complex relationship between text and practice, as we will see, is illustrated by the way he uses these cases to validate the efficacy of his remedies.

Formula Books from the Han to the Tang Period

The writing of formula books in China can be traced back to the Han period. The bibliographical section of *The History of the Han* places these books in the category of "classical formulas" (*jingfang*), which constitutes one of the four types of treatises on healing.[7] There are eleven titles in this group, most of which focus on treating specific types of illness, such as wind-induced fever and chills, internal injuries, and gynecological or pediatric disorders. It also includes a treatise on dietary taboos, indicating the awareness of food poisoning at the time. All of these texts, however, were lost long ago. In a different context, we find a collection of about three hundred formulas preserved in the Mawangdui medical manuscripts dating to the second century BCE. These texts provide simple cures, which often combine the use of drugs with spitting and incantations, to treat fifty-two types of maladies.[8] A smaller set of formulas was also discovered in manuscripts excavated from Wuwei and dating to the Eastern Han period. In these, the magical power of remedies is less prominent, suggesting regional differences in healing practice during the Han dynasty.[9] Poisons appear frequently in these formula collections: aconite of varying strengths (*wuhui, fuzi, tianxiong*) was one of the most often used medicines. The authors of these manuscripts remain unknown, and we find no trace of their voices therein.

During the Era of Division, medical culture flourished with the rise of hereditary medicine practiced by aristocratic families, especially in the south.[10] Formula books proliferated in this period. Although none of these works are extant in their entirety, many of their titles entered the bibliographies of the Sui and Tang official histories. *The History of the Sui*, for example, holds more than one hundred titles of formularies.[11] Significantly, many of these texts were ascribed to specific authors. These include the Han physician Zhang Zhongjing (150–219), the alchemist Ge Hong (283–343), the Daoist master Tao Hongjing (456–536), and several Buddhist monks. The rise of authorship indicates the effort of medical writers of various social backgrounds to produce formularies to enhance their reputation and establish authority. In particular, a number of these texts were compiled by the Xu family, who had practiced healing continuously for eight generations, suggesting the prominence of hereditary medicine during this period.[12] Moreover, ten titles carry the word "efficacy" (*yan* or *xiao*). Some of these texts were attributed to a single author or a family, such as Tao Hongjing or the Xu family. Others were collections of remedies from multiple sources, as suggested by the appearance of the term "collected efficacious formulas" in the title. The criteria according to which the efficacy of a formula was assessed is not made clear in the texts, yet it is evident that medical writers at the time valued the therapeutic outcome of their remedies.

The following seventh and eighth centuries witnessed the end of political division and the rise of the powerful Sui and Tang empires. In this new environment, the state became more active in compiling and circulating medical works, including formula books. For example, the Sui court issued a massive *Assorted Collection of Formulas from the Four Seas* (Sihai leiju fang), which contained 2,600 scrolls. Impressively comprehensive, the work probably served more to showcase the majesty of the empire rather than to guide medical practice. The court also sponsored an abridged version of the unwieldy book, which included only single-drug remedies in three hundred scrolls. It is more likely that this shortened text was used in practice.[13]

The Tang court also valued formula books and incorporated them into medical education. According to an eighth-century ordinance, students in the department of medicine at the Imperial Medical Office were required to study medical canons of acupuncture, pulse examination, and materia medica, as well as three others: a formula book of Zhang Zhongjing, *Formulas of the Lesser Grade*, and *Collected Efficacious Formulas*.[14]

Zhang was a physician during the Eastern Han dynasty known for treating "cold damage" disorders, a set of acute and often severe conditions characterized by fever. Although Zhang's status was substantially elevated in the Northern Song period (960–1127) thanks to the state's effort to systematize his writings on the treatment of epidemics, the Tang government in the eighth century already considered his works indispensable for medical learning. It is unclear which of Zhang's works the ordinance refers to—there are four formula books attributed to the Han physician in the bibliographical section of *The History of the Sui*, but suffice it to say that Tang medical training prized the remedies of a respected voice in the past.[15]

Second, *Formulas of the Lesser Grade* (Xiaopin fang) was a fifth-century work by Chen Yanzhi. It offered a collection of formulas for those who encountered medical emergencies where no expert care was available. In the preface, Chen describes formularies as works of a "lesser grade" compared to the theoretical texts, which he deems to be of a "greater grade." He further suggests a sequence for studying these texts: beginners should start with texts of a lesser grade to gradually reach the level of understanding that would allow them to grasp works of a greater grade. Empirical knowledge was a gateway to learning complex theories. With this goal in mind, Chen stresses the importance of understanding materia medica, especially knowledge of the properties of drugs that would inform their use in formulas. The Tang government chose this text for medical training probably because it effectively linked practical knowledge to doctrinal learning.[16]

The third text, *Collected Efficacious Formulas*, was likely produced based on the perceived effectiveness of its remedies, as indicated by the word "efficacious" in the title. The text could refer to one written by the sixth-century physician Yao Sengyuan because he compiled a book with exactly the same title. Yao came from an aristocratic family in the south that had been practicing medicine for many generations. Famous for his talents as a physician, Yao served as a high official at the courts of both the southern and northern dynasties. His formula book, which he compiled at the request of many who were seeking effective remedies, enjoyed lasting popularity, as Tang medical writers frequently cited his prescriptions for treating diverse disorders. The inclusion of this text in imperial education signifies the Tang court's attention to the efficacy of remedies, which could be detached from theoretical thinking.[17]

Sun Simiao and His Formula Books

None of the formula books discussed above are extant in their entirety. Nevertheless, several complete works of this genre from the early Tang period are still available, allowing for an in-depth analysis. In particular, *Essential Formulas* by Sun Simiao (581?–682) is significant, as it contains twenty-five medical cases scattered throughout the book, revealing how the physician integrated practice-based knowledge into his medical writing.

Sun, "the King of Medicines," was one of the most famous physicians in Chinese history; he collected a great number of drug remedies, some of which became standard treatments in the healing repertoire throughout imperial China and beyond.[18] Already a well-known figure in his lifetime, Sun gained more fame in the eleventh century, when the state enshrined his two formula books in the official canon. He was also deified during the Northern Song period, when the court granted to him the Daoist title of "the perfected" (*zhenren*).[19] Although the image of Sun as the greatest physician of all time would begin to dominate from the Song dynasty on, it is important to point out that during the Tang period, he was revered as a master who had versatile skills in medicine, alchemy, fasting, the cultivation of longevity, and divination. Rather than a medical specialist, Sun possessed broad knowledge of the arts of living.

Sun was born in the northwest, near the Tang capital Chang'an, sometime in the late sixth century.[20] Unlike some prominent physicians during the Era of Division, he did not come from an aristocratic family of medical heritage. He probably grew up in a comfortable setting, though, as both his grandfather and his father served as officials of different ranks in the northern dynasties.[21] According to the preface of his *Essential Formulas*, he obtained medical knowledge chiefly through self-study. When he was young, he had often been ill. Because visiting doctors was costly, he started to study medicine himself through extensive reading of the classics. At the age of twenty, feeling that he had grasped the essential knowledge of healing, Sun began to treat his relatives and neighbors, through which he gained practical experience. His reputation soon grew.

Based on his biographies in the two official histories of the Tang dynasty, it appears that Sun was not keenly interested in pursuing a political career; in his long life, he was asked by several emperors of a succession of dynasties to serve at court, but he declined the offers time and again. Understandably, in these biographies, he was placed in the category of either "[people possessing] methods and techniques" (*fangji*) or "recluses" (*yinyi*).[22] Yet beneath the façade of being a talented hermit uninterested in politics, he remained connected to the court. Summoned by Emperor Gaozong in 658, he took the position of assistant director in the Palace Drug Service, which offered technical guidance on the preparation of medicines for the imperial family. Given that this was the moment when the court was compiling *Newly Revised Materia Medica* (see chapter 4), it is possible that Sun was consulted in the making of the pharmacopoeia. During his stay in the capital, he was also socially active, offering medical service to court officials and befriending scholars who admired his wisdom.[23] According to a newly excavated tombstone that preserves the epitaph for one of Sun's sons, the physician "dwelled at the center of the court, and his aspiration extended to the faraway seas." The contrast encapsulates the image of a Sun who moved between public and

private spaces, and negotiated with political resources to enhance his reputation as a superb doctor and fulfill his pursuit of the arts of healing.[24]

Furthermore, Sun was familiar with Daoist and Buddhist teachings. He was
particularly interested in the techniques of life cultivation and spent two years
at Mount Taibai not far from the capital, learning the methods of refining *qi*
and nourishing the body. He also had advanced knowledge of alchemy, which
he put into practice. Sun's Buddhist knowledge came from his extensive reading
of scriptures and interaction with several eminent monks, from whom he
acquired unusual formulas and mastered the technique of ingesting water.[25]
Buddhist influence is also evident in his medical ethics: he embraced the idea
of treating patients compassionately regardless of their social status, echoing
Buddhist teachings of equality and universal salvation. This spirit is palpable
in Sun's formula books, where he offered varying remedies using expensive or
ordinary ingredients to patients of noble or humble origins, respectively.[26]

Sun compiled two formula books later in his life: *Essential Formulas* in the
650s and *Supplement to Formulas Worth a Thousand in Gold* (Qianjin yifang;
hereafter, *Supplement to Formulas*) in the 680s. The latter text, which he completed not long before his death, is more miscellaneous, incorporating a wide
range of healing methods, such as fasting, alchemy, and incantations. He also
included many formulas for prolonging life, probably because of his old age.[27]
Unlike the court-commissioned *Newly Revised Materia Medica*, Sun's two
formula books reveal no trace of the state's direct intervention. However,
given Sun's close ties to the court, it is conceivable that he had access to
resources in the imperial library to compile his books. The affinity is particularly evident in his *Supplement to Formulas*, in which he copied verbatim the
description of drugs from *Newly Revised Materia Medica*. The standardization of drug knowledge by the Tang government hence readily entered into
Sun's medical writings.[28]

Essential Formulas contains thirty scrolls.[29] The first scroll offers general
therapeutic guidelines, including diagnosis, prescription, and the preparation
of drugs. The following scrolls are organized by types of illness. In each of
them, Sun starts with a theoretical discussion of the illness, expounding its
causes, symptoms, and bodily dynamics. This is followed by a large number
of drug prescriptions that treat the illness, as well as a few moxibustion remedies at the end. Altogether, the book contains more than 4,200 drug remedies.
In the preface, Sun explains his purpose in compiling these formulas:

I find that all formula books are massive volumes. If one suddenly encounters an emergency, it is very hard to seek the remedy. By the time the formula is acquired, the illness has already become incurable. Alas! I agonize over the calamity of untimely death and lament the follies caused by crude learning. I then widely gathered various classics. I deleted the complicated formulas and made sure to keep the simple ones, thereby producing one book of *Essential Formulas Worth a Thousand in Gold for Emergencies*. Altogether it has thirty scrolls.[30]

Recognizing the difficulty of handling voluminous tomes, Sun selected "essential formulas" from earlier works that could be readily used in emergencies. This criterion evinces the practical orientation of his book: it was composed not to display scholarly erudition but to cure illness. The title of the book expresses the attitude well; he asserts that since a human life is extremely valuable, with its worth over a thousand in gold, the virtue of saving it by a formula even exceeds that value.[31] Sun was not alone in this aim. According to the bibliographical records, a number of physicians and scholar-officials during the Tang period compiled formula works whose titles contained "for emergencies." Easy use of remedies to treat acute conditions, therefore, was a widespread pursuit at the time.[32]

Although Sun emphasizes the practical function of his book, he still respects established doctrines. At the beginning of each scroll, he explains the nature and symptoms of the illness, starting with the set term "discussion" (*lunyue*), which is likely Sun's own voice. Such discussions are often framed in the conceptual schemes of yin and yang, the five phases, and *qi*, which characterize the illness as dynamic processes correlated with the environment.[33] Sun also frequently counts on authoritative voices to bolster his propositions. Among them, the words of Bian Que, a semimythical physician living in antiquity, appear most often—Sun cites him more than thirty times.[34] Other sources that appear in Sun's theoretical discussion include passages from the ancient physicians Zhang Zhongjing, Wang Shuhe, and Hua Tuo, as well as from the Han classics *The Divine Farmer's Classic* and *The Yellow Emperor's Inner Classic*. Sometimes he also cites more recent works, such as *Formulas of the Lesser Grade* (fifth century).[35] It is clear that Sun relied heavily on classical wisdoms in his conceptualization of illness.

Less obvious, though, is how Sun fit specific drug remedies into this theoretical framework. At the beginning of the book, he does include a section on the basic rules of making prescriptions, but the discussion is short and generic, primarily based on *The Divine Farmer's Classic*. For example, he presents the principle of opposites, namely, to use warming drugs to treat cold maladies and vice versa.[36] But the rule is probably too crude to explain the composition of many complex formulas in the book that contain multiple ingredients. Moreover, driven by his goal for easy use, Sun includes a large number of single-ingredient formulas that deploy ordinary substances, such as soil, foods, and feces, to treat emergencies.[37] Such remedies cannot be easily explained with the conceptual program that Sun inherited from classical texts. And he makes no effort to offer such an explanation. Therefore, despite the physician's attention to ancient medical principles, his formulas, which are abundant and eclectic, are largely detached from doctrinal teaching.

For whom did Sun write the book? Repeatedly, he uses the generic appellation "learner" (*xuezhe*) to address his readers. More specifically, he states in the preface that the book "may not be possible to be transmitted to scholarly groups, and I only wish to pass it on in private lines."[38] These "scholarly groups" (*shizu*) could refer to certain prestigious aristocratic families that had practiced medicine for generations or scholar-officials who were personally interested in medicine and exchanged medical knowledge within their circles. Given Sun's humble origins, his stated intention to keep his book within private confines—be it in his family or among his disciples—could have been a tactic to enhance the value of his work against powerful competitors. The idea of private transmission was not new—the phenomenon can be traced back to antiquity when medical learning often passed from masters to disciples in a secretive and ritualized fashion.[39] In fact, many formulas in Sun's book, especially those with claimed efficacy, end with the leitmotifs of "keep it secret," "do not transmit it," or "do not transmit it even for a thousand in gold."[40] Although it is hard to tell whether these are Sun's own words or what Sun copied from earlier sources, the frequent association of such expressions with his formulas indicates the physician's intention to limit their circulation.

That being said, Sun remained open to the court. In several medical cases that recount his own experience, he calls himself "your servant" (*chen*), the appropriate form of self-reference for a minister when speaking to the monarch. Given Sun's strong connection to the court, he could have borne the emperor in mind when he compiled the formulary. This intent would not necessarily conflict with his emphasis on private transmission; the value of his work precisely lay in its availability only to the highest powers. Although the text was not selected for imperial medical education, it gained recognition in Sun's official biography and the bibliographical record of the Tang dynasty.[41]

"Efficacious" Remedies in *Essential Formulas*

Besides the doctrinal teaching at the beginning of each scroll, Sun provides a large number of formulas that treat the illness under discussion. In general, the writing of each formula follows a set pattern. It starts with the name of the formula, often with the typical symptoms associated with the illness for which it is indicated. It then lists all the ingredients in the formula, specifying the dose for each one. Finally, it advises how to prepare and administer the formula. Sometimes, the description ends with a statement of the efficacy of the medicine. The size of the formulas in Sun's book varies greatly, ranging from single-drug remedies to enormous prescriptions that use as many as sixty-four ingredients. Almost all from the former group are applied topically to treat sores, swellings, and wounds. Those from the latter group, by contrast, often work as panaceas to eliminate obdurate maladies and restore the vitality of the body.[42] The following is an example that treats a gynecological disorder and triggers pregnancy:

> Formula of the White Vetch Pill from the magistrate of Jincheng. It cures blockage and stagnation of menses that leads to the inability to become pregnant for eighteen years. Upon ingesting this medicine for twenty-eight days, a woman will bear children.[43]
>
> White vetch (five *liang*), ginseng (three *fen*), southern asarum (three *fen*), bull dodder (three *fen*), achyranthes (two *fen*), asarum (five *liang*), magnolia bark (three *fen*), pinellia (three *fen*), adenophora (two *fen*), dried ginger (two *fen*), infected silkworm (three *fen*), gentian (two *fen*), pepper of Sichuan (six *fen*), angelica (three *fen*), aconite (six *fen*), saposhnikovia (six *fen*), purple aster (three *fen*).[44]
>
> Mix the above seventeen ingredients with honey to make into pills. First ingest three pills the size of a seed of the parasol tree. If the patient does not feel the effects of the medicine, slightly increase the dose to four or five pills. This medicine should not be ingested for long. The patient should stop using it when she suspects that she has become pregnant. Greatly efficacious.[45]

The formula uses seventeen drugs, mainly of herbal origins, to treat a menstrual disorder. Among them, three possess *du* (pinellia, pepper of Sichuan, and aconite). Sun recommends that the patient gradually increase the dose until she feels the effects of the medicine, indicating the importance of bodily sensations in gauging the therapeutic outcome.[46] It also warns against the excessive consumption of the medicine, probably due to the presence of the potent ingredients. A powerful medicine, in other words, must be cautiously administered.

Where did Sun obtain his formulas? The one above is attributed to the magistrate of Jincheng, a prefecture in the northwest (present-day Lanzhou) that was established in the Western Han period. It is unclear whether the magistrate was a contemporary of Sun or lived long before. In the latter scenario, Sun probably copied the formula from an earlier source.[47] Identification of a formula's originator, however, is rare in Sun's work; for the majority of his prescriptions, he simply wrote down their content without acknowledging the source. This is in sharp contrast to the theoretical sections of his book, in which he frequently cites ancient authors to buttress his discussion. Since Sun's work contains a massive number of formulas, he probably copied most of them from other texts, which the physician readily acknowledges in the preface. But the lack of mention of the origins of the formulas implies that he prioritized the practical value of healing over the scholarly production of knowledge.

What were the criteria for Sun to include a formula? In the introductory section on treating pediatric disorders, he first exposes the limitations of the formulas from the powerful Xu family, revealing his critical attitude toward aristocratic medicine. He then lays out the two basic principles for compiling his own formulas: to gather them widely from all schools of medicine, and to include those that prove "efficacious upon self-usage" (*zi jingyong youxiao*).[48] On the one hand, Sun's work is decidedly eclectic; it was compiled based on a comprehensive survey of available sources without subscribing to a particular lineage. On the other, Sun stresses the importance of personal experience in validating the efficacy of his formulas. In another section discussing hot diarrhea (*reli*), he declares that he could not record thousands of formulas that treat the disorder from ancient and contemporary sources. Instead, he picked only seven or eight among them that had proven efficacious.[49] Therapeutic efficacy therefore was a crucial criterion for the physician when selecting remedies.

Yet we must not hasten to associate the claimed efficacy of a remedy with Sun's own practice. In the sample formula presented above, the term "greatly efficacious" appears at the end, praising the success of the treatment. How do we make sense of it? Throughout *Essential Formulas*, we find many similar expressions attached to the end of prescriptions, which almost always include words for efficacy (*yan, xiao, liang*). Some of the most frequent phrases are "spectacularly efficacious," "spectacularly good," "extremely good," and "having efficacy." Other expressions, though not including the word "efficacy," convey a similar meaning, such as "no single failure upon trying ten thousand times" and "as if pouring hot water onto snow."[50] These "efficacy phrases" are terse, generic, and formulaic. They carry the rhetorical force of a boast rather than serving as evidence of the remedy's actual use.[51] A heightened attention to efficacy is already detectable in formula books during the Era of Division, as evidenced by the increasing appearance of the word in their titles. These earlier works also include "efficacy phrases" tagged to the end of some of their formula entries, undoubtedly serving the same rhetorical function.[52] Very likely, Sun incorporated these earlier formulas, including the set terms, into his book without voicing his own opinion. Efficacy was an artifact of copying.

Medical Cases in *Essential Formulas*

The most salient feature of *Essential Formulas* is the medical cases embedded in the prescriptions. No earlier formula books include such cases, making Sun's compilation a new phenomenon in the history of medical writing in China. Close study of these twenty-five cases illuminates the meaning of efficacy and the role of personal experience in the making of new medical knowledge.[53]

In general, each medical case appears at the end of a formula, in which Sun presents a specific situation to testify to the efficacy of the remedy. These cases contain some or all of the following components: the time, place, identity of the healer, identity of the patient, diagnosis, prescription, and therapeutic outcome. Although the majority of these narratives are based on Sun's own experience, this is not always so. For example, in a case of curing "the dragon illness" (*jiaolong bing*), Sun records that on the eighth day of the second month in 586, someone ate celery and contracted the illness. The symptoms resembled those of a condition called "abdominal bloating," with the face turning bluish yellow. Upon ingesting three liters of cooling foods and strong malt sugar, the patient spat out a dragon possessing two heads and a tail. It was a greatly efficacious cure.[54] The case confirms the efficacy of a simple food remedy to eliminate a pathological entity inside the body.[55] Revealingly, Sun did not identify who the patient was; he only used the generic phrase "someone" to refer to him or her, which suggests that he had no direct experience of the event described. He may have heard of the story from others and included it in his book to validate the formula. Efficacy could be disembodied knowledge bolstered by word of mouth.

The majority of the cases in *Essential Formulas* (twenty-one out of twenty-five), however, clearly show Sun's personal involvement. Among them, he treated others in eleven cases and himself in ten cases. In the former category, he reveals the identity of his patients in three cases, which include two local noblemen and a nun.[56] The patients in Sun's account usually do not have a voice—they are portrayed as passive recipients of the treatment. When they occasionally speak, their views are erroneous, often with serious consequences. In one case, a patient did not believe Sun's diagnosis of his illness as foot *qi* because he found no sign of swollen feet. The misjudgment cost the man his life. In another case, a patient became sick upon ingesting minerals, a popular practice for nourishing the body at the time, and died after trying numerous self-administered formulas. Without a capable physician, one's chances of surviving an intractable malady were slim.[57]

Presenting himself as one such capable physician, Sun boasts of his healing skills by highlighting his extensive experience; he points out in one case that he treated more than a hundred patients with the intransigent illness of "great wind" (*dafeng*).[58] Among his twenty-five medical cases, thirteen designate the date when the healing occurred, sometimes down to a particular day. For the cases that Sun himself was involved with, the dates range between the years 605 and 643, which correlates well with the years that were probably the prime of his life, suggesting that Sun's cases were built upon his own experience, rather than simply an artifact of his having copied earlier sources. With respect to the locations of healing, although Sun spent most of his life in the capital Chang'an and nearby regions, he also traveled to Jiangzhou (in present-day Jiangxi), Shuxian (present-day Chengdu), and Neijiang (in present-day Sichuan), where he attended a duke, practiced alchemy, and cured himself of a skin rash, respectively.[59]

The last aspect merits our attention, namely, self-healing. Sun regularly tried medicines on himself and used the experience as compelling evidence for a formula's efficacy; such instances appear frequently in the book (ten out of twenty-five cases). Sun's narrative of self-healing is varied. Sometimes, the situation was urgent and his use of the right formula proved to be life-saving. For example, when he was in Neijiang in 643, he became ill with a skin condition known as "vermilion poisoning" (*dandu*), a deep-red skin rash. The rashes first developed on his forehead and quickly spread to the rest of his body. He almost died. The county magistrate offered him various medicines, none of which worked. After seven days, Sun tried a single-drug formula of brassica paste, which cured him. He thus recorded the formula to make it widely known. Resolving a critical condition with a simple remedy undoubt-edly testified to its value.[60]

Moreover, Sun's medical cases often build on a narrative of trial and error. In one revealing example, he presents a formula that uses the cocklebur paste to treat "clove swellings" (*dingzhong*), ulcerous lumps shaped like cloves. Cocklebur (*cang'er*) was a *du*-possessing herb that already appeared in *The Divine Farmer's Classic*, where its fruit was valued for eliminating limb pain and nourishing the body. The authors of *Newly Revised Materia Medica* iden-tified more uses of the herb to treat seizures, poison in marrow, and venomous stings.[61] Although cocklebur was a well-recognized medicine during the Tang period, Sun's use of it to treat clove swellings was novel. Specifically, he directs the users to incinerate the roots, stems, and sprouts of the herb, mix the ashes with vinegar, and apply the paste to the swellings. Once the paste is dry, they should replace it with another fresh preparation, repeating the process until it eventually pulls out the root of the swellings. The medicine is "spectacu-larly good." Sun then relates that in 630, he suddenly had clove swellings at the corners of his mouth. He visited a person named Gan Zizhen, whose mother prepared a different paste for him, but the medicine did not work.[62] He then tried the cocklebur paste, which cured him immediately. Afterward he often made this medicine for patients, and none had failed to be healed. Among the thousand formulas that treat clove swellings, Sun avers, none of them is better—even the trusted formula from Granny Rong of Qizhou (pres-ent-day Jinan) is not as powerful as his.[63] By contrasting the efficacy of the cocklebur paste with the failure of another treatment, Sun underlines the sig-nificance of trial and error in finding excellent cures. The formula he singles out at the end, Granny Rong's, presumably a reputable remedy at the time, involves six ingredients and a long, complicated preparation process. Simple and effective, small wonder that the cocklebur paste became Sun's favorite to treat clove swellings.[64]

What illnesses appear in Sun's medical cases? Although the case studies are spread throughout the thirty scrolls of *Essential Formulas*, we find two clusters formed around specific conditions: the wind-induced disorders, especially foot *qi* (*juan* 7 and 8), and swellings and abscesses (*juan* 23). The first cluster concerns acute, life-threatening conditions that demand swift action; the second includes illnesses with manifest external signs. A successful treatment of a disorder in these clusters yields immediate and unambiguous outcomes—the patient survives, the ulcers disappear—which clearly showcases the efficacy of the remedy.

Notably, Sun often prescribed potent medicines in his medical cases. In twelve of the twenty cases that involved drug therapy, he utilized *du*-possessing substances of herbal, mineral, and animal origin, including aconite, pinellia, croton, orpiment, and bovine bezoar. These drugs were often deployed to treat severe and obstinate conditions, such as hot, poisonous diarrhea and *gu* poisoning.[65] Sun also traveled to Shuxian to obtain the best materials for his alchemical practices. Fully aware of the danger of one key ingredient used in alchemy, realgar (an arsenic compound), he cautions that one must detoxify the potent mineral before using it for making elixirs.[66]

One of the most frequently prescribed potent medicines in Sun's formulas was aconite. The drug was considered particularly effective for treating sudden turmoil (*huoluan*), an acute condition caused by improper diet leading to the entanglement of pure and turbid *qi* in the stomach and intestines.[67] In one case, Sun recommends a formula that employs ten herbs, including two possessing great *du*—aconite and arisaema (*huzhang*)—to cure the severe disorder and prevent it from recurring. The ingredients are ground into powder, mixed with honey to make pills the size of a parasol tree seed, and taken with alcohol twenty pills a time, three times a day. Sun then continues with a story:

> During the Wude period [618–626], there was a virtuous nun named Jingming. She suffered this illness for a long time. Sometimes the illness erupted once a month, sometimes more than once a month. Every time the illness erupted, she almost died. At the time, great physicians at court such as Jiang, Xu, Gan, and Chao failed to recognize the illness. I treated it as sudden turmoil and prescribed this formula, which cured her. I thus recorded the formula.[68]

The story emphasizes Sun's ability to correctly diagnose the patient. Revealingly, Sun contrasts his superb skills with the clumsiness of the court physicians, who, despite their high position, were unable to discern the illness. Many of these physicians came from medical families of aristocratic origin who entered the imperial medical bureaucracy during the early Tang period.[69] Sun did not belong to this select group of social elites, though he frequently interacted with them while staying in the capital (the aforementioned Gan Zizhen, from whom he sought treatment, might have been the same court physician named Gan in this story of the nun). He was generally critical of their healing expertise, often calling them foolish, coarse, or clumsy.[70] The disparaging tone implies an uneasy tension between medical practitioners of distinct social origins at the time. By pointing out the mistakes of his noble yet inferior contemporaries, Sun tried to carve out a space beyond hereditary and court medicine, elevating his reputation as a superb healer based on the evidence of his practice.

These case reports of Sun's successful healing of both himself and his patients suggest that he had an excellent grasp of the relationship between the symptoms of an illness and the corresponding rationale for designing a formula to treat it. In other cases, however, he admits that his understanding of how a remedy worked was limited. This brings us back to the opening episode. In a section on panaceas, Sun depicts Genkwa Powder as a powerful medicine that can cure all illnesses of wind cold, the accumulation of phlegm, concretions and aggregations, and intermittent fevers, as well as those conditions that myriad physicians fail to cure.[71] After a lengthy explanation of the various methods of preparing and deploying the cure-all, he reveals that the formula did not actually appear in any of the books he had read. Rather, he obtained it from a Buddhist monk named Jingzhi over thirty years before.[72] During his days, no eminent physician sanctioned the use of the peculiar medicine, yet upon trying it, Sun found it spectacularly effective. He further reflects:

> The way this formula uses drugs does not follow regular orders at all, and the rules of its ingestion are far beyond human reasoning. Yet as for treating emergencies, its efficacy is extraordinary. I then realized that the efficacy of spectacular things is not bound by common rules. The supreme principle of resonance cannot be fathomed by intelligence. This also resembles the situation when a dragon cries, clouds rise; when a tiger roars, the wind comes into

being. This is without understanding why it is so—even sages cannot discern the reason.[73]

What is striking in this passage is Sun's ready recognition of the inadequate understanding of why the medicine works (*buzhi suoyiran*). Even sages, he avows, cannot comprehend the logic of the highest principle. This comment is in sharp contrast to his theoretical discussion of illnesses at the beginning of each scroll, which heavily relies on ancient wisdom and established doctrines. Here, however, his perspective is more open: there are things in the world whose ways of working are beyond human understanding. Yet as long as they can effectively treat emergencies, Sun finds no reason not to include them in his collection.[74] This practical sentiment is not just associated with large, complex formulas. In another case, Sun tried several remedies to treat sores that were caused by the urine of earwigs, but to no avail. He then learned the unusual method of drawing the shape of the insect on the ground, taking the soil enclosed by its abdomen, mixing it with saliva, and smearing the paste onto the sores. This simple remedy swiftly cured him, though he confessed that "myriad things under heaven resonate with each other, and I do not fathom the reason."[75] Despite this, he cherished the formula because of its undeniable efficacy. For Sun, empirical knowledge outweighed doctrinal learning.

The practical orientation of Sun's medical cases is also indicated by how he treated patients of different social origins. Likely due to Buddhist influence, Sun embraced the spirit of treating all people equally, whether the person was "noble or ordinary, poor or rich, old or young, beautiful or ugly, enemy or friend, Chinese or barbarian, stupid or wise."[76] This ethical principle required a physician to treat patients regardless of their social status—but this does not mean that the same remedy was appropriate for everybody. For example, in the section on treating cold diarrhea, Sun offers two formulas for the nobles, both to restore the vitality of the Spleen.[77] The first, the Spleen-Warming Decoction, is a generic prescription to treat either cold or hot diarrhea, using rhubarb, cinnamon, aconite, dried ginger, and ginseng to induce draining in the stomach. The second, the Spleen-Strengthening Pill, is specific for cold diarrhea. It contains fifteen ingredients, including stalactite, coptis, ginseng, dried ginger, cinnamon, and aconite, that aim to nourish the Spleen to facilitate its full recovery. However, Sun notes that it was hard for the poor to prepare these formulas, likely because of the cost of certain ingredients.[78]

Moreover, the two formulas work in concert: the first to eliminate the illness, the second to nourish the body and restore its strength. The latter requires sufficient rest with a proper regimen—a remedy that is compatible with the leisurely lifestyle of the nobility. Not just money but time was a luxury that the poor did not necessarily possess.[79]

Conversely, Sun considers certain remedies inappropriate for the nobles. In a formula that treats welling abscess (*yongzhong*), Sun proposes making a paste out of a chicken egg and fresh human feces and applying it to the pus. He comments that the formula is filthy, so it should not be applied to the nobles. Yet as for its power to cure this illness, the medicine is second to none. Other formulas, by contrast, just follow the protocols and abide by the rules; hence people should be aware of this unique remedy, which could treat them effectively in case of emergency.[80] Sun considers certain ordinary substances—human excrement in this case—too filthy for elites but acceptable for the less privileged. Medicines were social substances.[81] Yet the efficacy of the formula was beyond doubt despite its unusual ingredient. Comparing it with conventional formulas that better fit established frameworks but were less effective, Sun makes it clear that he prefers utility to conformity.

Conclusion

What does Sun's *Essential Formulas* tell us about the relationship between text and experience in Tang China? His book contains over four thousand prescriptions, so it is hard to imagine that he tested all of them himself. Rather, he followed a long tradition of copying formulas from earlier and contemporary sources, though he rarely specified the titles of these texts. The frequent appearance of the "efficacy phrases," which are mechanical, repetitive, and nonspecific, signals that such copying served to rhetorically promote his remedies. That being said, Sun's text is not merely an artifact of replication but reveals something important about empirical knowledge. In particular, his twenty-five medical cases, which are concrete and detailed, underscore the value of personal experience in his assessment of formulas. Although Sun cherished doctrinal principles and the voices of ancient authorities, he recognized their limitations and prioritized the efficacy of remedies based on his own experience, even in cases where the logic of a formula escaped his understanding. Admittedly, the scattered narratives in

Sun's work are modest in scale compared to later compilations that are devoted to medical cases. Yet as the first formula book that incorporates such cases in Chinese history, the text exhibits the fledgling consciousness of using practice-based knowledge to validate therapeutic efficacy.

To appreciate this new feature of Chinese medical writing, it is necessary to position Sun's text in the evolution of two medical genres, both with a practical bent. The first are formula books (*fangshu*), which already emerged in antiquity and remained a thriving genre throughout imperial China and beyond. The second are medical cases (*yi'an*), which appeared sporadically in early sources and only started to blossom as an independent genre beginning in the sixteenth century. Intriguingly, medical cases (*observatio*) in Europe also proliferated at the same time, leading to the rise of a new "epistemic genre," a concept developed by the historian of medicine Gianna Pomata, which reveals distinct cognitive processes of generating empirical knowledge based on direct observation and firsthand experience.[82] This comparative insight illuminates the reading of Sun's *Essential Formulas*. Different from commentary texts such as materia medica, which faithfully copy the structure and content of the ancient classics, formula books are more eclectic, flexible, and open, incorporating remedies from diverse sources and of disparate social origins. Sun's innovation of inserting medical cases into his collection of formulas, which resembles texts of *experimenta* that appeared in late medieval Europe, adds further weight to the practical orientation of the genre.[83] Using these examples to showcase the efficacy of his formulas, Sun promotes a new mode of knowledge production that is rooted in personal experience.[84]

Finally, it is important to point out that within the genre of formula books, different texts reveal subtle epistemic differences. The eighth-century *Arcane Essentials from the Imperial Library*, for instance, also contains a massive number of formulas. Yet unlike *Essential Formulas*, the text specifies the source of each of its six-thousand-odd prescriptions, many of which were copied from Sun's writing, and includes no accounts of the author's own experience. Revealingly, Wang Tao, the author of the book, was a scholar-official who had keen interest in medicine but probably did not engage in medical practice beyond self-healing. As the title indicates, he compiled the formula book based on a thorough survey of medical works in the imperial library, which is in contrast to Sun's emphasis on the practical use of his remedies to treat emergencies.[85] Hence the ways that scholar-officials produced medical knowledge and wrote about their experiences (or lack thereof) were related to but distinct from those of physicians like Sun. The two groups frequently exchanged knowledge of healing and sometimes debated the proper use of certain formulas. The dynamic interplay was broadcast in their heated discussion on one of the most controversial drugs in medieval China, Five-Stone Powder, the subject of the next chapter.

PART III

Enhancing the Body

CHAPTER 6

Alluring Stimulant

Since the beginning, the Great Powder has been a medicine hard to manage.

—*FORMULAS OF THE LESSER GRADE* (FIFTH CENTURY)

THE HISTORY OF THE SOUTHERN DYNASTIES RECOUNTS A STORY IN which a physician treated his patient according to an unusual method: Fang Boyu, a general at the Southern Qi (479–502) court, ingested scores of doses of a medicine to vitalize his body but enjoyed no benefit. Instead, he developed chills and had to wear thick clothes in summer. The physician Xu Sibo, upon diagnosis, announced that the general suffered from "dormant heat" (*fure*), which could be released by water. This therapy, the physician insisted, must be given in winter. They waited until the eleventh month of the year, when Xu asked two people to hold the general tight on a stone with his clothes off. They then poured a great amount of cold water on his head, so much that he lost consciousness. Despite pleas from the general's family to stop the brutal treatment, Xu requested that yet more water be poured on the lifeless patient, who eventually started to move, with warm *qi* rising from his back. Soon he sat up, complaining about intolerable heat in his body and asking for a cold beverage. After drinking some cool water, he was cured. From then on, his body constantly emanated vital heat, and he became plump and strong.[1]

This dramatic tale reveals a singular characteristic of the medicine that the general ingested: it generated massive heat inside the body. If kept latent, such heat would cause problems, manifesting in the chills that the patient suffered initially. Once properly released, as triggered by Xu's harsh therapy of cold stimulation, the heat would erupt and become a source of bodily nourishment. The key to using the medicine was thus to prudently release and manage the heat it induced, maximizing its benefits.

The medicine that had first troubled the general was Five-Stone Powder (Wushi San), which refers to its five major mineral ingredients. This was alternatively called the Great Powder (Dasan) or Cold-Food Powder (Hanshi San), the latter name describing the necessity of consuming cold food to balance the heat it induced. The powder enjoyed remarkable popularity in medieval China, with a fad for the drug persisting from the third century until the late Tang period. With its promise of not just curing sickness but also invigorating the body and illuminating the mind, it was particularly appealing to literati, who consumed it as part of a carefree, idiosyncratic way of living. Alongside numerous accounts that extolled the virtues of the powder, just as many deplored its devastating effects on the body, including causing unbearable pain, noxious ulcers, lunatic impulses, and even death, and offered treatments to mitigate the damage. To be sure, Five-Stone Powder was as popular as it was controversial, which fueled impassioned discussions among physicians and scholars about the value of the medicine, its potential dangers, and above all, the proper way of managing the powerful stimulant.

The abundant depictions of the afflictions caused by Five-Stone Powder in standard histories, medical works, and literary productions from the Era of Division to the Tang dynasty have compelled modern scholars to focus on the debilitating harm the drug caused both individuals and society. Despite its promise to heal, these scholars argued, the "side effects" of the powder were extreme. Portrayed in this negative light, it was nothing but poison; opium was often invoked as a point of comparison.[2] A close reading of discussions of the medicine in medieval China, however, tells a different story. Physicians and scholars enthusiastically endorsed the medicine for its power of both curing illness and enhancing life. They readily recognized the suffering it could cause, but instead of blaming the inherent toxicity of the drug, they pointed to the erroneous ways of channeling the heat it induced out of the body. The powder was, first and foremost, extremely difficult to deploy. Those who used it incorrectly, or ingested it for wrong purposes, were doomed to suffer, if not die. The considerable difficulty involved in employing the drug safely provoked animated debates among physicians and scholars, and may also account for the eventual decline of its appeal toward the end of the Tang dynasty.

A Drug of Remarkable Appeal

The widespread popularity of Five-Stone Powder is often attributed to He Yan, a scholar-official living in the third century. According to *A New Account of the Tales of the World* (Shishuo xinyu), a fifth-century collection of scholarly anecdotes, He once said, "Ingestion of Five-Stone Powder not only cures sickness but also makes one feel that the spirit is open and bright."[3] The commentary on the text cites the work of the fifth-century physician Qin Chengzu, who explains that the powder's formula originated during the Han period but was rarely used. It was He who discovered its marvelous effects, attracting numerous users and inaugurating the craze.[4]

What was the special allure of Five-Stone Powder in medieval China? He Yan lived in the tumultuous period of the early third century, when the Han dynasty collapsed and three aristocratic powers, often referred to as the Three Kingdoms (220–280), divided the country. Raised in the palace of the Kingdom of Wei in the north and later clinging to a powerful general at court, he enjoyed the political fortunes and social prestige of a nobleman. Later sources, however, do not portray him as a man of noble character: obsessed with his physical beauty, he lived an unrestrained and licentious life, and Five-Stone Powder, along this line of thought, was an accomplice to his sexual indulgence.[5]

Yet He's own words tout the drug's ability to illuminate the mind, alluding to his intellectual pursuit. In fact, the aristocrat was a leading figure in a philosophical movement called Mysterious Learning (Xuanxue) that arose in the early third century. Together with another thinker Wang Bi (226–249), He revisited Daoist classics and offered fresh interpretations that tied ancient philosophical thinking to political governance. At the heart of their thoughts was the concept of "mystery" or "darkness" (*xuan*); followers of the Mysterious Learning school traced all phenomena and actions in the cosmos back to this spontaneous and inscrutable nothingness. Significantly, these thinkers tried to apply their ideas to the state-sanctioned Confucian ideology by elucidating the dialectical relationship between nonaction and action, and stressing a way of ruling that followed the spontaneous pattern of nature.[6]

The rise of Mysterious Learning in the third century coincided with a changing political and social landscape. With the collapse of the Han dynasty, the orthodox status of Confucian ideology was substantially weakened, allowing for the revival and reinvention of other types of philosophical thinking that had hitherto remained marginal. In the following three centuries, except for a brief moment of unification during the Western Jin dynasty (266–316), the political division that persisted between the north and the south resulted in constant wars, social turmoil, and the loss of countless lives. It is not surprising that in this volatile environment, the Daoist ideas of nothingness and nonaction offered solace for those inclined to make sense of harsh realities. Such aspirations were, however, limited. Despite He's attempt to apply his philosophy to state policy, his execution as the result of a brutal court rivalry in the mid-third century only testified to how futile his efforts were in a time of chaos and uncertainty.[7]

Such power struggles became the norm in the succeeding centuries, increasingly forcing the followers of Mysterious Learning to turn away from state affairs and embrace a spontaneous, carefree way of living that centered on the cultivation of the self. A group of third-century literati whose behavior was perceived to be idiosyncratic if not utterly bizarre was the Seven Worthies of the Bamboo Grove (Zhulin Qixian). These scholars, essayists, and poets shunned politics, defied social norms, and followed their impulses, aligning themselves with the spontaneous rhythms of nature. They became famous for their unconventional conduct: wild drinking, loud singing, mocking funeral rituals, and walking around naked. It was a time of high individualistic energy.[8]

It is in this context that we can better understand the social character of Five-Stone Powder. In an often-cited lecture delivered in the early twentieth century, writer and social critic Lu Xun situated the consumption of the drug in the intellectual milieu of the Era of Division and suggested that many types of strange behavior associated with social elites at the time were the direct effects of the powder they regularly ingested as part of their uninhibited life. They walked around naked to release the immense heat generated by taking it, wore loose clothes and wooden sandals so as not to rub the ulcers induced by the powder, and often had erratic emotions—short temper, easy agitation, and even madness, all signs of the drug's untoward influence on the mind. Although Lu Xun may have exaggerated its effects as part of his condemnation of the episode, his remarks point to the important social life of the drug that accounted for its extraordinary popularity.[9]

The linking of Five-Stone Powder to eccentric behavior—an image depicted by some later commentators, who blamed libertines for cultural decadence and moral failing—emphasized that the drug was consumed for self-indulgent pleasure. The negative portrayal of He Yan by these scholars and physicians was as much a critique of a flawed individual as a reproof of the cultural trend that he embodied.[10] Yet upon a closer look at the sources, we find that most discussions about the drug centered on its medicinal uses. The third-century scholar Ji Han, for example, wrote a rhapsodic poem extolling its virtues, which he claimed had cured his infant son of an acute case of vomiting and diarrhea. After other formulas failed, the father gave the powder to his child and it "saved him from the severe trouble and restored his spirit afresh."[11] The famous calligrapher Wang Xizhi (303–361) also ingested the powder to treat his chronic ailments. Its effect on his body, though, was more ambiguous. In a series of letters that he wrote to his relatives and friends, he described his experiences of taking the drug: sometimes it markedly improved his condition, and other times the heat released by the powder caused him pain and distress. These letters also reveal that not just the celebrated calligrapher but also his family members and acquaintances took it to combat illnesses. Sharing their experiences in epistolary exchanges, they tried to work out the best methods for using the powerful drug to alleviate their suffering.[12]

Besides curing sickness, there was more to the appeal of Five-Stone Powder, namely, invigorating the body and prolonging life. Wang, for example, reported that a certain Five-Color Stone Paste Powder offered by his friend made his body feel so light that he moved as though flying.[13] The aforementioned physician Qin Chengzu hailed the drug as "the best of medicinal preparations and the leader of all formulas." Although the powder couldn't utterly transform one's body, he claimed, it was second to none for the enhancement of life.[14] His contemporary Huiyi, a Buddhist monk from the north, expressed this view more explicitly: "Five-Stone Powder is among the superior drugs. It can prolong life and harmonize one's inner nature. How could it be that it only cures sickness?"[15] Notably, a number of Buddhist monks during the Era of Division ingested the powder or wrote about its proper use, possibly attracted by its promise of purifying the mind and nourishing life.[16]

The enticing benefits that Five-Stone Powder offered, however, were coupled with its ever-present danger. The third-century scholar and medical compiler Huangfu Mi (215–282) enumerated people during his days who suffered the ill effects of the powder: Wang Liangfu from the east developed ulcers on his back, Xin Changxu from the west was tormented by festers along his spine, six relatives of Zhao Gonglie from the southwest died, and Huangfu's own cousin was afflicted by the shrinking of his tongue into the throat. The tragedies resulting from the use of the powder were widespread.[17]

Besides inflicting physical pain, Five-Stone Powder could also devastate the mind. In 409, Emperor Daowu of the Northern Wei dynasty (reigned 386–409) was ill and began to take the powder. He soon became distressed and flustered, alternating between extremes of anger and joy. Sometimes he talked to himself incessantly; sometimes he stopped eating for days. Annoyed by their peccadilloes, he began killing his officials on a whim. The drug eventually ended his life: one of his sons, wishing to protect his mother from this erratic behavior, took the initiative of murdering his paranoid father.[18] Three centuries later, a similar fate befell An Lushan (703–757), the rebellious general who ravaged the Tang empire: he suffered mental instability and physical agonies from ingesting the powder, leading to his premature death.[19]

No better example illustrates the danger of Five-Stone Powder than the story of Huangfu, who left a vivid account of his own experience of the powerful drug. At the age of thirty-five, he contracted a wind-induced malady, which caused half of his body to become paralyzed. He then started ingesting the powder, only to find that instead of curing his incapacitating condition, it aggravated it: he had trouble swallowing food, sudden fever and chills, and insomnia, and became easily frightened and confused. To end the unbearable pains, he once tried to kill himself using a knife, only to be saved by his watchful family. Upon pondering, he forced himself to eat cold food and drink cool water, and survived the dramatic episode. But the miserable scholar never recovered from the lingering effects of having used Five-Stone Powder, effects that persisted for the rest of his life. It is perhaps not surprising that he offered a lengthy discussion of it based on his own experience of having misused this potent stimulant.[20]

The many accounts of the deleterious effects of Five-Stone Powder from the third to the eighth century have led some modern scholars to condemn the drug outright. One estimated that hundreds of thousands of people suffered or died from taking the powder during this period, making it the most deadly substance in premodern China.[21] Although its toxicity cannot be denied, this appraisal is probably an exaggeration. In particular, we need to pay attention to its rhetorical use, which served specific social and political functions. For instance, Huangfu, like many of his contemporaries, favored a hermetic life and tried to eschew public service. Yet as an erudite scholar, he soon drew attention from Emperor Wu of the Western Jin dynasty, who summoned him several times to serve at court. To dodge the request without causing trouble, Huangfu submitted an elaborate response in which he highlighted his implacable suffering not just from the original wind illness that had tormented him for nineteen years but also from the Five-Stone Powder that had intensified his pain over the past seven years. With such a debilitated body, he lamented, it was impossible for him to serve. The emperor eventually gave up on the recluse. Although it is unlikely that Huangfu completely fabricated his illness, given the amount of detail he provided, he nonetheless used it skillfully to avoid political engagement.[22]

In other cases, entirely fabricated malingering is more evident. *The History of the Jin* recounts an episode in which the scholar-official He Xun (260–319), when called upon by a rebel leader, claimed that he had contracted an illness that had impaired his limbs, paralyzing him. He then ingested Five-Stone Powder, presumably to treat the illness, but the result was worse: he disheveled his hair and exposed his body in public, clear signs of insanity. The hyperbolic performance appears to have been a strategic move for He to escape the undesirable service: an unruly body triggered by the drug could no longer function in its expected political space.[23]

In addition, ingesting Five-Stone Powder—as private treatment or public performance—was an act in defiance of social norms. Excessive drinking, too, was a quintessential characteristic of the unorthodox behavior of many social elites during the Era of Division. The combination of alcohol and Five-Stone Powder was common and became emblematic of the eccentric and carefree spirit of the time. Ruan Ji (210–263), one of the Seven Worthies of the Bamboo Grove, was particularly famous for his uninhibited drinking. Contrary to the Confucian rule of avoiding drinking and eating meat during mourning, at his mother's funeral he steamed a fat boar and shamelessly drank alcohol. Liu Ling (221–300), another member of the group, even composed an essay on the virtues of alcohol. In a well-known story, after immoderate drinking, he was found completely naked in his room. When the visitors reproached him for his erratic behavior, he retorted, "I take heaven and earth as my house, and the rooms of that house as my clothes and pants. Why do you people enter my pants?"[24]

There is no direct evidence that these social iconoclasts ingested Five-Stone Powder, but scholars have made the tantalizing suggestion that since drinking warm alcohol was part of the practice of channeling the power of the drug, it is possible that the two activities were linked.[25] The fourth-century writer Ge

Hong observed that vulgar people during his time often ate and drank immoderately during funerals, using the excuse of needing to enhance the effects of the powder. For him, this was truly a deplorable state of affairs.[26] Altogether, Five-Stone Powder opened up a social space that allowed for non-conformist behavior driven by varied motives.

Minerals and Heat

Determining the composition of Five-Stone Powder is a complex issue, as multiple formulas were associated with the name. The term "Five-Stone" already appeared in Han sources. *The Divine Farmer's Classic* places many mineral drugs in the top group that are useful for strengthening the body and prolonging life. Among these we find five types of clay, each described as being of a different color: green-blue, red, yellow, white, and black. With regular ingestion, they can "replenish marrow, enhance *qi*, make one plump and strong, prevent hunger, lighten the body, and extend life." The text further explains that these five minerals, with their respective colors, replenish the five viscera correspondingly.[27] These five colors also perfectly match those defined in the five-phase system, a conceptual scheme that correlated the body with time, space, and the cosmic rhythms.[28] There is no mention of Five-Stone Powder in this text, but the symbolism of the five colors offers an important clue to understanding the composition of the drug.

The grouping of five minerals also appears in a Han commentary on the ancient classic *Rites of Zhou*, which delineates the imagined bureaucracy of the Zhou dynasty (see chapter 1). In a section that describes the royal medical administration, the text specifies that physicians who specialize in treating lesions deploy five potent drugs. The Han scholar Zheng Xuan (127–200) identified these as the following five minerals of distinct colors: chalcanthite (*shidan*, green-blue), cinnabar (*dansha*, red), realgar (*xionghuang*, yellow), arsenolite (*yushi*, white), and magnetite (*cishi*, black). He further elucidated that after firing these minerals for three days and three nights, the resulting soot could be collected and applied to the lesion, which would remove any putrefied flesh. This topical use of the minerals, though telling in its own right, was probably different from the ingestion of Five-Stone Powder.[29]

More discussions related to something called "Five-Stone" emerge in physicians' documents from the Han period. In the twenty-five medical cases of the physician Chunyu Yi (fl. ca. 180–154 BCE) that are preserved in

Historical Records, we find the following episode. Chunyu encountered a medical officer from the east who prepared and ingested "Five-Stone" to treat his illness caused by internal heat. The physician considered it a grievous mistake, because the powerful minerals would trigger the circulation of malignant *qi* in the body, which would in due course coagulate and lead to the formation of abscesses. Just as Chunyu predicted, the patient died from an eruption of ulcers. Erroneous use of "Five-Stone," the case warns, could result in a calamitous outcome.[30] Although the case doesn't reveal the ingredients of "Five-Stone," its potent nature and the symptoms it induced resemble those of Five-Stone Powder seen in later sources. The episode also reveals Chunyu's knowledge of mineral drugs. Elsewhere in the text, he provides a list of medical works that he received from his master and carefully studied to advance his healing skills. One of them is titled *Spirit of Stones* (Shishen), a lost book that probably discusses the medical use of minerals. Such knowledge of mineral drugs in early China likely informed the creation of Five-Stone Powder.[31]

Archeological finds provide further material evidence for the early use of minerals. Five types of mineral were discovered in the tomb of Zhao Mo (reigned 137–122 BCE), the second ruler of the Nanyue kingdom (204–111 BCE) in the far south: amethyst, sulfur, realgar, ochre, and turquoise.[32] Except for the last one, all the substances are found in *The Divine Farmer's Classic*, indicating their medical value for royal consumption. The combination of minerals, though, is unique in that it does not follow the color pattern of the five-phase system, reflecting a local variance of the set principle.[33]

These various accounts of "Five-Stone" in early sources indicate the widespread use of mineral drugs for healing. Although they share certain features with the namesake powder that became immensely popular later, they are probably not the same. The earliest reference for the composition of Five-Stone Powder appears in the Han medical text *Essential Synopsis of the Golden Cabinet* (Jingui yaolüe), in which we find two formulas that could be the precursors of the popular drug. The first is called Amethyst Cold-Food Powder (Zishi Hanshi San), which is recommended to treat "cold damage" disorders. This complex formula, which employs five minerals, seven herbs, and one animal-derived substance, aims to use the heating power of the medicine to strengthen the viscera so as to dispel malignant influences that have penetrated the body.[34]

The second formula, called Mr. Hou's Black Powder (Houshi Heisan), contains fourteen ingredients that overlap considerably with those in the first one. A marked difference is that it uses only one mineral, kalinite (*fanshi*), and many more herbs (twelve in total), which is why it is alternatively called "Herbal Cold-Food Formula." The powder offers to treat limb paralysis induced by "great wind," and overwhelming cold in the heart that results in deficiency. The text further instructs that one should ingest it with warm alcohol and only eat cold food afterward, so as to retain the drug in the abdomen and facilitate its power. These guidelines are similar to the procedures for handling Five-Stone Powder.[35]

Huangfu Mi, in his commentary on the origin of Five-Stone Powder, identifies the above two formulas as the likely precursors of the drug.[36] Based on this information, the historian Yu Jiaxi, in his pioneering study of the history of the powder, has argued that He Yan combined the two prescriptions and created a powerful tonic that he consumed to recover from exhaustion caused by sexual indulgence.[37] This is a possible scenario, yet we need to be aware that just like the advent of varied compositions for "Five-Stone" during the Han period, multiple formulas for Five-Stone Powder circulated in the following centuries.[38] Attributing the creation of the powder to He Yan, as I have suggested before, has much to do with his eccentric behavior that was denounced by later scholars. At least one other origin story is given: according to *The History of the Jin*, Jin Shao, a talented physician who excelled in materia medica and the study of medical classics, invented the formula of Five-Stone Powder; scholar-officials at the time all ingested it and enjoyed extraordinary effects. This brief account, in contrast to that of He Yan, focuses on the marvelous power of the medicine to heal.[39]

This is a point that merits our attention. Already in *Essential Synopsis of the Golden Cabinet*, the two formulas that anticipated Five-Stone Powder are deployed to combat specific disorders of "cold damage" and "great wind," respectively, which induce fever and paralyze the body. Because of the cold nature of these conditions, the text recommends the heating medicines— the majority of the ingredients in these formulas have warming properties— to dissipate the cold and restore the vitality of the body. Compared to some later physicians and scholars who lauded the powder for its exceptional life-extending virtue, the perceived value of these formulas in the Han medical text was quite restricted.

Further scrutiny of these two formulas reveals a puzzle: none of the minerals therein possesses *du* as defined by the materia medica literature, and the only *du*-possessing herbs are aconite, dysosma, and platycodon, which were regularly used in classical Chinese pharmacy. How, then, do we explain the many accounts of the powder's unmistakable capacity to cause harm? A variant of Mr. Hou's Black Powder gives a clue. Preserved in the eighth-century *Arcane Essentials from the Imperial Library*, the prescription made a minor, but significant, modification of the original—it added two more minerals: stalactite (*zhongru*) and arsenolite (*yushi*), the latter referring to arsenic ore.[40] The danger of arsenolite was recognized early on in Chinese medicine. Tao Hongjing solemnly warned in the fifth century, "Ingested for long, it causes convulsion of tendons." He further advised, "Refine it by fire for one hundred days, and ingest the amount of one tip of the jade-knife [0.2 g]. If taken without prior refinement, it kills people and the hundred beasts."[41] Because of its violent power, the formula in *Arcane Essentials* specifies that one must wrap the mineral with mud and fire it for half a day before adding it to the medicine. Without a doubt, arsenolite was a dangerous substance.

It is possible that after the creation of the precursor formulas for Five-Stone Powder in the Han dynasty, arsenolite was added at certain point during the Era of Division, which substantially enhanced the drug's force. An inadvertent substitution may have also happened: in early Chinese sources, the character for kalinite (*fan*), which is a mineral without *du*, is sometimes written interchangeably with the character for arsenolite (*yu*), implying that arsenic might have been used more frequently in Chinese history than we originally thought.[42] Some of the symptoms triggered by Five-Stone Powder in fact resemble those of arsenic poisoning: abdominal pain, digestive troubles, pain in the limbs, deterioration of vision, skin eruptions, convulsions, and mental disorders, among others.[43] Moreover, arsenic could also induce tonic effects: it could improve one's complexion and revitalize the body (at least temporarily), and, above all, act as a potent aphrodisiac.[44] This echoes certain portrayals of the drug's devotees—we are reminded of He Yan's notoriety for sexual indulgence. In medical sources, the potential of a drug for use as an aphrodisiac is often expressed in terms of its capacity for strengthening the Kidneys, which are associated with sexual power. For example, according to the seventh-century *On the Origins and Symptoms of All Illnesses*, the regular consumption of the powder could induce a condition called "strengthen the center" (*qiangzhong*), manifesting as prolonged erections and the leakage of semen, which would cause all kinds of trouble as one aged. Temporary pleasures sow the seeds of lasting agonies.[45]

Many stories about Five-Stone Powder describe the immense heat the body emanated upon ingesting it, the proper discharge of which was crucial to healing. Withholding the heat inside the body, by contrast, caused troubles. Therefore, the proper care of the body upon taking the drug to "disperse the powder" (*jiesan*) distinguished cure from malady, although the line between them was very thin. Pei Xiu (224–271), a statesman of the Western Jin dynasty, was killed after taking the powder by having so much cold water poured onto his body that it extinguished his vital heat.[46] The fifth-century general Fang Boyu, in the story that opens this chapter, also endured the pouring of a vast amount of cold water onto his body, yet the outcome could not be more different: Fang recovered and remained vigorous. Assuredly, to "disperse the powder" was a delicate matter.

How could Five-Stone Powder generate massive heat? This is an intricate issue given the complex composition of its ingredients. A typical formula of the drug contains a subset of the following minerals: amethyst, quartz, red clay, stalactite, limonite, sulfur, and kalinite or arsenolite. The materia medica literature defines the majority of these minerals as drugs with warming properties.[47] For example, Tao Hongjing, in his *Collected Annotations*, states that arsenolite, a mineral of great heat, could prevent water from freezing. Such a substance, properly prepared, could dissolve frigid and congealed stagnation in the body. Naturally, warming drugs counter cold maladies.[48]

Yet the administration of warming minerals is no easy task, as elucidated by the fifth-century *Formulas of the Lesser Grade* (Xiaopin fang).[49] In a section devoted to Five-Stone Powder, the author Chen Yanzhi contrasts the power of herbs with that of minerals as follows: upon ingestion, herbs quickly manifest (*fa*) a force that is easy to subdue while minerals slowly manifest a force that is hard to subdue. Hence while one can promptly benefit from the effects of herbs, one must be more patient with minerals. Chen further explains:

Regarding the nature of minerals, their essential *qi* correlates with the five phases and replenishes the five viscera; their dregs are the same as dust and soil. But sick people suffer depleted blood and *qi*, hence are not able to potentiate the minerals. These minerals then deposit and turn into hard stagnation. If the essential *qi* of these minerals is not manifested, they are as cold as ice. Sick people ingest minerals hoping these substances will immediately produce heat upon entering the abdomen. If they don't feel the heat, they ingest even more. Without seeing the effect of minerals right away, they claim that they fail to obtain the force of the drug. When the drug manifests its power later, they don't consider it to be the effect of minerals, and hesitate to take actions to manage these minerals. They then treat the condition as something else, which often causes harm.[50]

This is a rare passage in medical sources in medieval China that ponders the relationship between the materiality of drugs and their effects on the body. The unique nature of minerals, in Chen's eyes, is that "their material is cold yet their nature is warming."[51] Having entered the body, they can release their intrinsic heat, which manifests as the circulation of their essential *qi*, strengthening the viscera. Importantly, this process depends on the state of the body: a sick person is too weak to potentiate the essential *qi* of minerals, and the accumulation of cold minerals inside the body will ultimately cause troubles. The use of herbs in the powder and drinking warm alcohol might have helped stimulate the latent stones. Time also matters; one has to wait patiently to allow the minerals to manifest their power, and when the effects begin to appear, take shrewd action to channel the heat out of the body. Those who misjudge the initial dormancy of the drug and hastily ingest more doses are doomed to suffer. Fang Boyu, in our opening story, is one such impatient zealot who took an excessive amount of Five-Stone Powder. The worsened situation was only reversed by a dramatic method that managed to release the "dormant heat."

To further understand Five-Stone Powder's heating power, we must contemplate a word that frequently appears in the writings about it: *fa*. The primary meaning of the word, according to a first-century dictionary, is "to shoot an arrow."[52] In the context of Five-Stone Powder, the word implies the activation of the drug and the subsequent release of its heat. If the heat remains "unshot," problems arise. A typical symptom is the extreme coldness of the body resulting from the accumulation of the inactive drug. *Fa* hence points to its potentiation, which is tied to bodily sensation. Yet *fa* could also carry a negative sense, especially in the discussion of the drug's adverse effects. In Sun Simiao's *Essential Formulas*, for instance, the Tang physician somberly points out the untoward manifestations of the power of the drug as a result of its mismanagement, causing pain in the head and the formation of ulcers on the back. Although the medicine's force is certainly released, Sun considers the effects damaging due to the misguided discharge of heat. He then recommends the proper ways of managing the powder and various methods to palliate the injuries it induces. Mishandling the drug's power could yield more punishing a result than not initiating that power at all.[53]

Debates on Five-Stone Powder

The immense heat produced by Five-Stone Powder, the intricate interplay between its mineral and herbal ingredients, and the dynamic process of the powder's action on the body all point to the extraordinary difficulty of handling the potent drug. As a result, many physicians and scholars from the third through the eighth century took pains to discuss its proper use and various remedies to assuage its harm, evidenced by the emergence of a large number of writings dedicated to this topic throughout the period. The Sui and Tang bibliographical records, for example, include two dozen titles that offer either theoretical discussion of how the powder works or formulas that treat the injuries it could engender. Written by a diverse group of people, including scholar-officials, hereditary healers, and Buddhist monks, these treatises encompass a wide array of views and methods that kindled animated debate on the proper understanding and use of the drug.[54]

At the core of these discussions was not whether the drug should be taken or not but *how* it should be taken. No one rejected it outright. But even those who enthusiastically endorsed the powder offered sober warnings. The fifth-century physician Qin Chengzu, for instance, after extolling the drug's superior healing powers, admonished that "water can carry the boat yet can also capsize it; the powder can protect life yet can also end it." He further commented that ignorant people in his day could not grasp its subtlety, leading to countless disasters.[55] His contemporary, the monk Huiyi, made the point even more clearly: "If one obtains its proper management, the drug can cure sickness and nourish life; if one loses the way of controlling it, the drug can kill. Should we not be cautious? The harm is due to the mistake of the user, not the manifestation of the drug."[56] Proper administration was key to obtaining its benefits.

Already in the third century, when the fad of consuming the powder had just taken off, different opinions on how to manage the drug arose. Huangfu Mi was one of the earliest to advocate the cooling method. Soon after taking the powder in three doses, he advises, users should use cold water to wash their hands and feet. This will stimulate the drug's *qi* and result in a slight numbing sensation. Then, they should take off their clothes and use cold water to bathe, further activating the drug. Subsequently, when the body is felt to be cooling, their heart will become open and bright, resulting in the cure of all illnesses. The alternative name of the drug, Cold-Food Powder, encapsulates this cooling approach. Furthermore, Huangfu counsels in detail how the method might be adjusted for patients of different ages and constitutions, and for different maladies. For example, young and old people should take reduced doses, and a person whose body is already replete, in a state of healthy fullness, should avoid it altogether.[57]

However, Huangfu's contemporary Cao Xi, an aristocrat of the Wei kingdom, held a different view. In his *Formulas That Disperse Cold-Food Powder* (Jie Hanshi San fang), Cao champions a warming method of managing the drug. That is, one should wear more clothes upon ingesting the powder and actively walk to provoke sweating, which will carry the heat out of the body. Those with weak constitutions, he further warns, should not use cold water to release the potential of the powder, because exposing the body to sudden coldness will inevitably lead to "cold damage" disorders. Cao also uses his own experience of taking the drug for more than forty years to support his method.[58] Later medical writers during the Era of Division often juxtaposed the contrasting views of Huangfu and Cao to highlight the intricacy of managing the powder. Some sided with Huangfu, as the idea of using cooling methods to dissipate bodily heat made intuitive sense, while others contended that one should not be constrained to one particular rule but remain flexible according to the specific condition for which the drug was deployed.[59] Tao Hongjing upheld the latter view:

> In the past, there were people who ingested Cold-Food Powder. Upon inspecting the ancient method, they poured two hundred jugs of cold water onto their body, and immediately dropped to the ground, lifeless. There were also those who followed the method of sweating. They set up fire at the four corners of a narrow room, and died straight away. To tend the body in accord with the current situation, isn't it based on the individual? To look to past examples, isn't it even worse than "waiting at the stump"?[60]

The two types of action that Tao depicts correspond to the cooling and warming methods that Huangfu Mi and Cao Xi advocated, respectively. By criticizing the rigid application of these established procedures, Tao underscores the importance of adjusting the way of managing the drug for individual bodies and specific circumstances.

Among these various opinions, one is particularly striking, as it offers a novel interpretation of the interplay between the minerals and the herbs in the powder. In his *Formulas for Dispersing the Powder by Duo Treatment* (Jiesan duizhi fang), the Buddhist monk Daohong (fl. fourth or fifth century) lists a number of matched pairs of minerals and herbs: stalactite and atractylodes, sulfur and saposhnikovia, quartz and aconite, amethyst and ginseng, red clay and platycodon. Each pair targets a specific organ and triggers unique sensations, manifesting the power of Five-Stone Powder. For instance, stalactite and atractylodes target the Lungs, which connect to the head and the chest. When atractylodes stimulates the power of stalactite, the chest feels stifled with shortness of breath; when stalactite stimulates the power of atractylodes, headache arises, with pain in the eyes. When this happens, Daohong advises, one must quickly take a decoction of scallion and pickled beans to alleviate the disturbance. The dynamic interaction between the minerals and the herbs in the powder gives rise to distinct bodily signs that call for further swift intervention to prevent the cure from becoming its own serious problem.[61]

Yet this novel explanation of the drug's action was challenged by other medical writers. Chen Yanzhi, in his *Formulas of the Lesser Grade* (fifth century), launches a spirited critique of Daohong's unconventional interpretation despite its popularity at the time. He asserts that the idea of "duo treatment," as proposed by the monk, appears in none of the writings on the powder he has checked. He further muses that if one follows Daohong's theory, it is hard to explain the combination of trichosanthes (*gualou*) and dried ginger in the powder, as the two herbs are in a relationship of "mutual hatred" (*xiangwu*, see chapter 2), as defined in the materia medica literature. He then recommends that one should follow Huangfu Mi's method but remove trichosanthes from the formula to avoid antagonistic effects. Since Chen's work pays keen attention to integrating materia medica knowledge into the use of formulas, it is not surprising that his critique of Daohong's unconventional idea is guided by established pharmacological writings.[62]

The debate on Five-Stone Powder continued in the Tang period, but with the focus shifted to the type of illness that the drug was supposed to treat. Sun Simiao discusses the matter extensively. In his *Supplement to Formulas*, we find one formula called Life-Restoring Five-Stone Powder (Wushi Gengsheng San), which resembles the prescriptions of Five-Stone Powder in the preceding centuries, but with a notable change—it replaces arsenolite with sulfur (*shi liuhuang*). The substitution has been interpreted as Sun's effort to improve the formula by curbing its toxicity.[63] This may not be the case though.

After all, according to medical writings at the time, sulfur was as potent as arsenolite, and the ingestion of this mineral was not benign, as a number of high-profile cases during the Tang dynasty attested to its danger.[64] The modified formula seems to have less to do with reducing toxicity than with the specific conditions it treats.

Sun's formula contains fifteen ingredients: five minerals, nine herbs, and one animal product. This composition is likely derived from the two precursor formulas for Five-Stone Powder in *Essential Synopsis of the Golden Cabinet*, as their ingredients overlap substantially. Yet Sun prescribes it for a different purpose. That is, he considers the powder particularly effective in curing "the five exhaustions and seven injuries of men, and those who are bedridden due to depletion and weakness."[65] The drug, the physician stresses, is only for intractable conditions that cannot be cured by other means. Hence the name, Life-Restoring Five-Stone Powder, revealing its power to make one live again. Such a powerful drug should not be used at random. Sun alerts the reader:

> Once the illness is developed, one must be diligent in applying tonic medicines. Hence, I establish the formulas of supplementing and nourishing the body. These formulas all concern the sort of drugs like Five-Stone, Three-Stone, and Great Cold-Food Pill/Powder. Only in the situations of fully developed depletion and exhaustion, bedriddenness caused by paralysis, or proximity to death with no one to resort to should one use these drugs. They can truly revive dead people. Normal people without sickness should not rashly handle them. One should be extremely cautious about not violating this rule.[66]

Sun's vigilance about Five-Stone Powder and similar drugs, to wit, that they be saved only for recalcitrant, life-threatening conditions, contrasts sharply with the habitual ingestion of the powder for enhancing life and illuminating the mind by the many enthusiasts I have previously discussed.[67]

These accounts of Sun solve a puzzle that has baffled modern scholars. In his earlier work, *Essential Formulas*, he openly condemns Five-Stone Powder, declaring that he would rather take the deadly poison of gelsemium (*yege*) than ingest the dangerous drug. He also exhorts that whenever one encounters the formula for the powder, one should burn it immediately.[68] This harsh criticism seems to contradict the inclusion of the same formula in his later work. It is possible that Sun changed his attitude over time, but if we pay attention to the context of his denouncement, another interpretation comes up.

Sun's discussion of Five-Stone Powder in *Essential Formulas* appears in a section where he enumerates methods of countering mineral poisons. At the beginning of the section, curiously, Sun announces that, "if people don't ingest minerals, various things [in the body] won't do well."[69] Specifically, he believes that certain minerals, especially stalactite, possess great power to nourish life. He even cites his own experience as testimony: When he was thirty-eight or thirty-nine, he once ingested five or six *liang* (200–240 g) of stalactite. Since then, he had deeply experienced the benefits of the mineral.[70] Hence Sun did not oppose the use of minerals altogether; he instead assigned different minerals for distinct uses. In treating obdurate illnesses, Five-Stone Powder was a viable choice; in the case of nourishing life, stalactite would serve the purpose.

This latter practice indicated a significant change that had occurred between the Era of Division and the early Tang period: stalactite replaced Five-Stone Powder as a prime tonic for life cultivation.[71] Stalactite's benign nature may account for this change—it was defined as a drug without *du* in the materia medica literature, but this didn't mean that one could consume it capriciously. Sun warns that if the mineral is harvested from the wrong sites, it can kill more effectively than the feathers of the *zhen* bird.[72] Moreover, the use of the mineral also hinges on constitution and age. People who are already "plump and replete with fair flesh," Sun admonishes, should avoid the drug entirely. Only those over thirty can ingest it. The older one is, the more frequently one can consume the substance: one dose every three years for those over fifty; one dose every two years for those over sixty; one dose every year for those over seventy. Therefore, Sun not only identifies disparate uses for different minerals but also underscores the proper use of them in specific circumstances.[73]

Conclusion

The tale of Five-Stone Powder, one of the most popular and controversial drugs in Chinese history, illustrates the extraordinary difficulty of handling a potent medicine. In earlier studies, scholars have tended to portray it in a negative light—its toxic ingredients, its violent insult to the body, and the numerous recorded injuries and even deaths it induced all make the powder appear to be a destructive poison. These scholars have often compared the powder with opium, the notorious drug that decisively shaped recent Chinese history, as a way to expose the social ills caused by these substances.[74] Yet several critical features distinguish the two. First, they trigger different effects on the body. Whereas opium is a sedating narcotic that induces drowsiness and lethargy, Five-Stone Powder was a potent stimulant that energized the body and excited the mind. Second, although opium is well-known for being addictive, no evidence suggests that Five-Stone Powder possessed the same potential. None of its ingredients are physically addictive, and no sources disclose cases of users ingesting the drug habitually. This doesn't, however, negate its social addictiveness, that is, a persistent desire to follow the fashion of consuming the powder as a way of acquiring or maintaining social status.[75] Third, in comparison with the wide circulation of opium through all strata of society in the nineteenth century, the consumption of Five-Stone Powder was restricted to the group of social elites.[76] This is not surprising given the complexity of the formula and its usage, which demanded significant time and resources.

Above all, the most pronounced distinction between the two drugs is the different ways they were understood socially. Unlike the opprobrium heaped on opium as a vicious poison that ruined individual lives and tore apart the social fabric, the perception of Five-Stone Powder was never entirely condemnatory. In fact, the majority of physicians and scholars in medieval China valued the powder though they were fully aware of its dangers. This prompted vibrant debates, which centered on two issues. First, from its emergence in the Han period, Five-Stone Powder had been deployed to treat specific illnesses. Later physicians, such as Sun Simiao, narrowed the drug's use to only treating intractable conditions and saving patients who were on the verge of death. In this context, his famous denunciation of the powder was less about its inherent toxicity than its use for the wrong purpose: one should not take it habitually to cultivate life. To his dismay, many enthusiasts, lured by inflated promises, took it indiscriminately. This haphazard consumption of the powder as an all-purpose magic tonic rather than a precision medicine led to numerous tragedies.

Second, discussions of Five-Stone Powder stress the difficulty of using the drug, especially the delicate procedures for stimulating its power and channeling the heat it generated safely out of the body. What was unique about the powder was that ingesting it was merely the beginning; afterward patients needed to closely monitor their sensations and then undertake a series of carefully planned measures to release the drug's heat to benefit the body. If the heat was confined within the body, great harm could arise. However, interpreting these injuries as "side effects" of the powder, as suggested by earlier scholars, misses the point.[77] In modern biomedicine, side effects are perceived as the *inevitable* adverse outcome of a pharmaceutical product; the assumption is that any drug therapy induces both the intended primary (positive) effects and the unintended side (negative) effects, so great effort has been made to minimize the latter so as to reduce the toxicity of medicines.[78] Tellingly, there is no concept of side effects in classical Chinese medicine. A clear distinction between the two opposing effects—an intended effect as distinguished from unintended effects—does not hold in many traditional healing cultures, because the outcome of therapy is often interpreted as dynamic, systemic, and processual. In such systems, healing takes place in multiple stages, each of which is manifested by distinct bodily signs and each of which in turn requires careful management by the physician or patient.[79] In the use of Five-Stone Powder, physicians regarded the injuries caused by the potent drug as the untoward result not of "side effects" but of mismanagement. If one handled it and its effects correctly, harm would be avoidable. This was no easy task, as attested to by the painful experiences of Huangfu Mi and many others. The extreme difficulty of using the drug might explain its ultimate disappearance from Chinese society.

The popularity of Five-Stone Powder as long as it lasted lay in its promise of revitalizing the body and illuminating the mind. There was yet another set of drugs in medieval China that aimed for an even higher goal, nothing less than the transformation of the body and the attainment of immortality. Often called elixirs, these numinous medicines were also made of potent minerals but resulted from complex alchemical preparations. The final chapter investigates these marvelous substances in detail, focusing on alchemists' various interpretations of *du* as well as how they incorporated the bodily experience into the understanding of these powerful materials.

CHAPTER 7

Dying to Live

If a medicine does not cause dizziness, it cannot cure illness. Initially it induces minor discomforts; later it is greatly efficacious.

—*THE RECORD FROM THE STONE WALL OF THE GREAT CLARITY*

(EIGHTH CENTURY)

LI BAOZHEN WAS GETTING OLD. HAVING SERVED THE COURT AS A general for a decade, he could boast remarkable military exploits. He still remembered the glorious days when he heroically quelled the rebellion in the north and saved the empire from collapse. Over the course of his life, he had defeated numerous enemies and gained fame and riches. But his body had become emaciated, undoubtedly due to his long and arduous service. Now, at the age of sixty-two, he was facing the only enemy that he could not defeat: death.

Or could he? Recently he had been approached by a *fangshi* named Sun Jichang, who offered him an elixir that promised the transcendence of death.[1] He also had recurrent dreams in which he rode on a crane and soared into the sky. Inspired by this clear omen, Li took the pellets from Sun and ingested twenty thousand of them. Shortly thereafter he suffered a hardened abdomen, became unable to eat, and fell into unconsciousness for many days. A Daoist adept showed up and used lard and "grain lacquer" to purge him.[2] The general soon regained consciousness, only to see Sun reproach him, "You almost transcended. Why did you give up?" Persuaded, Li took another three thousand pellets of Sun's elixir and died soon after. The year was 794, in the mid-Tang period.[3]

Li's death from elixir poisoning was dramatic but by no means unique. During the Tang dynasty, many enthusiasts, including five emperors, ingested elixirs and died.[4] This is the moment in Chinese history when the popularity of taking elixirs reached its apex. Often called "outer alchemy" (*waidan*), the practices required setting up elaborate devices and following sophisticated procedures so as to produce numinous medicines that promised not only to transmute base metals into silver or gold but also, and more importantly, to elevate one's very body to higher states of being.[5] The ideas and practices of *waidan* had a strong connection to Daoism, and the majority of alchemical writings are found in Daoist treatises. The ingredients employed in the operations were primarily minerals, including mercury, arsenic, sulfur, and lead. Li's death, we may infer, likely resulted from the lethal effects of these potent substances.

The history of Chinese alchemy is a rich topic that has piqued the interest of generations of scholars. Early scholarship, epitomized by Joseph Needham and his collaborators' monumental *Science and Civilisation in China*, focuses on the material aspects of the practice, especially their chemical achievements as seen through the lens of modern science.[6] Later scholars, including Nathan Sivin and Fabrizio Pregadio, have paid more attention to the theoretical frameworks of alchemical operations, highlighting the centrality of cosmological thinking and ritual procedures that provided elixir practices with rich meanings.[7] Few works thus far, however, have addressed the medical implications of Chinese alchemy, especially the issue of elixir poisoning. There are two exceptions, though. One early essay surveys the relevant sources on this issue, highlighting the danger of ingesting elixirs.[8] A later study positions the practice in a Daoist context and offers a more sympathetic analysis of Chinese alchemists' daring pursuit, revealing their fearless conviction that taking powerful medicines could bring transcendence.[9] It is remarkable that in spite of the tension between material danger and spiritual aspiration in the understanding and practice of elixirs, engagement with outer alchemy was persistent. From its inception in the Han period to its ultimate decline toward the end of the Tang period, the practice lasted for more than a millennium. How do we explain this enduring passion for elixirs given their manifest perils?

The key to answering this question lies in the perception of *du* in Chinese alchemy. Just like its paradoxical meaning expressed in medical sources, the

word connoted potency that could both transform the body and cause serious injuries, if not death. Different alchemists over time offered varied interpretations of *du* that on the one hand justified the ingestion of powerful
elixirs and on the other fostered new methods to tame their power to reduce
harm. Relatedly, Chinese alchemists readily observed and sometimes experienced the violent effects of elixirs on the body, which critically informed
their understanding of these potent substances. Their different explanations
of "the elixirated body," that is, a body upon taking an elixir, demonstrate
how somatic signs manifested the power of elixirs, and as a result both justified and contested their ingestion.

Furthermore, a few words to clarify two important terms in Chinese
alchemy. The first is "elixir" (*dan* or *yao*), which refers to an alchemical product. The English word likely derives from the Greek word *xērion*, dry powder
for healing wounds. In medieval times, the word entered Arabic as *al-iksīr*,
and then in Latin as *elixir*, which often designated "the philosopher's stone,"
a magical substance that European alchemists produced to transmute metals
or prolong life. Starting in the sixteenth century, the word also acquired the
meaning of a tincture or a tonic. Evidently, "elixir" in the Greco-Arabic world
had diverse meanings that crossed the boundary of alchemy and medicine.[10]
We find a similar phenomenon in China. *Dan* or *yao* regularly signifies
alchemical products, but it can also denote medicines. In fact, *yao* is the standard word for referring to all kinds of medicines in Chinese pharmacy. The
translation of *dan* or *yao* as "elixir" in the alchemical context thus captures
the broad meaning of these words, encompassing substances of diverse properties and purposes.

The second term is "transcendence" (*xian*), which was the ultimate goal of
Chinese alchemists. There is a variety of related expressions in Daoist and medical sources, including "long-living" (*changsheng*), "achieving transcendence"
(*chengxian*), and "deathlessness" (*busi*). Although *xian* has been often translated as "immortality," there are some important differences. Above all, *xian*
carries a strong sense of elevating the body to higher states of being that could
not only extend one's life span but also perhaps bypass death altogether.[11]
Compared with the clear distinction between moderate and radical exten-
sion of life in Europe, longevity and immortality constituted a continuum in
China, encapsulated by the idea of *xian*.[12] Furthermore, unlike the concept
of immortality in Western Christianity that implied a disembodied soul and
a fixed state in Heaven for all eternity, *xian* entailed multiple levels of bodily

existence often imagined in a hierarchy in which transcendents (those who have become *xian*) could rise or fall depending on their spiritual cultivation, moral conduct, and social position. Hence spatially, the terrestrial and celestial worlds form a continuum in which one's life span is correlated to one's level of ascension. Grasping this dynamic sense of *xian* will help us understand how alchemists of different sects promoted their own visions of transcendence through distinctive means of transforming the body.[13]

Theoretical Foundations

The origins of Chinese alchemy can be traced back to antiquity. One famous episode is the avid search for elixirs by the first emperor of China, Qin Shi Huang (reigned 221–210 BCE), who dispatched scouts to the remote islands east of his empire to look for transcendents and obtain wondrous drugs that could prolong his own life, but to no avail. Elixirs during this period were usually conceived of as magical versions of ordinary edible plants, such as mushrooms and fruits, that grew on distant mountains and islands and were extraordinary-looking.[14] In the Han period that followed, the attention shifted to man-made elixirs, especially those produced from gold. Emperor Wu (reigned 141–87 BCE) is famous for his passionate pursuit of elixirs. He once summoned a *fangshi* named Li Shaojun, who proposed transmuting cinnabar into gold and then molding the gold into vessels. Eating food carried by these vessels, Li averred, would enhance the emperor's life. The alchemical element is noticeable in this story, but intriguingly, it is contact with gold rather than its ingestion that promised longevity. Moreover, this material touch was only an intermediate step, helping the emperor live long enough to have visions of the otherwise invisible transcendents living on remote islands. Ritual worship of these deities would ultimately result in his escape from death.[15]

The episodes of Qin Shi Huang and Emperor Wu are two of the few cases of elixir pursuit in extant sources of early China. In general, references to alchemy are sporadic and obscure in antiquity.[16] More systematic alchemical writings emerged in the fourth century, exemplified by the works of Ge Hong (283–343), one of the most famous alchemists in Chinese history.

Ge grew up in a family in the southeast that had served in the imperial administration for generations. Ge himself, when he was young, took up governmental service during the Western Jin dynasty (266–316) and participated in suppressing a rebellion in the south. His chief interest, though, was the cultivation of long life and the pursuit of the Dao. When he was fourteen, he followed the famed master Zheng Yin, who transmitted alchemical methods to him. Later in his life, he became keenly interested in making elixirs. In 331, learning that cinnabar was found in the southern district of Jiaozhi (in present-day northern Vietnam), he traveled southward to seek the crucial ingredient. Eventually, he withdrew to Mount Luofu (near present-day Guangzhou) and died there.[17]

There is no evidence that Ge actually practiced alchemy, which is likely due to the prohibitive cost of compounding elixirs.[18] Yet his writings on the rationale and methods of the art were central to guiding alchemical practices in the following centuries. Before he headed to the south, Ge completed a book that summarized his thoughts on a wide range of techniques of culti-vating life and achieving transcendence. The book, *Inner Chapters of the Master Who Embraces the Unhewn* (Baopuzi neipian; hereafter *Inner Chapters*), is a key source for exploring early Chinese alchemical theories.

In this work, Ge makes it abundantly clear that ingesting elixirs is the best way to prolong life and the only way to transcend death. In particular, he regards gold and cinnabar as the drugs for transcendence. He calls them "the great drugs" (*dayao*) in comparison to "the little drugs" (*xiaoyao*) that are made from herbs, claiming that "even cinnabar of low quality is far better than herbs of high quality."[19] The hierarchy is based on his reasoning that while herbs decay easily, minerals last much longer, and gold and cinnabar, being the most robust minerals, hold up as long as heaven and earth.

Why can ingesting enduring substances prolong life? This is because, Ge proposes, the body seeks external things to strengthen itself, like using fat to nourish fire or smearing the feet with verdigris (the patina of copper or bronze) so they won't deteriorate once entering water.[20] In a passage describ-ing a specific formula for preparing gold, Ge further relates that "once the gold liquid enters the mouth, the whole body becomes golden."[21] The material-ity of gold is thus transferred to the body, making it as robust and enduring as gold itself. This rationale assumes that a thing of utterly different nature can interact with the body and drastically transform it. Embedded in this belief is the ancient philosophy that stresses the changeability of all things in the cosmos.[22]

Besides the transfer of material persistence, Ge notes additional benefits of an elixir on the body: "Once gold and cinnabar enter the body, they moisten the nourishing *qi* and the defensive *qi*. The benefit is not merely like that of applying verdigris externally."²³ The nourishing *qi* (*rong*) and the defensive *qi* (*wei*) are two types of *qi* circulating in the body. According to *The Yellow Emperor's Inner Classic*, the nourishing *qi* is the essential *qi* of water and grain, which circulates throughout the viscera; the defensive *qi* is the ferocious *qi* of water and grain, which circulates inside the skin and in the partings of the flesh. A smooth movement of both types of *qi* is crucial for life.²⁴ Ge affirms that elixirs, when ingested, can moisten both kinds of *qi*, facilitating their flow and preventing stagnation. The statement reveals a different way of understanding an elixir's power: it averts death by sustaining the perpetual circulation of *qi* in the body.

Elsewhere in *Inner Chapters*, Ge demonstrates his broad knowledge of healing in the domains of breath control, bodily exercise, fasting, and sexual cultivation. Although Ge considers all of these inferior to elixir-taking, he believes that they are useful techniques for sustaining health and prolonging life. Moreover, throughout his life, Ge actively sought medical formulas to treat illnesses and handle emergencies. Before finishing *Inner Chapters*, he had already compiled a voluminous formula book titled *Formulas in the Jade Case* (Yuhan fang). The text is lost, but a selection of easy-to-use remedies for treating urgent conditions has survived. The work, titled *Formulas for Emergencies to Keep at Hand* (Zhouhou beiji fang), was influential, as many of its prescriptions were cited by later medical texts.²⁵

Given Ge's extensive knowledge of medicine, we might expect him to offer a discussion of the harmful effects of elixirs in his works. But he does not. Throughout *Inner Chapters*, Ge highlights the benefits of elixirs, claiming their superiority to all other methods for obtaining transcendence. As Ge strove to persuade readers of the unique power of elixirs and launched vigorous critiques of competing methods, such as ritual sacrifice and shamanistic practice, any mention of the harms of alchemy may have undercut his goal.²⁶ Nevertheless, the potential danger of ingesting elixirs did not go entirely unheeded. In a passage on building up the bodily constitution, Ge warns, "I am worried that before a ladle of benefit has been solidified, one proceeds with a cauldron of exhaustion. Before the holding of foundation has been achieved, one attacks [the body] with potency (*du*) of ice and frost."²⁷ *Du* here underscores the power of "ice and frost," a particular type of elixir. Potency matches the word "attack" (*gong*), which implies strength and violence. In Ge's eyes, elixirs are powerful. The robust nature of minerals promises to forge a strong body, but this very robustness can also cause injuries. To avert the danger, one must pay attention to time; only after the body is solidly built can one safely ingest elixirs. For Ge, to obtain this foundation involves first and foremost the cultivation of the body by various techniques of breath control, therapeutic exercise, and taking herbal medicines. He considers these to be lifelong practices requiring dedication and perseverance, which explains why he planned to make elixirs only in the last years of his life. He had much to do before.

Ge's mention of *du* reveals that the use of elixirs is contingent on the state of the body. The context of taking the numinous drug is as important as its content. Another key factor prior to elixir-taking is the cultivation of morality. Ge declares that if one hasn't done enough good deeds, one cannot benefit from an elixir for transcendence. Conversely, if someone performs good deeds without ingesting an elixir, although he cannot become a transcendent, he can still avoid disasters leading to sudden death. Virtuous conduct is thus another prerequisite for enjoying the full benefit of an elixir.[28]

Alchemy in Practice

Although Ge Hong's writing was foundational for alchemical theories in China, no robust evidence shows that he actually ever made an elixir. In the following centuries, however, the situation changed as more alchemists put the alluring idea into practice and presented their refined products to the court to gain imperial patronage.[29] Emperor Ai of the Eastern Jin dynasty (reigned 361–365), for example, began ingesting such elixirs at the age of twenty-four. Following an overdose, he was rendered no longer able to understand the affairs of his country. One year later, he died.[30] Other emperors were more cautious. Emperor Daowu of the Northern Wei dynasty (reigned 386–409) established an office devoted to making elixirs, yet before taking any himself, he would test substances on criminals condemned to death. Many of them died. Given this discouraging outcome, the emperor himself refrained.[31] Emperor Wenxuan of the Northern Qi dynasty (reigned 550–559) was also hesitant to take elixirs, despite his great interest. He once summoned a certain Zhang Yuanyou to compound a well-known elixir. Instead of ingesting it, the emperor kept it in a jade box and declared, "I still desire pleasures in this human world, so I cannot fly to heaven now. I will wait until I am about to die to take it."[32]

Evidently, rulers from the fourth to the sixth century adopted various strategies to handle elixirs. But before they decided on what to do with one, they needed to have it prepared first by an alchemist, most of whom, such as Zhang Yuanyou, left little trace in history.[33] Fortunately, we have more sources on the practice of another adept, who also prepared elixirs for the court. This is Tao Hongjing (456–536), a key figure in the history of medicine and the history of Daoism in China.

Besides his extensive knowledge of drugs (see chapter 1), Tao was keenly interested in alchemy. A native of the southeast, where Ge Hong had lived two centuries earlier, Tao was readily exposed to the alchemical knowledge that circulated in the region. At the age of ten, he read Ge's *Biographies of Divine Transcendents* (Shenxian zhuan), a hagiography of masters who had achieved transcendence, often by taking elixirs. At twelve, he read the fourth-century alchemist Qie Yin. He was greatly inspired by these works.[34]

In 492, at the age of thirty-six, Tao resigned from his official position at the Southern Qi court (479–502) and retired to Maoshan, near present-day Nanjing, where he dedicated himself to Daoist practices and the compilation of several treatises, including the materia medica text *Collected Annotations*. During the first decade of his life as a recluse, there is no evidence that Tao practiced alchemy. The situation changed in 502, though, when Emperor Wu of the Liang dynasty (reigned 502–549) established a new regime in the south. Although Tao lived in the mountains, he did not entirely cut off connections to the outside world, instead maintaining good relations with the court and offering valuable advice for state affairs at the emperor's request. As a result, he gained the reputation of being "the chancellor in the mountains."[35] The new emperor was also interested in elixirs and requested Tao to compound one for him.

Imperial sponsorship was central to Tao's alchemy, because certain ingredients were costly and difficult to acquire. Hence Tao did not start the practice until he had gained full support from Emperor Wu, who granted a lavish supply of gold, cinnabar, laminar malachite, and realgar.[36] With all the resources at hand and with the help of three disciples, Tao made a series of attempts between 505 and 519 to compound an elixir in Maoshan.[37]

The elixir that Tao tried to make is called Reverted Elixir in Nine Cycles (Jiuzhuan Huandan), and its preparation involved a ninety-day operation, with seven cycles of heating. The required ingredients were the seven minerals of kalinite (*fanshi*), laminar malachite (*cengqing*), quartz (*bai shiying*), cinnabar (*dansha*), realgar (*xionghuang*), orpiment (*cihuang*), and mercury (*shuiyin*). Tao first made an earthenware crucible that consisted of two dome-shaped halves connected by their mouths; it could hold three and a half pecks (about ten liters) of starting materials. Near an east-flowing stream, he then built a chamber that was forty feet long and twenty feet wide, and had a four-foot-high foundation. He constructed the stove at the center of the chamber, with an iron stand to hold the crucible nine inches from the stove.

After all these preparations, he started the operation, adding into the lower half of the crucible one pound of kalinite, three pounds of laminar malachite, two pounds of quartz, ten pounds of cinnabar, four pounds of realgar, and five pounds of orpiment. He then poured six pounds of mercury over the ingredients. After this, he covered it with the other half of the crucible and luted the two parts tightly. He placed the well-sealed container on the iron stand, lit the fire underneath, and kept the fire six inches from the bottom of the crucible for nine days and nine nights. He then gradually built up the fire over time so that it reached different levels of the crucible: three inches below its bottom, three inches above its bottom, three inches above its belly, five inches above its belly, and one inch under the seal of its two halves. At each level, the heating lasted for nine days and nine nights. He then extinguished the fire and allowed the crucible to cool for ten days. Afterward, he lit the fire again so it reached the level of half an inch under the seal of the crucible and maintained it for thirty-six days. Altogether, the operation took ninety days. He then stopped the fire and let the crucible cool for seven days before opening it and collecting the product adhering to its upper half. He had made an elixir.[38]

At the beginning of 506, Tao completed his first trial of compounding the Reverted Elixir in Nine Cycles. When he opened the crucible, however, he did not see the desired product. He repeated the whole operation once more, but still with no success. Tao blamed the failures on the unfavorable environment of Maoshan, where a recent flood of pilgrims had corrupted the sacred place. The lack of isolation from the mundane world, in his view, was a serious problem for the work of alchemists. To improve the situation, he left Maoshan in 508 and traveled around the southeast to find a better place for his alchemical mission.[39]

The History of the Sui offers a different explanation for Tao's failures.[40] Many of his ingredients came from northern regions, which at the time were controlled by a separate (Northern Wei) regime. The great difficulty of obtaining these materials from the north forced people in the south to use substitutes that were easier to acquire but of inferior quality. For example, one important ingredient in Tao's operation was realgar, an arsenic compound that came from the valley of Wudu in the northwest (in present-day Gansu). Because the northern regime was powerful, the flow of realgar from Wudu was cut off, making the material hard to obtain.[41] In his *Collected Annotations*, Tao notes that the price of authentic realgar during his days was equivalent to that of gold, due to the difficulty of obtaining it. He also observes that servants of aristocratic families often stole cinnabar and amethyst from their masters and sold the purloined goods at high prices on the market, suggesting a great demand for such materials at the time.[42] Although there sporadically existed markets that sold medicinal materials along the border, and there is record of some drug smuggling from the north to the south, alchemical practices often demanded large amounts of substances and repeated trials, for which these unstable channels may not have offered sufficient supply. Material constraints thwarted Tao's ambition.[43]

But how did Tao know that he had failed to make the elixir? In fact, Tao seemed close to his goal; every time he opened the crucible, he saw a product with the color of "frosty aurora" (*shuanghua*), which convinced his disciples that it was a success. Tao disagreed, insisting that all supreme elixirs should radiate variegated colors. For example, the Elixir of Langgan displayed thirty-seven types of color, the Elixir of Quchen one hundred different colors. And the aurora of the Elixir of Golden Liquid of Great Clarity resembled "the falling stars that fly to the moon and the clouds embroidered with nine colors." In the case of the Reverted Elixir in Nine Cycles, he would expect it to display nine colors of sublimated essence, with flowing light radiating brightly. But what he actually obtained after years of effort possessed a cloudy aurora whose color and shape resembled "frost and snow" (*shuangxue*) without variegated colors. For Tao, this was a clear sign of failure.[44]

The biography of Tao further cites a text referred to as *Instructions on Elixirs* (Danjue) to explain his assessment: "If a completed elixir does not radiate variegated colors, it is an elixir with *du*. One who ingests it will 'die temporarily' (*zansi*). Then, in a moment, he will rise and disappear."[45] Similar to its meaning in medical works, the concept of *du* in Chinese alchemy was also paradoxical. On the one hand, the elixir could trigger a momentary death, and the body would eventually vanish, a sure sign of transcendence. On the other hand, due to its imperfect preparation, the monochromatic elixir couldn't enable the highest level of transcendence, a goal that Tao strove for. In 519, fourteen years after he initiated the alchemical operation, Tao received a revelation. A deity descended and informed him of the futility of his elixir-making undertaking. The deity plainly told him that no one ascended to heaven in broad daylight by ingesting elixirs. Five years later, after seven attempts, Tao halted the enterprise altogether.[46]

Unlike some of his fellow alchemists, Tao never ingested a potent elixir.[47] His extensive drug knowledge, manifested in his *Collected Annotations*, might have directed him to take a more cautious attitude toward potent minerals.[48] More influential, though, is the crucial role that Tao played in the formation of a new sect of Daoism in fifth-century southeast China. Called "the Highest Clarity" (Shangqing), this new movement emphasized techniques of bodily cultivation, such as meditation, breathing, and inner visualization, to achieve transcendence.[49] Although they still recognized the wonder of alchemy, Highest Clarity adepts believed that the supreme level of accomplishment would be that of "the perfected" (*zhenren*), whose transcendence would be superior to that achieved by taking elixirs. Importantly, one could only reach the level of the perfected by practicing Highest Clarity techniques.[50] As a central figure in the early development of the Highest Clarity, Tao, after he retired to Maoshan, devoted himself to formulating its texts and practicing its bodily techniques. This does not mean that he denied the power of elixirs altogether, and it is probably not true that his alchemical practices were the exclusive result of imperial coercion. But he remained more cautious than some of his fellow alchemists. For Tao, there was no rush to ingest these potent drugs, since they were not the only means—and certainly not the best means—for achieving transcendence.

Taming Elixirs

Despite the rise of alternative paths to transcendence in Tao's time, alchemy in China persisted and even flourished in the following centuries. This is partly due to the increased accessibility of alchemical ingredients, facilitated by the Sui-Tang unification. Easy access to minerals reduced their price dramatically. For instance, realgar, a key alchemical ingredient, cost as much as gold in Tao's days. But during the Tang period, it could be easily obtained in the northwestern Wudu region and carried to the capital. Its price was "as low as that of tiles and stones"—not even worth the cost of transport.[51] The reduced price of ingredients made alchemy more affordable, contributing to its popularity. In addition, the expansion of the Tang empire to the western regions fostered trade along the Silk Road and the importing of substances from foreign lands. New minerals flowed into the empire, some of them highly valued by alchemists. Lead from Persia, for example, was considered superior to that from China for compounding elixirs.[52] Tang alchemists also treasured asbestos (*buhui mu*) from Persia, which was often used to detoxify mercury.[53] These new materials enriched alchemists' arsenals, galvanizing them to explore new ways of making elixirs.[54]

Because of lowered prices and the diversification of ingredients, alchemy was no longer a privileged enterprise for emperors and became possible for interested aristocrats and literati. As a result, we find writings by many Tang elites about their alchemical experience—even the famous poet Li Bai (701–762) dabbled in the practice.[55] Besides textual evidence, archeological finds also testify to the popularity of alchemy during the Tang period. Among them is an excavation from a site in Chang'an, the Tang capital, where two earthen jars containing more than a thousand items were discovered. The site has been identified as the residence of Li Shouli (672–741), a cousin of Emperor Xuanzong (reigned 712–756). Dating to the end of the eighth century, these items, likely owned by Li's descendants, offer a rich view of the material culture of Tang aristocrats.[56]

Among the miscellaneous items in the jars were dietary utensils, decorations, coins, and instruments for preparing medicines, as well as cinnabar of seven types probably for conducting alchemy. They were brilliant purple cinnabar, large-piece brilliant cinnabar (figure 7.1, left), brilliant crumbled cinnabar, red-glowing cinnabar, inferior brilliant cinnabar, cinnabar, and pit cinnabar. These fine differentiations, based on the quality of the material, indicates the rising connoisseurship of this key alchemical ingredient during the Tang period. In addition, the collection also contained four silver, pomegranate-shaped jars that were likely employed as heating vessels in alchemy (figure 7.1, right). In fact, traces of burning are still visible on the exterior of these jars. These substances and artifacts provide us with a concrete sense of alchemical practices in Tang China.

The flourishing of alchemy during the Tang dynasty led to the proliferation of texts on both the theoretical and technical aspects of the practice. These texts discuss the potency of the ingredients more extensively and present

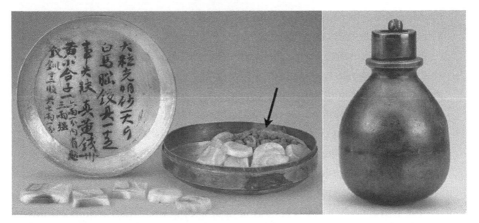

FIGURE 7.1. Cinnabar and an alchemical utensil from a Tang aristocratic family. An arrow points to one of the seven types of cinnabar: large-piece brilliant cinnabar (746 g). In the foreground and in the container are tile-shaped pieces of gemstone agate. The characters written on the lid describe the name and amount of the cinnabar and other items in the box. On the right is a silver jar in a pomegranate shape (height: 9.3 cm; diameter: 3.05 cm; weight: 845 g). Images from Qi and Shen, *Huawu da Tang chun*, 151, 153. Courtesy of Wenwu Press, Beijing.

various methods to curb their power.[57] An important treatise on this subject is *Instructions on the Scripture of the Divine Elixirs of the Nine Tripods of the Yellow Emperor* (Huangdi jiuding shendan jingjue; hereafter *Instructions on the Scripture*). The twenty-scroll text consists of a core (the first scroll) on alchemical methods that was probably produced during the Han period, followed by elaborate instructions added in the seventh century. The author(s) of these instructions is unknown, but given the repeated use of the term "your servant" (*chen*) throughout the text, a typical self-reference when addressing the ruler, it is possible that the treatise was presented to the court to solicit imperial interest.[58]

Overall, *Instructions on the Scripture* considers most minerals for making elixirs potent. The text claims that the various top-level minerals mostly contain potent *qi* (*duqi*). Hence things made from them would be harmful, like drinking the alcohol laced with *zhen* to quench thirst and consuming poisonous meat to avert hunger. One desires benefits but is instead badly damaged.[59] The statement clearly refers to the drug classification system according to which the materia medica literature was then organized. Yet while the majority of the top-level minerals in Chinese pharmacy were defined as nonpotent, the alchemical treatise regarded these materials as possessing potent *qi*, which could quickly injure the body. To produce a safe elixir, the text implied, one had to subdue its puissant ingredients.

Another example was cinnabar, an essential ingredient in the making of elixirs. From the Han period on, Chinese alchemists had been recognizing its potential to change into mercury and then back to cinnabar again. This unique transformation between a vermillion solid mineral and a white metallic fluid made them prime substances for alchemists.[60] Consequently, cinnabar and mercury were often discussed together in alchemical and medical sources. *Collected Annotations* places them one after another in the top group, stressing their value for enhancing life. Curiously, this materia medica text defines mercury, but not cinnabar, as possessing *du*.[61] *Instructions on the Scripture* challenges this view:

> People see in materia medica texts that cinnabar does not possess *du*, so they say that it does not injure people. They do not know that mercury is derived from cinnabar and possesses great *du*. Hence materia medica texts say: "Mercury is the spirit of cinnabar and emerges out of it." If the branch possesses *du*, how does the root not too?[62]

This appears a plausible reasoning, given how the two substances were intimately connected.[63]

The danger of minerals prompted Tang alchemists to develop a variety of methods to mollify their potency. For example, *Instructions on the Scripture* offers a series of guidelines for preparing mercury, the "pivot of elixirs."[64] First, it recommends heating. Here the technical term *fuhuo* invites scrutiny. Scholars have translated it as "fixed by fire," referring to a heating technique that prevents the evaporation of volatile minerals.[65] But there is a second meaning to the term. Given the frequent use of "fiery poison" (*huodu*) in alchemical writings to designate the heating power of certain minerals, *fuhuo* may also mean "subdue fire." The technique of *fuhuo* then seeks not only to preserve the ingredients but also to make them less potent. The heating often takes a long time, with assorted substances added in sequence. In one method, an adept starts with boiling mercury in a solution of crude halotrichite (*huangfanshi*) until the solution completely evaporates. He then boils pulverized magnetite (*cishi*) in water and pours the liquid onto the ashes of burned cow dung and burned asbestos. This is followed by boiling the prepared mercury in the resulting solution for one day and one night. He continues boiling the product with vinegar for another day and night, with alcohol and honey for a further day and night, and with butter for three days and three nights. Finally, he steams it with millet for three days and three nights. After this long process, mercury becomes "utterly devoid of poison, so one can use it for making myriad elixirs, the ingesting of which confers transcendence."[66]

The use of vinegar (*zuowei*) in this method is noteworthy. In pharmacological writings, vinegar often serves as an antidote that can "kill malevolent poisons." Alcohol and honey could be used to similar ends.[67] But vinegar was special in alchemical practices because it was one of the three yang drugs that were deemed essential for eliminating poison in mercury and lead.[68] A central rationale for alchemy during the Tang period was to reverse the cosmic unfolding inside a crucible, and to return differentiated forms of matter to their original oneness. This oneness was often imagined as a state of pure yang, before undergoing a series of yin-yang differentiations.[69] Using yang drugs, by this logic, would add yang force into the alchemical ingredients and facilitate their return to the state of pure yang. In this regard, time was also important. *Instructions on the Scripture* emphasizes that one must prepare mercury at the time of yang, namely, on the odd days of the year, during the odd hours of the day. In particular, the fifth day of the fifth month and the seventh day of the seventh month were the best times for the practice, as they were the hottest yang times in the summer. If one failed to observe these rules, the poison in mercury would not be eliminated and the resultant elixir would be fatal.[70]

In addition to taming elixirs during their preparation, Tang alchemists were also cautious about how to ingest these powerful drugs. In particular, they paid keen attention to dosage. *Instructions on the Scripture* warns that if one takes an elixir in the amount of one tip of the jade-knife (0.2 g), one will die temporarily for half a day or so and then come back to life as if waking up from sleep, a condition that the text considers extremely dangerous. To avert the danger of overdose, the text advises that one must follow formulas and instead use the size of half a millet grain as the measurement, which is one sixty-fourth of the jade-knife dose.[71] This sensitivity to dosage echoes Chinese physicians' cautious attitude in pharmaceutical practice; for example, *The Divine Farmer's Classic* recommends the size of a millet grain as the starting point for administering potent drugs.[72] The similarity indicates shared knowledge of dosage control between alchemical and medical texts.

Moreover, the term "temporary death" (*zansi*) merits attention. We encountered this term in Tao Hongjing's biography, where it signals transcendence—not the highest accomplishment in Tao's view but a level of transcendence nonetheless. In the Tang text, however, the term implies a state of coma, a condition that reminds us of the opening episode, where the general fell into a similar state of unconsciousness after taking an elixir. The amount he ingested, twenty thousand pellets, clearly indicates overdose, which led to his collapse. This change in the meaning of "temporary death," from a sign of transcendence to a symptom of bodily crisis, reveals a heightened awareness of the danger of elixirs during the Tang period.

Elixirated Bodies

It is evident that *Instructions on the Scripture* relies on bodily signs to gauge the proper use of elixirs. This attention to their effects on the body was not new in the Tang period; throughout the long history of Chinese alchemy, many adepts noted the often violent impact of their refined drugs on the body and offered various interpretations. Study of these elixirated bodies offers a revealing view of the power of medicines through the lens of self-transformation.

In the early years of alchemy, an elixirated body often evoked wonder and awe. One biographical record recounts that in the last days of his life on Mount Luofu, Ge Hong sent a letter to his friend Deng Yue, in which he wrote of a plan to depart soon to distant lands to seek a master. Deng hastened to Mount Luofu to see his friend off, only to find that Ge had already died. Though no longer alive, Ge's face still had the hue of the living and his body was supple. When his corpse was carried, it felt extremely light, as if there was nothing there but his clothes. People said that Ge had become a transcendent by "corpse deliverance" (*shijie*).[73]

Shijie is a term, often found in early Daoist hagiographies, that depicts the death of an accomplished master. The body of the master vanishes soon after his death, only leaving some paraphernalia behind, such as clothes, swords, and talismans. The master then reappears somewhere far away, roaming under a different name. Early Daoist texts often explain *shijie* as a process similar to how a snake molts its skin or a cicada leaves behind its shell, which implies metamorphosis. The analogies signal that the master's death is only apparent; he has actually achieved transcendence.[74]

Yet it merits our attention that Ge Hong considered *shijie* an inferior way to obtain transcendence. In his *Inner Chapters*, he cites a certain *Classic of*

Transcendents to the effect that those who raise their bodies and ascend to the void are superior masters, those who roam in famous mountains are mid-level masters, and those who die first and metamorphose later, namely attaining *shijie*, are only inferior masters.[75] In this hierarchy, those who have achieved transcendence through *shijie* still linger in the human world. Ge further explains that the dose of an elixir determines the obtainable level of transcendence: taking half a dose, one remains in the human realm; with a full dose, one ascends to the celestial world. But then wouldn't everyone choose the latter? Not necessarily. Ge points out that because the bureaucratic work in heaven is so taxing, especially for the new transcendents, many prefer to stay below for some time to enjoy the carefree life of the human world.[76] Achieving *shijie* thus offers its own advantages.

Other sources present *shijie* differently. *The History of the Song* (fifth century) recounts a story of a general named Sun Liang who, in 472, asked a Daoist master to make an elixir for him. The alchemist produced the elixir but had not yet eliminated its "fiery poison" (*huodu*). Ignoring the master's warning, Sun enthusiastically ingested the elixir. Upon eating a full meal, he felt that "his heart became agitated as if being pierced" (*xin dong ru ci*), and he died soon after. Later, people saw him riding a white horse to the west with scores of followers, which was a clear sign of *shijie*. In this episode, *shijie* still promised transcendence, but at a price: a painful sensation induced by the heating power of the elixir.[77]

The agonies of the elixirated body also appear in the writings of Tao Hongjing. In his *Declarations of the Perfected* (Zhen'gao), a Daoist compendium based on a series of celestial revelations that circulated in the southeast during the fourth century, he describes a certain Leaving Your Belt Behind Powder by the Perfected of Grand Supreme (Taiji Zhenren Yidai San):

> Upon ingesting one tip of the jade-knife of the white powder, one suddenly feels piercing pain in the heart. In the following three days, he has a craving for water. Having drunk a full *hu* of water, his *qi* is exhausted.[78] The exhaustion of *qi* is death. After the burial, his corpse disappears, leaving only the clothes behind. He has become a transcendent, releasing his belt in broad daylight.[79]

Similar to Sun's case, the elixir induced violent bodily sensations: severe pain in the heart and intense thirst, the latter probably caused by the heat released by the elixir. Compared to the depiction of *shijie* in Daoist hagiographies, which highlights the extraordinary *look* of the body and its miraculous disappearance *after* death, the examples above shift the focus to the *experience* of the body *before* death. This altered perception of the elixi-rated body stresses the paradox of *du*: the power of an elixir is manifested in the painful bodily experience it induces, though this does not hinder its ulti-mate goal of potentiating transcendence.

But despite their alluring promise, the torments triggered by powerful elixirs made the journey to transcendence a daunting one. As a result, we find records of alchemists who did not dare to ingest elixirs. In his *Declarations of the Perfected*, Tao tells a story in which four adepts made an elixir together. Two of them ingested it and died. The other two were frightened and decided not to take the elixir—only to realize later that their fellows had become transcendents. The theme of the tale—overcoming an apparent death to achieve transcendence—is typical of Daoist hagiographies of the time, but it clearly shows misgivings about elixir-taking among alchemists.[80]

Later Tang alchemical texts offer more detailed descriptions of the bodily experience of elixir-taking. Particularly relevant is a treatise titled *The Record from the Stone Wall of the Great Clarity* (Taiqing shibi ji; here-after *The Record from the Stone Wall*), compiled in 758 or 759 by a certain Master Chuze based on a late sixth-century source.[81] The text contains a col-lection of alchemical formulas together with the rules of ingesting elixirs and descriptions of their effects on the body. Distinctively, it depicts the various elixirs as capable not only of triggering transcendence but also of curing myriad illnesses. A section titled "Sensations and Stirrings upon Ingesting Elixirs" (Fudan juechu) observes:

> After ingesting the elixir, one feels his body and face itching as if worms are crawling there. His hands and feet are swollen. He finds that food stinks, and eating makes him nauseated and vomit. His four limbs are weak. Sometimes he has diarrhea; sometimes he vomits. He has headache and pain in the abdo-men. One should not take these signs amiss. They manifest the efficacy of the elixir to eliminate illnesses.[82]

This is a vivid account of the violent effects of the elixir on the body, includ-ing pain, fierce draining, and confusion of the senses. Compared to earlier records that highlight heart pain, the account here depicts the elixir's forceful impact all over the body, experiences that are not considered pathological but signs of therapeutic efficacy. To support this interpretation, the text cites an ancient aphorism on potent drugs: "If a medicine does not cause dizziness, it cannot cure illness."[83] The violent responses provoked by an elixir do not signal pathology but testify to its healing power.

To elucidate this point, *The Record from the Stone Wall* further correlates bodily experiences with the curing of specific illnesses. The text predicts that fifteen days after ingesting an elixir, one should feel an unusual sensation in the body followed by vomiting fluid that is mostly mucus and saliva. This is when a latent illness in the abdomen, between the Spleen and the Lungs, is manifested. In another case, one develops headache and dizziness, with dry lips and a burning face, and the eyes shed tears and mucus runs from the nose, all of which reveal a latent illness of "hot wind." In yet another case, the elixir loosens the bowels and provokes frequent urination, the ceaseless draining of pus and blood, and the purging of various worms. In this case, an illness of the triple *jiao* has been brought to the surface.[84] And the list goes on. In the end, the text reassures readers that they should not mistake these powerful reactions for anything other than manifestations of the circulation of the elixir's *qi*. As one obtains the power of the numinous medicine, these experiences signify the agitation of the illness.[85] The word "agitation" (*dong*) implies that the illness is latent in the body, only to be brought out of dormancy by the potent elixir. Many of the effects—vomiting, mucus, tears, diarrhea, and worms—indicate the purging of harmful material. These intense experiences are thus understood as a process of purification, that is, the agitation and elimination of dormant pathological agents so as to heal the body.[86]

What did the purification of the body have to do with transcendence? Transcendence is the ultimate goal, which *The Record from the Stone Wall* fully recognizes. Earlier narratives often portray the effects of an elixir on the body as excruciating and extreme, leading to quick death. In this text, an elixir could still induce intense reactions, but not immediate demise, likely due to careful preparation and dosage regulation, as discussed above. As a result, one would have time to experience the unfolding effects of the elixir and contemplate its impact on the body; the perception of the elixir as a healing agent might well be a product of this prolonged experience. Eliminating latent illnesses purifies the body, which paves the way for one's eventual transcendence.

Finally, although *The Record from the Stone Wall* interprets the sensations of an elixirated body in a positive light, these effects could become pathological if they persist too long. An uncomfortable bodily experience should only last temporarily; after the malady is removed, one should begin to feel normal again. For example, the text counsels that if one still vomits and endures diarrhea eight days after taking the elixir, one should then alleviate the symptoms by applying cooling therapies, such as eating cold porridges and washing the body with cold water.[87] These methods resemble those for managing Five-Stone Powder (see chapter 6). In both cases, potent minerals were used to cure sickness, and the experience of the body became a crucial marker for monitoring and managing the therapeutic outcome of the medicine.

Conclusion

Scholars have often situated the ideas and practices of elixir-taking within a significant transition in Chinese religious history, which was characterized by a shift of focus from outer alchemy to inner alchemy. Inner alchemy refers to a variety of meditative techniques that shared the language and goals of outer alchemy but replaced consuming substances with the cultivation of *qi* in the body. These two types of practice coexisted early in history, but after the tenth century, inner alchemy became the dominant form of attaining transcendence among Daoist practitioners.[88] Elixir poisoning probably played an important role in this transition, as suggested by alchemists' various, and sometimes contentious, ways of explaining the power of elixirs. Such power was often understood through the paradox of *du*, for which different alchemists offered distinct interpretations.

The effects of *du* in Ge Hong's writing hinged on the precondition of the body: only after an adept had built a robust constitution could he enjoy the benefits of a potent elixir. For Tao Hongjing, on the other hand, an elixir with *du*, marked by its monochromatic hue, resulted from the lack of prime ingredients or from ritual pollution. Despite its inferior quality, such an elixir could still promise a low level of transcendence. By contrast, Tang alchemists took care to emphasize the danger of ingredients such as mercury. *Du* in their works connoted the heating power of these minerals, which had to be adequately tamed. As a result, they developed a series of methods to detoxify the ingredients, moderate the dose, and manage the effects of elixirs.

Moreover, accompanying the different understandings of the power of an elixir were the varied perceptions of an elixirated body. For Ge Hong, the robust materiality of an elixir could be readily transferred to the body, making it similarly strong. Such an imperishable body elicited wonder and drew admiration, and its miraculous disappearance in the form of *shijie* further enhanced the appeal of the elixir. Other sources, such as those compiled by Tao Hongjing, depict the experience of *shijie* as acutely painful, making some alchemists hesitant to ingest the elixir. Undaunted devotees, however, took the experience as a necessary step toward their ultimate transcendence. Furthermore, certain Tang accounts of elixir-induced sensations were framed in a therapeutic light; elaborate and specific, they include vomiting, diarrhea, and purging worms. These violent experiences, though, were interpreted approvingly, as signs of purifying the body and potentiating its transformation.

Finally, it is important to point out that alchemists such as Ge Hong, Tao Hongjing, and Sun Simiao were also well versed in medicine and wrote influential medical texts.[89] Admittedly, their medical writings focus on curing illness and sustaining health rather than seeking transcendence. Nevertheless, certain knowledge was relevant for both types of pursuit. For example, the potency of minerals, well recognized in medical works, was a foundation from which alchemists could fathom the power of elixirs. In many ways, alchemists' handling of elixirs was similar to how physicians managed potent drugs such as Five-Stone Powder: both generated intense heat inside the body, both required careful administration, and both could easily turn into deadly poisons. Although the practices of ingesting elixirs and Five-Stone Powder died out by the end of the Tang period, the therapeutic use of potent minerals, and potent substances in general, lived on and remained vital to Chinese medicine for centuries to come.

Conclusion

In ancient times, incompetent physicians killed people. Nowadays incompetent physicians don't kill people, but they don't save people either. They leave them between not dead and not alive. The patient's illness deepens over time, leading to death eventually. . . . Those who prescribe medicines today tend to offer indiscriminate and static remedies. They cannot detect the illness clearly, nor can they treat it aggressively. This is why the illness cannot be cured.

—GU YANWU, *RECORD OF DAILY LEARNING* (1695)

OUR JOURNEY THROUGH POISONS IN MEDIEVAL CHINA HAS, I HOPE, made clear the importance of potent substances in classical Chinese pharmacy and beyond. The paradox of *du* and its repercussions in many corners of society reveals how this key concept was embodied in pharmaceutical techniques, political agendas, and religious aspirations. At the core of these diverse expressions of *du* lay the idea of transformation, which was manifested in the following three aspects.

First, classical Chinese pharmacy, from its inception during the Han period, encompassed a wide range of substances, each of which possessed great transformative capacity. No medicine was characterized by a fixed essence or a set effect; in the proper context, any material, even some of the most poisonous, could be harnessed for healing. The idea of the remarkable malleability of drugs, rooted in the ancient philosophical mode of perceiving all things in the cosmos as ceaselessly changing, was central to pharmaceutical practices in medieval China. Drugs in the pharmacy of this period, especially those possessing *du*, were judiciously prepared and deployed to moderate their potency: dosing, roasting, combining with other substances, attending to the nuances of the changing condition of the patient, and precision in ritual procedures all mattered. This variety of techniques had already emerged during the Han period and became more elaborate in the pharmaceutical writings of the fifth century as a result of physicians' growing concern about the quality of ingredients and the safe use of drugs. The prominence of poisons in classical Chinese pharmacy thus reveals the centrality of techniques of intervention for transforming these powerful substances.

Second, in addition to the fluid materiality of the medicines themselves, knowledge of medicines was also subject to transformation as it moved across different political and social spaces. Seventh-century China witnessed the active engagement of the Sui and Tang courts in standardizing drug knowledge and regulating medical practice by producing authoritative texts and establishing new institutions and laws. Yet such knowledge was not solidified by imperial edicts; once reaching local communities, it underwent marked changes contingent on the availability of resources and the needs of local actors. Moreover, knowledge of medicines from the ancient classics was not stable either; it was readily adapted by physicians who were interested in the efficacy of remedies and relied on their own experience to assess the utility of formulas. The making of new medical knowledge was then a dynamic negotiation between political authority and local demands, between textual authority and practical concerns.

Third, medicines, upon ingestion, could profoundly alter the body. This alteration involved not just the restoration of the body to its normal condition, in the case of curing sickness, but also the transformation of the body into higher states of being. This latter pursuit of life enhancement constituted a distinctive feature of Chinese pharmacy and Daoist religion. Poisons figured prominently in this endeavor yet presented a paradox for alchemists and physicians alike: the alluring promise of their power to radically change the body and transcend death was entwined with their ever-present threat to cut life short. Significantly, the elixirated body, manifesting fierce and painful sensations caused by numinous medicines, offered both warning and reassurance for devoted users. Investigating poisons in this context illustrates the importance of bodily experience in mediating the understanding and deployment of medicines.

Furthermore, by situating the study of poisons in the medical, political, and religious cultures of medieval China, this book traces the changing landscape of Chinese medicine via an examination of disparate groups of actors engaged in medical practice and the production of new drug knowledge.

During the Era of Division, physicians from aristocratic families practiced medicine continuously over generations and produced influential pharmacological texts. In particular, the southeastern region became the nucleus of such activities, where a variety of medical and alchemical texts circulated within an intimate network of local elites. In the seventh century, the center of medical activities shifted to the northwestern region, where the unified Sui and Tang empires established their courts. In this favorable political environment, the state assumed an active role in standardizing drug knowledge, regulating the use of poisons, and creating new medical institutions to recruit capable healers. The situation changed in the mid-eighth century, when the An Lushan Rebellion considerably weakened the central government. As a result, the locus of engagement in medicine shifted again from the state to scholar-officials, who became increasingly involved in the making and spreading of pharmaceutical knowledge.

This last transition merits elaboration. The engagement of scholar-officials in medicine was not entirely new in the late Tang period. Su Jing, the director who oversaw the production of *Newly Revised Materia Medica* (659), and a number of other compilers involved in the imperial project came from this group (see chapter 4). Wang Tao, the author of the formula collection *Arcane Essentials from the Imperial Library* (752), was also one such figure (see chapter 5). These cultural elites were avidly interested in medicine but did not practice the art of healing to earn a living. Yet starting in the ninth century, more literati, often those who had been frustrated in their political careers, participated in learning medicine, collecting formulas, and sharing useful knowledge of healing with their friends. Liu Yuxi (772–842), who appears in the story that opens this book, was a revealing example. Having been involved in an ambitious but short-lived project of political reform at court, Liu was banished to the far south in the early ninth century, where he collected formulas, often based on his own experience, that he hoped could protect him from the dangers of the new physical environment.[1] His autobiographical story discussed at the beginning of this book delivers a key lesson on the medical use of poisons, the history of which I then probed throughout the rest of the chapters. Importantly, Liu's story also offers a political message: he concludes at the end that just as medicines must be used judiciously to cure the body, a leader should adopt forceful and flexible policies to rule the country.[2] The exiled scholar used medicine as a vehicle to advocate his political views.

Liu was not alone in his engagement of medicine for both therapeutic and political purposes. Several of his contemporaries also took part in passionate discussions of medicine. They often focused on the contentious issue of ingesting potent minerals for life cultivation, a practice particularly popular among literati at the time. Liu Zongyuan (773–819), for instance, was enthusiastic about stalactite and had sophisticated knowledge of its morphological varieties and different source locations. In a letter he wrote to his brother-in-law, he demonstrated this detailed knowledge and criticized those who were fixated on single sources they believed to yield the best stalactite. There was also a political message in Liu's letter: the strategy of selecting capable people for government should not be restricted to specific regions but rather be based on their inherent skills and qualities.[3] Han Yu (768–824), the leading literary figure of the time, consumed sulfur in his senior years to invigorate his body, a practice frowned upon by his contemporary Bai Juyi (772–846), a famous poet who also wrote enthusiastically on medicine.[4] Yet despite his interest in certain minerals, Han Yu condemned the practice of unbridled ingestion of elixirs. In an epitaph he wrote for his grandson-in-law, who died of elixir poisoning, he lambasted the craze, blaming it for numerous deaths. Revealingly, the scholar considered the agonizing experiences induced by elixirs to be pathologies rather than signs of healing. In fact, he directly refuted therapeutic explanations, like those we have seen in *The Record from the Stone Wall* (see chapter 7), calling them lamentable excuses. An elixir, in his eyes, was nothing but a lethal poison.[5]

Although a comprehensive study of the medical writings of Tang scholars requires future research, I hope these episodes offer a glimpse into the diverse understandings of medicines held by the literati of the ninth century—understandings that were often entangled with their political views. From this perspective, the ninth century marked a new era of Chinese medicine, with the rise of scholar-officials as major producers and circulators of medical knowledge. This engagement became more pronounced in the following Song period (960–1279), when increasing numbers of literati, having failed to enter officialdom, took up alternative careers as practitioners of medicine.[6]

The literati's active involvement in medicine persisted into late imperial times. But that would be a different moment in the history of Chinese pharmacy, one with waning state interest in producing pharmacological texts, the development of an empire-wide pharmaceutical trade, and the penetration of materia medica knowledge into popular culture.[7] The practice of employing poisons for healing, however, remained a vital one. The acclaimed sixteenth-century *Systematic Materia Medica*, for instance, introduces a section of *du*-possessing herbs, including fifty-one powerful plants with diverse medical uses.[8] The administration of these potent substances was a matter of intense debate given their entwined efficacy and danger. The commentary of the eminent seventeenth-century scholar Gu Yanwu (1613–1682), cited in the epigraph, is one such example. Gu's criticism of medical practice in his time underscores the value of potent medicines—often left unexploited by doctors of the day—to aggressively eradicate illnesses rather than leaving them untreated for the sake of safety. Using poisons in spite of their dangers was a risk that a good doctor had to take. It merits our notice that Gu's remark had political overtones: he concluded at the end of his essay that selecting officials should adhere to the same rules as those for prescribing medicines. That is, it is better to appoint a specific group of capable people rather than indiscriminately assigning positions to many.[9] Gu's writings thus follow a long tradition of using medicine as an instrument to convey political messages.

Given the robust tradition of the medical use of poisons throughout imperial China, we may wonder where today's idea of Chinese drug therapy as mild and benign came from. The answer lies in a refashioning of Chinese medicine in the modern era. With the introduction of Western biomedicine and the rise of scientism in China in the nineteenth and early twentieth centuries, classical Chinese medicine experienced a serious crisis that called its legitimacy into question. During this tumultuous period, advocates for Chinese medicine vigorously negotiated with the state and initiated a series of measures to transform their medical practices and reinstate their authority.[10] The emphasis on the benign naturalness of Chinese drug therapy was hence a strategic rhetoric that highlighted the unique benefits of Chinese medicine, thereby securing its legitimacy against the dominance of modern biomedicine. Furthermore, the dynamics between Chinese and Western medicine shifted in the second half of the twentieth century: the globalization of Chinese medicine meant that it was increasingly perceived as a promising alternative to biomedicine and its attendant shortcomings. This perception often romanticized Chinese medicine as offering a cogent critique of biomedicine, a critique that came at the expense of admitting the heterogeneity, diversity, and complex internal dynamics of multiple traditions of Chinese medical practice developed across vast expanses of time and place. This romanticized impression has carried on to our own time.[11]

But we cannot reduce Chinese medicine to an idealized, unchanging other; we must treat it seriously as an intricate and dynamic system of ideas and practices deeply rooted in history. We cannot just dwell on the striking differences between Chinese and Western medicine; we must also contemplate their meaningful resonances that might illuminate our understanding of medicine today. Poisons offer an excellent perspective for this purpose: my historical inquiry of these potent substances provides fresh insights into our view of contemporary pharmaceutical practice both in China and beyond.

Chinese pharmacy today continues to deploy various potent substances, such as aconite, cinnabar, and snake gallbladders. Informed by Western toxicology, these drugs are, in general, under tight regulation and administered with extreme caution, an attitude we have seen in some of the physicians presented in this book. What was new in the twentieth century is that, with the rise of Western biomedicine, some medical researchers in China, in a strategic move to modernize Chinese medicine, endeavored to incorporate classical pharmacological knowledge into biomedical research in order to develop new remedies. A project widely touted as a success of the program of "the integration of Chinese and Western medicine" (*zhongxiyi jiehe*) was spearheaded by Tu Youyou (1930–) and her research team, who in the 1970s successfully isolated artemisinin from an herb commonly used in classical Chinese pharmacy, artemisia (*qinghao*). The drug proved highly effective to treat malaria, which won her a Nobel Prize in Physiology or Medicine in 2015.[12]

What is less known, but of equal significance, is the story of Zhang Tingdong (1932–), a Harbin hematologist with training in both Chinese and Western medicine. During the 1970s, Zhang led a team in a series of studies of a formula developed by a local practitioner of Chinese medicine. The formula, which contained arsenic, mercury, and toad venom, was popular in the countryside because of its power to treat several types of cancer. Eventually, Zhang's team identified arsenic trioxide as the key ingredient that was particularly effective for treating patients of acute promyelocytic leukemia (APL). The discovery, which remained obscure for two decades, gained international recognition in the 1990s. Today, arsenic trioxide has become the most effective drug for combatting APL. In this telling example, a potent drug with a long history of use in Chinese pharmacy was successfully translated into modern chemotherapy.[13]

Yet promising news of the successful use of poisons in biomedicine today should not conceal the dark side of these materials. Reports of medical accidents caused by drugs in classical Chinese pharmacy have emerged both in China and in Western countries in recent decades, manifesting the danger of certain medicines and the need to regulate their production and administration. One high-profile case during the 1990s concerned the ingestion of a compound drug called Gentian Liver-Draining Pill (Longdan Xiegan Wan). The formula, which first appeared in a seventeenth-century medical text, uses ten herbs, including one called aristolochia (*mutong*). The herb contains aristolochic acid, which has been shown to induce kidney failure, bladder cancer, and liver cancer. Incidents involving the drug in China, Taiwan, and Europe prompted new biomedical research, public debates, and lawsuits, bringing the issue of safety in classical Chinese pharmacy to the fore. The scientific community strongly recommended a categorical ban on the drug, because the laboratory evidence clearly shows its harm to the body. Its defenders, on the other hand, stressed that it was the use of the pill to treat the wrong patients and conditions, its long-term consumption, and above all, a mistaken substitution for one of the ingredients in its formula that turned the medicine into a poison.[14] In fact, as this book demonstrates, concern about the safe use of medicines has always occupied practitioners' minds since medieval times. It seems that the debate over this controversial pill will not be settled anytime soon.

Furthermore, by highlighting the hazy boundary between poisons and medicines in classical Chinese pharmacy, this book intimates some compelling resonances between premodern Chinese and modern Western pharmaceutical practices. Just like the Chinese character *yao*, which has carried a range of meanings throughout history, the English word "drug" can refer to either a curative medicine or an illicit substance.[15] But where do we draw the line between the two? The turbulent history of marijuana use and legislation in the United States is revealing. Condemned and criminalized by the government throughout the twentieth century due to its perceived damage to physical and mental health, the controversial plant has gained recognition in recent decades as a valuable medicine and as a benign recreational substance, leading ultimately to its decriminalization in many states.[16] Accompanying this change, the medical community has shown renewed interest in the potential that some currently illegal psychedelic drugs may have to treat anxiety, addiction, and depression.[17] No drugs are inherently destructive; in the right contexts, they may have potential for transformation into beneficial agents.

Nonetheless, with the rise of the pharmaceutical industry and the proliferation of its products, especially those for the treatment of mental illnesses in the late twentieth century, our bodies have encountered drugs on an unprecedented scale.[18] As estimated by the National Center for Health Statistics, almost half of Americans have used at least one prescription drug in the past thirty days, and nearly a quarter of the population has used three or more.[19] This high exposure to pharmaceutical products, in many cases without sufficient public education and effective governmental regulation, has engendered some serious problems, among which licit drug abuse is a conspicuous one. The recent opioid epidemic in the United States is one striking example. Promoted by pharmaceutical companies in 1990s for the relief of chronic pain, opioid medications, when not administered with extreme caution, can become highly addictive, resulting in severe if not lethal consequences. In 2017 alone, more than 47,000 Americans died of opioid overdose, prompting the government to declare a public health emergency.[20] To solve the problem, coordination between medical practitioners, researchers, and policymakers will be required. At a more fundamental level, the episode again manifests the paradox of drug therapy: handled improperly, a promising medicine can become a deadly poison.[21]

What is a medicine? We have traveled to some of the earliest recorded periods of Chinese history to look for answers, returning to our own time, where we see both parallels and divergences. This much seems clear: medicines are fluid substances that defy rigid categorizations as curative or harmful, good or bad, legal or illegal. In a sense, it makes little difference whether a medicine is from a seventh-century Chinese doctor's apothecary, from a plastic bottle in a modern Chinese pharmacy, or from a product catalog of an American pharmaceutical company. The lesson is the same: no essential, absolute, or unchanging core exists that determinately characterizes a medicine; its effects in practice are always *relational*, contingent on technological interventions, sociopolitical conditions, and bodily experiences.

Ultimately, these reflections on medicines invite us into the intimate and complex relationship between the human self and the world. Medicines, a special kind of materiality, become a crucial mediator between the two. Our confidence in the power of these substances to improve us is always entwined with our anxiety about the dangers that they may bring. Despite this uncertainty, the poison-medicine paradox has empowered us to relentlessly experience, understand, and harness things in the world. We turn poisons into healing agents, adapt these substances to particular situations in our times and places, and even fundamentally transform ourselves to live afresh. It is through these ceaseless changes that potent medicines relieve our suffering, enhance our body, and underpin our perpetual quest for a better life.

GLOSSARY OF CHINESE CHARACTERS

Note: Chinese characters for authors and book titles cited in the notes can be found in the bibliography.

An Lushan 安祿山
anmo 按摩

badou 巴豆
Bai Juyi 白居易
bai shiying 白石英
banxia 半夏
bencao 本草
bencao daizhao 本草待詔
bian 變
Bian Que 扁鵲
buhui mu 不灰木
busi 不死
buzhi suoyiran 不知所以然

cai song zhi jia 採送之家
caiyao shi 採藥師
cang'er 蒼耳
Cao Xi 曹歙
cengqing 曾青
cezi 側子
changsheng 長生
Chao Yuanfang 巢元方

chaoji shi 朝集使
chen 臣
Chen Yanzhi 陳延之
chengxian 成仙
chong 蟲
chonggou 重鈎
Chu Cheng 褚澄
Chunyu Yi 淳于意
cihuang 雌黃
cishi 慈/磁石
cong 蔥

dadu 大毒
dafeng 大風
dan 丹
dandu 丹毒
danggui 當歸
Danjue 丹訣
dansha 丹砂/沙
daogui 刀圭
Daohong 道弘
daoyin 導引
Dasan 大散

177

dashu 大書
dayao 大藥
de 德
Deng Yue 鄧嶽
dingzhong 丁腫
dong 動
dongliu shui 東流水
du 毒
Duan Yi 段翳
Dugu Tuo 獨孤陁
duheng 杜衡
Dunhuang 敦煌
dunjia 遁甲
duqi 毒氣
duyao 毒藥

Erya 爾雅

fa 發
fan 燔
Fan Wang 范汪
Fang Boyu 房伯玉
fangji 方技
fangshi 方士
fangshu 方書 (formula books)
fangshu 方術 (methods and arts)
fangzhong 房中
fanshi 礬石
fen 分
feng 風
Fudan juechu 服丹覺觸
fuhuo 伏火
fuju 咬咀
fure 伏熱
fushui 服水
fuzi 附子

Gan Zizhen 甘子振
gansui 甘遂
Ge Hong 葛洪
gong 攻
gouwen 鉤吻
gu 蠱
Gu Yanwu 顧炎武

gualou 栝蔞
Guangji fang 廣濟方
Guangli fang 廣利方
guchong 蠱蟲
gudu 蠱毒
guduo xi 骨咄犀
gui 桂 (cinnamon)
gui 鬼 (demon)
guijiu 鬼臼
guizhu 鬼疰/注
guqi 穀漆

Han Kang 韓康
Han Yu 韓愈
Hanshi San 寒食散
He Xun 賀循
He Yan 何晏
hou 厚
Houshi Heisan 侯氏黑散
Hua Tuo 華佗
huanfang 患坊
huangfanshi 黃礬石
Huangfu Mi 皇甫謐
huangjing 黃精
Huayin 華陰
hufen 胡粉
Huiyi 慧義
huo 惑
huodu 火毒
huoluan 霍亂
huzhang 虎掌

Ji Han 嵇含
Ji Zixun 薊子訓
jian 煎
Jiankang 建康
Jianyao 鑒藥
jiaolong bing 蛟龍病
jiaoqi 腳氣
Jie Hanshi San fang 解寒食散方
jiesan 解散
Jiesan duizhi fang 解散對治方
jiji 及己
jin 堇

Jin Shao 靳邵
jin'an 謹案
jingfang 經方
jingshi 靜室
jingyan 經驗
Jinya San 金牙散
jiu 酒
Jiuzhuan Huandan 九轉還丹
jiuzi 酒漬
jiyan fang 集驗方

Kong Zhiyue 孔志約
kuhu 苦瓠

langdang zi 莨菪子
langdu 狼毒
Lei Xiao 雷斆
li 狸
Li Bai 李白
Li Baozhen 李抱真
Li Shaojun 李少君
Li Shouli 李守禮
Li Ziyu 李子豫
liang 良
liangyao 良藥
Liangzhou 梁州
liao 療
liaoshi 蓼實
Liu Ling 劉伶
Liu Yuxi 劉禹錫
Liu Zongyuan 柳宗元
Longdan Xiegan Wan
　龍膽瀉肝丸
longgu 龍骨
lunyue 論曰

mafen 麻蕡
maogui 貓鬼
Maonü 貓女
Maoshan 茅山
Mawangdui 馬王堆
Mensi 門司
mubiezi 木鱉子
mutong 木通

naosha 硇砂
neidan 內丹
niuhuang 牛黃
nüqing 女青

paozhi 炮炙/製
Pei Xiu 裴秀
pishuang 砒霜

qi 氣
qian 遷
qiangzhong 強中
Qie Yin 郤愔
Qin Chengzu 秦承祖
qinghao 青蒿
qiqing 七情

ranshe dan 蚺蛇膽
reli 熱痢
renshen 人參
rong 榮
Ruan Ji 阮籍

sanjian 三建
sanjiao 三焦
Shangdang 上黨
shanghan 傷寒
Shanghan zabing lun 傷寒雜病論
Shangqing 上清
shangyao dianyu 尚藥典御
Shangyao Ju 尚藥局
Shazhou 沙州
Shennong 神農
shenxian 神僊
Shenxian zhuan 神仙傳
shenyan 神驗
shenyan fang 身驗方
shexiang 麝香
shi 實
shi liuhuang 石硫黃
shidan 石膽
shihu 石斛
shijie 尸解
Shike 噬嗑

shiren 市人

Shishen 石神

shizu 士族

shu 熟

Shuanggudui 雙古堆

shuanghua 霜華

shuangxue 霜雪

shuisu 水蘇

shuiyin 水銀

Sihai leiju fang 四海類聚方

Su Jing 蘇敬

Sun Jichang 孫季長

Sun Liang 孫亮

Sun Simiao 孫思邈

Taiji Zhenren Yidai San 太極真人遺帶散

Taiqing 太清

Taiyi Beiji San 太乙備急散

Taiyi Shu 太醫署

Tao Hongjing 陶弘景

Tianshi Dao 天師道

tianxiong 天雄

Tu Youyou 屠呦呦

tugong 土貢

waidan 外丹

Wang Bi 王弼

Wang Shuhe 王叔和

Wang Tao 王燾

Wang Xizhi 王羲之

Wanwu 萬物

wei 衛 (defensive)

wei 味 (flavor)

Wei Boyang 魏伯陽

wu 巫

wudi 午地

Wudu 武都

wugu 巫蠱

wuhui 烏喙

Wushi Gengsheng San 五石更生散

Wushi San 五石散

wutou 烏頭

Wuwei 武威

wuxin 五辛

xian 仙

xiangfan 相反

xiangsha 相煞

xiangshi 相使

xiangwei 相畏

xiangwu 相惡

xiangxu 相須

xiao 效/効

xiaodu 小毒

xiaoyan fang 效/効驗方

xiaoyao 小藥

xin dong ru ci 心動如刺

xionghuang 雄黃

xu 虛

Xu Ani 徐阿尼

Xu Shen 許慎

Xu Sibo 徐嗣伯

Xu Zhicai 徐之才

Xuanxue 玄學

xuezhe 學者

yan 驗

yang 養

Yang Su 楊素

Yang Xiu 楊秀

yangsheng 養生

yao 藥

Yao Sengyuan 姚僧垣

yaojia 藥家

yaoyuan 藥園

Yaozang Ju 藥藏局

ye 冶

yegan 射干

yege 冶/野葛

yi boshi 醫博士

yi du gong du 以毒攻毒

yi'an 醫案

Yiji ling 醫疾令

yijing 醫經

yin zhen zhi ke 飲鴆止渴

yinyi 隱逸

yishi 醫師

Yizhou 益州

yongzhong 癰腫

youdu 有毒
Yuanhua San 芫花散
Yuhan fang 玉函方
yushi 礜石
Yuzhou 鬱洲

zansi 暫死
Zhang Tingdong 張亭棟
Zhang Yuanyou 張遠遊
Zhang Zhongjing 張仲景
Zhao Mo 趙昩
zhendu 鴆毒
Zheng Xuan 鄭玄
Zheng Yin 鄭隱
zhenmu wen 鎮墓文
zhenniao mao 鴆鳥毛

zhenren 真人
zhi 治 (manage)
zhi 炙 (roast)
zhong'e 中惡
zhongru 鐘乳
zhongsong 塚訟
zhongxiyi jiehe 中西醫結合
Zhou Ziliang 周子良
zhu 煮 (boil)
zhu 疰/注 (infestation, pouring)
Zhulin Qixian 竹林七賢
zi jingyong youxiao 自經用有效
Zishi Hanshi San 紫石寒食散
zisu 紫蘇
zuodao 左道
zuowei 左味

NOTES

INTRODUCTION

1 Liu Yuxi, *Liu Yuxi ji*, 6.76–77.
2 Fan Ka-wai, "Liu Yuxi yu *Chuanxin fang*," 111–44.
3 Sun, *Qianjin yifang*, 1.6.
4 Nappi, *Monkey and the Inkpot*, 50–68.
5 Kaptchuk, *Web That Has No Weaver*, 372; Scheid, *Chinese Medicine in Contemporary China*, 108; Hilary Smith, *Forgotten Disease*, 13–19.
6 Lo, *Potent Flavours*.
7 Appadurai, ed., *Social Life of Things*; Miller, ed., *Materiality*; Daston, ed., *Things That Talk*; Findlen, ed., *Early Modern Things*.
8 Porkert, *Theoretical Foundations of Chinese Medicine*; Lu and Needham, *Celestial Lancets*; Barnes, "World of Chinese Medicine and Healing," 284–333.
9 The issue of transformation in Chinese pharmacy has been explored in Carla Nappi's study of a sixteenth-century pharmacological text chiefly through the lens of natural history. See Nappi, *Monkey and the Inkpot*. The transformative power of medicines is not unique to Chinese pharmacy, as it figures in other healing traditions as well. See Whyte, van der Geest, and Hardon, eds., *Social Lives of Medicines*, 5–6.
10 In the same vein, focusing on three medical writings in the seventh and eighth centuries, Kuo Ho-Hsiang has examined the historical meanings of *du* in these sources. See Kuo, "Sui-Tang yiji zhong guanyu du de xin renshi."
11 Mou, "Duyao kukou," 437–38; Kawahara, *Dokuyaku wa kuchi ni nigashi*; Li Ling, "Yaodu yijia," 28–38; Huo, "'Du' yu zhonggu shehui."
12 Arnold, *Toxic Histories*.
13 Arnold, *Toxic Histories*, 209. Orpiment is an arsenic ore.

14 It is entirely possible that the knowledge of the medical use of poisons was
    exchanged between China and India in the premodern period. One telling exam-
    ple is the claim by Sun Simiao cited earlier, which he ascribed to Jīvaka, the
    "Medicine King" of India, indicating the influence of Indian pharmacological
    thought on Sun's work. See Liao Yuqun, *Renshi Yindu chuantong yixue*, 281–84.
    On the history of Jīvaka in China, see Salguero, "Buddhist Medicine King in Liter-
    ary Context," 183–210.

15 Collard, *Crime of Poison in the Middle Ages*; Whorton, *Arsenic Century*; Parascan-
    dola, *King of Poisons*.

16 Rinella, *Pharmakon*. Jacques Derrida has noted how the dual meanings are mani-
    fested in Plato's works, though his main goal is to use *pharmakon* to demonstrate
    the instability of writing. See Derrida, "Plato's Pharmacy," 61–171.

17 Beck, trans., *De Materia Medica*.

18 Collard and Samama, eds., *Le corps à l'épreuve*; Grell, Cunningham, and Arriza-
    balaga, eds., *"It All Depends on the Dose."*

19 Gibbs, *Poison, Medicine, and Disease*.

20 No medical works devoted to poisons and antidotes appeared in China until the
    late sixteenth century, possibly influenced by European medicine. One such text
    is *Formulas to Counter a Hundred Poisons* (Jie baidu fang) compiled by Gao Lian
    (1573–1620).

21 Beck, *De Materia Medica*, 281 (IV 77); Riddle, *Dioscorides on Pharmacy and Medi-
    cine*, 65–66.

22 The appellation is given by Tao Hongjing in his *Collected Annotations on the Classic
    of Materia Medica* (Bencao jing jizhu, ca. 500). See Tao, *Bencao jing jizhu*, 5.344.

23 For further discussion on this comparison, see Yan Liu, "Poisonous Medicine in
    Ancient China," 437–39.

24 Liao Yuqun, "Zhongguo chuantong yixue de 'chuantong' yu 'geming,'" 217–23;
    Goldschmidt, *Evolution of Chinese Medicine*, 199. Throughout this book, I use
    "classical Chinese medicine" or "classical Chinese pharmacy" as shorthand terms
    to refer to medical or pharmaceutical traditions before the nineteenth century.

25 Yamada Keiji, "Formation of the *Huang-ti Nei-ching*," 67–89; Harper, "Physicians
    and Diviners," 91–110; Li Jianmin, *Sisheng zhiyu*; Lo, "Influence of Nurturing Life
    Culture on the Development of Western Han Acumoxa Therapy," 19–51; Hsu,
    Pulse Diagnosis in Early Chinese Medicine.

26 Chen Yuanpeng, *Liang Song de "shangyi shiren" yu "ruyi"*; Despeux, "System of
    the Five Circulatory Phases and the Six Seasonal Influences (*wuyun liuqi*)," 121–
    65; Goldschmidt, *Evolution of Chinese Medicine*; Hinrichs, "Governance through
    Medical Texts and the Role of Print," 217–38; Chen Yun-ju, "Accounts of Treating
    Zhang ("miasma") Disorders," 205–54.

27 The definition of the medieval period in China remains a contested issue due to
    the different historical experiences of China and Europe. The debates are also
    linked to the issue of the starting point of Chinese modernity, which some schol-
    ars have dated as early as the tenth century (see discussion below). This book is
    not a place to adjudicate these debates. Rather, I use the term as shorthand to

refer to the period from the post-Han to the mid-Tang (third to eighth century). See Brook, "Medievality and the Chinese Sense of History," 145–64; Knapp, "Did the Middle Kingdom Have a Middle Period?," 8–13; and Holcombe, "Was Medieval China Medieval?," 106–17.

28 Dien and Knapp, eds., *Cambridge History of China*, vol. 2.

29 Fan Xingzhun, *Zhongguo yixue shilüe*, 57–96.

30 Fan Ka-wai, *Dayi jingcheng*.

31 Nathan Sivin's early study of Sun Simiao's alchemy remains an important reference. See Sivin, *Chinese Alchemy*. For a recent survey of medicine in this period, see Fan Ka-wai, "Period of Division and the Tang Period," 65–96.

32 Fan Ka-wai, *Liuchao Sui-Tang yixue zhi chuancheng yu zhenghe*; Fan Ka-wai, *Dayi jingcheng*; Fan Ka-wai, *Zhonggu shiqi de yizhe yu bingzhe*.

33 Li Jianmin, *Lüxingzhe de shixue*; Lin, *Zhongguo zhonggu shiqi de zongjiao yu yiliao*; Lee Jen-der, *Nüren de Zhongguo yiliao shi*; Chen Hao, *Shenfen xushi yu zhishi biaoshu zhijian de yizhe zhi yi*.

34 Lo and Cullen, eds., *Medieval Chinese Medicine*; Chen Ming, *Shufang yiyao*; Despeux, ed., *Médecine, religion et société dans la Chine médiévale*; Chen Ming, *Zhonggu yiliao yu wailai wenhua*; Iwamoto, *Tōdai no iyakusho to Tonkō bunken*.

35 Unschuld, *Medicine in China*, 17–28; Harper, *Early Chinese Medical Literature*, 98–109.

36 My periodization is informed by Li Jianmin, *Lüxingzhe de shixue*, 33–94.

37 Studies on the Tang-Song transition are voluminous. Representative works are: Lau, "Hewei 'Tang-Song biange'?," 125–71; Bol, *Neo-Confucianism in History*; von Glahn, *Economic History of China*, 208–54; Tackett, *Origins of the Chinese Nation*.

38 This is the famous "Naitō hypothesis" advanced by the Japanese sinologist Naitō Konan in the early twentieth century. On the summary of the hypothesis and its influence, see Miyakawa, "Outline of the Naitō Hypothesis," 533–52; Smith and von Glahn, eds., *Song-Yuan-Ming Transition in Chinese History*; and Zhang Guangda, "Neiteng Hunan de Tang-Song biange shuo jiqi yingxiang," 5–71.

39 Goldschmidt, *Evolution of Chinese Medicine*; Hinrichs, *Shamans, Witchcraft, and Quarantine*; Lei, *Neither Donkey nor Horse*; Andrews, *Making of Modern Chinese Medicine*; Taylor, *Chinese Medicine in Early Communist China, 1945–1963*.

40 From a comparative perspective, the role of the state in regulating medicine was less pronounced in medieval Europe than it was in China during the same period. In the early medieval period (fifth to tenth century), monasteries were the major sites of the production for medical writings; in the late medieval period (eleventh to fifteenth century), universities took a leading role in generating scholarly works on medicine. See Siraisi, *Medieval and Early Renaissance Medicine*.

41 Goldschmidt, *Evolution of Chinese Medicine*, 19–136; Fan Ka-wai, *Beisong jiaozheng yishuju xintan*; Brown, *Art of Medicine in Early China*, 110–29.

42 For important studies of manuscript culture in medieval China, see Tian, *Tao Yuanming and Manuscript Culture*; Nugent, *Manifest in Words, Written on Paper*; Yu Xin, *Zhonggu yixiang*.

43 Lo and Cullen, *Medieval Chinese Medicine*; Despeux, *Médecine, religion et société dans la Chine médiévale*.

44 Unschuld, *Medicine in China*.

45 Pomata, "Observation Rising: Birth of an Epistemic Genre," 45–80.

46 An example of the former is Tao Hongjing's *Collected Annotations on the Classic of Materia Medica*. In his commentary, Tao offers elaborate explanations of drugs, often based on his own observations or other people's words. See Chen Yuanpeng, "*Bencao jing jizhu* suozai 'Taozhu' zhong de zhishi leixing," 184–212. An example of the latter is Wang Tao's *Arcane Essentials from the Imperial Library* (Waitai miyao fang, 752). In this text, Wang specifies the source of every formula, revealing his scholarly effort to compile medical information based on existing books. See Gao, *Waitai miyao fang congkao*, 906–55.

47 Zheng Jinsheng, *Yaolin waishi*, 96–99; Akahori, "Drug Taking and Immortality," 73–98.

48 Tambiah, *Magic, Science, Religion, and the Scope of Rationality*.

49 Yates, *Giordano Bruno and the Hermetic Tradition*; Webster, *Paracelsus*; Biller and Ziegler, eds., *Religion and Medicine in the Middle Ages*; Horden, "What's Wrong with Early Medieval Medicine?," 5–25.

50 There is a large body of literature that examines this topic. Of particular importance are Sivin, "On the Word 'Taoist' as a Source of Perplexity," 303–30; Strickmann, *Chinese Magical Medicine*; Lin, *Zhongguo zhonggu shiqi de zongjiao yu yiliao*; Stanley-Baker, "Daoists and Doctors"; and Salguero, *Translating Buddhist Medicine in Medieval China*.

51 Bynum, "Material Continuity, Personal Survival, and the Resurrection of the Body," 51–85; Duden, *Woman beneath the Skin*; Schipper, *Taoist Body*; Kuriyama, *Expressiveness of the Body and the Divergence of Greek and Chinese Medicine*.

52 Kieschnick, *Impact of Buddhism on Chinese Material Culture*; Copp, *Body Incantatory*; Steavu, "Paratextuality, Materiality, and Corporeality in Medieval Chinese Religions," 11–40.

53 A collection of anthropological studies offers insights into this issue. See Yu Shuenn-Der, ed., *Tiwu ruwei*.

54 For an excellent study of the irreducible physicality of the body in medieval Christianity, see Bynum, "Why All the Fuss about the Body?," 1–33.

CHAPTER 1: THE PARADOX OF *DU*

Epigraph: Liu An et al., *Huainanzi*, 9.292.

1 Sima, *Shiji*, 55.2037.

2 Mou, "Duyao kukou," 437–38.

3 On the previous discussions of the etymology of *du*, see Unschuld, "Zur Bedeutung des Terminus *tu* 毒," 165–83; Obringer, *L'aconit et l'orpiment*, 25–26; Shi Zhicheng, "Zhongguo gudai duzi jiqi xiangguan cihui kao," 1–9.

4 Xu Shen, *Shuowen jiezi*, 1b.15, 5b.111.

5   In an early study of *du*, the historian Yu Yan contends that the definition of "thickness" for *du* implies a negative sense of harmfulness. I interpret *hou* as a neutral word that could indicate either harm or benefit. See Yu Yan, "Duyao bian," 1–4.

6   This graph of *du* is the prevailing way of writing the character in excavated manuscripts from the Qin and Han periods. Information from the Multi-function Chinese Character Database (http://humanum.arts.cuhk.edu.hk/Lexis/lexi-mf /search.php?word=%E6%AF%92, accessed August 1, 2020).

7   Xu Shen, *Shuowen jiezi*, 1b.18. The earliest appearance of the character *fu* is in *The Book of Odes* (Shijing), which refers to an unsavory vegetable that one can eat to stave off starvation. See *Maoshi zhengyi*, 11.794.

8   Unschuld, "Zur Bedeutung des Terminus *tu* 毒," 169–70.

9   The English word "toxic" is derived from the Greek word *toxon*, which means "bow," or *toxikon*, which means "pertaining to a bow," indicating a similar involvement of poisons in hunting or warfare. See Stevenson, *Meaning of Poison*, 3–4. On the arguably earliest evidence of using poisons in hunting activities (24,000 years ago), see d'Errico et al., "Early Evidence of San Material Culture," 13214–19. On the military use of poisons in ancient China, see Bisset, "Arrow Poisons in China. Part I," 325–84.

10 Boltz, *Origin and Early Development of the Chinese Writing System*.

11 Gu Yewang, *Songben yupian*, 25.467.

12 I thank Constance Cook for sharing her unpublished research on reading the oracle bone graph of *du*. See her "Exorcism and the Spirit Turtle," forthcoming.

13 Xu Shen, *Shuowen jiezi*, 1b.24.

14 Nylan, *Five "Confucian" Classics*, 202–52.

15 *Zhouyi zhengyi*, 3.121; Shaughnessy, *I Ching*, 110–11, 146–47.

16 See Tōdō, *Kanji gogen jiten*, cited in Unschuld, "Zur Bedeutung des Terminus *tu* 毒," 166. The ancient pronunciations of *du* and *shu* are *[d]ˤuk and *[d]uk, respectively. Information acquired from the Baxter-Sagart reconstruction of Old Chinese (http://ocbaxtersagart.lsait.lsa.umich.edu/, accessed August 1, 2020). Relatedly, James Matisoff has interpreted the original meaning of *du* as "a pregnant woman revolted by food" (https://stedt.berkeley.edu/~stedt-cgi/rootcanal.pl /etymon/2202, accessed August 1, 2020). This interpretation, though, requires further evidence. I thank Laurent Sagart for bringing Matisoff's interpretation to my attention.

17 *Zhouyi zhengyi*, 2.60–61.

18 *Du* meaning "govern" only appears in the commentary section of *The Classic of Changes*, which is a later addition. This suggests that this meaning developed later, possibly during the Warring States period (476–221 BCE).

19 *Laozi jiaoshi*, 51.204.

20 Nylan, *Five "Confucian" Classics*, 168–201, esp. 182–85; Chin, *Zhongguo gudai de yixue, yishi yu zhengzhi*, 291–352.

21 *Zhouli zhushu*, 5.127.

22 *Zhouli zhushu*, 5.136–38.

23 *Zhouli zhushu*, 5.138–39.

24 Li Jianmin, *Huatuo yincang de shoushu*, 18–20.

25 *Huangdi neijing suwen jiaozhu*, 13.180. Other examples of this meaning of *duyao* can be found in 12.174–75, 25.353–55, 76.1142–43, and 77.1156–57.

26 *Huangdi neijing suwen jiaozhu*, 22.329–30.

27 Wang Chong, *Lunheng jiaoshi*, 66.949–60. A French translation of the chapter was rendered by Frédéric Obringer, in his *L'aconit et l'orpiment*, 275–83.

28 On the relationship between *du*, fire, and heat during the Han period, see Li Jianmin, *Lüxingzhe de shixue*, 112–15. Wang was not the first person who linked *du* to words. In a collection of excavated manuscripts dating to the third century BCE, we find a similar connection in a legal context, where powerful words are believed to disrupt social harmony. See Hulsewé, *Remnants of Ch'in Law*, 206–7.

29 Zheng Jinsheng, *Yaolin waishi*, 7–10.

30 Beck, *De Materia Medica*.

31 Liu An et al., *Huainanzi*, 19.629–30.

32 On the historical role of the sages in Han medical texts, see Chin, *Zhongguo gudai de yixue, yishi yu zhengzhi*, 56–70.

33 Ban, *Hanshu*, 12.359, 25b.1257–58. For important studies on the origins of the materia medica genre in China, see Yamada Keiji, "Hongzō no kigen," 454–73; and Liao Yuqun, *Qi Huang yidao*, 124–52.

34 Wang and Zhang, *"Shennong bencao jing" yanjiu*.

35 Unschuld, "Ma-wang-tui *Materia Medica*," 11–63; Harper, *Early Chinese Medical Literature*, 98–109.

36 Among ancient works on natural history in China, the third-century *Record of Comprehensive Things* (Bowu zhi) by Zhang Hua is particularly important. The text has been lost, but fragments of it, including a short section on drugs, are preserved in later sources. See Zhang Hua, *Bowu zhi jiaozheng*, 4.47–48.

37 Fuyang Hanjian Zhengli Zu, "Fuyang hanjian *Wanwu*," 36–47; Hu and Han, "*Wanwu* lüeshuo," 48–54; Li Ling, "Liandanshu de qiyuan he fushi zhuyou," 323–30.

38 Chin, *Zhongguo gudai de yixue, yishi yu zhengzhi*, 157–210; Brown, *Art of Medicine in Early China*, 89–109.

39 Ban, *Hanshu*, 30.1776–80.

40 The Han text has long been lost, but its content has been preserved in later materia medica sources, based on which a number of modern reconstructions have been produced. In my analysis, I rely on Shang Zhijun's edition to examine the text.

41 *Shennong bencao jing jiaozhu*, 1.1–3. The translation is mine in consultation with Unschuld, *Medicine in China*, 19; Lloyd and Sivin, *Way and the Word*, 232–33; and Wilms, *Divine Farmer's Classic of Materia Medica*, 2–3.

42 *Huangdi neijing suwen jiaozhu*, 2.31–32.

43 Kohn, ed., *Taoist Meditation and Longevity Techniques*; Sakade, ed., *Chūgoku kodai yōjō shisō no sōgōteki kenkyū*.

44 I must point out that the classification of drugs based on their *du* is not absolute in *The Divine Farmer's Classic*. For example, there are some *du*-possessing drugs

in the top group, which I will examine in part III. In addition, many top-level drugs, in addition to their life-enhancement properties, can also cure sickness. However, rarely can we find an example in the text where a bottom-level drug can promote longevity. In other words, top-level drugs tend to be versatile, while those at the bottom are more restricted to treating illness.

45 *Huangdi neijing suwen jiaozhu*, 5.82–91. Viscera as defined in Chinese medicine cannot be reduced to anatomical organs in modern biomedicine but are functional units that act in concert in the body. Because of this, I capitalize the organ names in English to signal this difference. See Sivin, *Traditional Medicine in Contemporary China*, 124–33.

46 Scholars hold different views on this point. Some believe that, in order to maintain consistency between the preface and the rest of the text, the *du* status of each drug is specified in *The Divine Farmer's Classic*. Others have contended instead that this information was added later. These scholars point to a strong piece of evidence from a commentary text to buttress their claim (more on this in the following section). Moreover, there are other characteristics of drugs that are outlined in the preface but not specified in the main text. I am thus inclined to agree with the view that the definition of *du* for each drug is a later addition. See *Shennong bencao jing jizhu*, 609–11; and *Shennong bencao jing jiaozhu*, 1–8.

47 Li Jianmin, *Lüxingzhe de shixue*, 33–94; Fan Ka-wai, *Liuchao Sui-Tang yixue zhi chuancheng yu zhenghe*, 96–108.

48 Lin, *Zhongguo zhonggu shiqi de zongjiao yu yiliao*; Salguero, *Translating Buddhist Medicine in Medieval China*; Pregadio, *Great Clarity*.

49 Tao, *Bencao jing jizhu*, 1.30. *Fan* in the title likely refers to Fan Wang, a fourth-century officer of the Eastern Jin who excelled at medicine. See Fan Xingzhun, *Zhongguo yixue shilüe*, 59.

50 Wei Zheng et al., *Suishu*, 34.1040–50. For Tao Hongjing's biography, see Yao Silian, *Liangshu*, 51.742–43; Li Yanshou, *Nanshi*, 76.1897–1900; and Wang Jiakui, *Tao Hongjing congkao*, 313–76.

51 Tao, *Bencao jing jizhu*, 1.1–6.

52 Liao Yuqun, "Kaoding *Mingyi bielu* jiqi yu Tao Hongjing zhushu de guanxi," 261–69.

53 The specification of the *du* status for individual drugs is already seen in the third-century *Materia Medica of Wu Pu* (Wu Pu bencao), which is extant only in fragments. Unlike *Collected Annotations*, the book simply juxtaposes accounts on each drug from disparate sources without a synthesis. See Wu, *Wu Pu bencao*.

54 Chen Hao, *Shenfen xushi yu zhishi biaoshu zhijian de yizhe zhi yi*, 97.

55 Iwamoto, *Tōdai no iyakusho to Tonkō bunken*, 83–86.

56 It is also possible, based on Iwamoto Atsushi's research, that the Tang court modified Tao's writing system when they copied his work, making the precise recovery of Tao's original text impossible. See Iwamoto, *Tōdai no iyakusho to Tonkō bunken*, 85–86.

57 The earliest complete text of materia medica that is still extant to us is the *Materia Medica Prepared for Emergency, Verified and Classified from the Classics and*

Histories (*Jingshi zhenglei beiji bencao*, eleventh century, often abbreviated as *Zhenglei bencao*), compiled by Tang Shenwei during the Northern Song dynasty. This is the text that modern scholars have used to reconstruct the whole texts of *The Divine Farmer's Classic* and *Collected Annotations*.

58   Tao, *Bencao jing jizhu*, 1.3.

59   Tao, *Bencao jing jizhu*, 1.6; Mayanagi, "Three *Juan* Edition of *Bencao jizhu* and Excavated Sources," 306–21.

60   The second-century scholar Zheng Xuan, in his commentary to the ancient text *Rites of Zhou*, defines five types of drugs based on their natural category (herbs, trees, worms, stones, and grains). See *Zhouli zhushu*, 5.132. Scholars have offered various explanations for Tao's novel organization of drugs, including Indian influence, possibly facilitated by the transmission of Buddhism (Liao Yuqun, "Yindu gudai yaowu fenleifa jiqi keneng dui zhongguo yixue chansheng de yingxiang," 56–63), and influence from Confucian writings where "natural categories" are invoked to assist political governance and offer moral guidance (Yamada Keiji, *Honzō to yume to renkinjutsu to*, 67–72). To understand Tao's organizational scheme, it is also necessary to align this medical text with his Daoist writings. Tao seems fascinated with the number seven: both of his Daoist works, *Declarations of the Perfected* and *Secret Instructions for Ascending for Perfection*, contain seven scrolls. He claims that this organization corresponds to the seven stars of the Northern Dipper (aka the Big Dipper) that guide earthly patterns. Worshipping the Northern Dipper was an important Daoist ritual in premodern China. The numerological significance of seven in *Collected Annotations* is thus consistent with the cosmological thinking that undergirds his Daoist works. See Tao, *Zhen'gao* (HY 1016), 19.3a; and Mollier, *Buddhism and Taoism Face to Face*, 134–73.

61   This calculation does not include the 178 drugs that "have names but are not used anymore" and the 81 drugs whose *du* statuses are not specified. Out of the 108 *du*-possessing drugs, 23 are new in *Collected Annotations*. From a comparative perspective, among major pharmacological treatises produced in Greek antiquity, about 10 percent of the drugs are perceived to be toxic. See Touwaide, "Les poisons dans le monde antique et byzantin," 268.

62   The precise correspondence between the name of a drug in Chinese pharmacy and its modern referent is often difficult to identify due to the various, sometimes conflicting descriptions of the medicine across different sources. Throughout this book, I use either the common names in English to translate these substances when possible, or sometimes in the case of plants, the name of the genus instead of the species in order to leave some ambiguity granted by the sources. My identification of drugs is guided by Sivin, *Chinese Alchemy*, 272–94; Shiu-ying Hu, *Enumeration of Chinese Materia Medica*; and Wilms, *Divine Farmer's Classic of Materia Medica*.

63   Tao, *Bencao jing jizhu*, 2.130, 148–51, 154–55, 168, 175.

64   Tao, *Bencao jing jizhu*, 5.344. The "attached offspring" refers to the side tubers of the herb. See the more detailed discussion of aconite in chapter 2.

65 According to Frédéric Obringer's calculation, 10 percent of prescriptions in an eighth-century formula book use aconite. See Obringer, *L'aconit et l'orpiment*, 121–22.

66 Tao, *Bencao jing jizhu*, 5.327–29, 335–36, 354–55, 374.

67 Tao, *Bencao jing jizhu*, 6.441–42.

68 Tao, *Bencao jing jizhu*, 6.389.

69 Tao, *Bencao jing jizhu*, 6.449.

70 The idiom signals the use of a measure that appears to temporarily solve an urgent problem but actually leads to disasters. See Fan Ye, *Hou Hanshu*, 48.1616.

71 For a study of the *zhen* bird, see Mayanagi, "Chintori," 151–85. Could a bird's feathers be so poisonous? For a modern biological study, see Dumbacher et al., "Homobatrachotoxin in the Genus *Pitohui*," 799–801.

72 Tao, *Bencao jing jizhu*, 7.499; Li Hui-lin, "Origin and Use of Cannabis in Eastern Asia," 51–62.

73 Tao, *Bencao jing jizhu*, 7.510.

74 Liu An et al., *Huainanzi*, 9.291–95. A similar passage can be found in 10.319–22. On the use of medical discourse for political persuasion in ancient China, see Brown, *Art of Medicine in Early China*, 21–62.

75 Liu An et al., *Huainanzi*, 3.79–129.

CHAPTER 2: TRANSFORMING POISONS

Epigraph: Lü et al., *Lüshi chunqiu jishi*, 25.661.

1 Ban, *Hanshu*, 97a.3966.

2 On this division, see Latour, *We Have Never Been Modern*; on the perception of nature in the East Asian context, see Vogel and Dux, *Concepts of Nature*; and Marcon, *Knowledge of Nature and the Nature of Knowledge*, 16–21.

3 Arnold, *Colonizing the Body*; Lei, *Neither Donkey nor Horse*.

4 The quote is from Paracelsus's *Seven Defensiones*, III, cited in Gibbs, *Poison, Medicine, and Disease in Late Medieval and Early Modern Europe*, 201. For a collection of essays on this topic in European history, see Grell, Cunningham, and Arriza-balaga, eds., *"It All Depends on the Dose."*

5 *Shennong bencao jing jiaozhu*, 1.8.

6 Tao, *Bencao jing jizhu*, 1.19–20.

7 Tao, *Bencao jing jizhu*, 1.36–37. On the change of weight systems from the Han period to the Era of Division, see Guo, *San zhi shisi shiji Zhongguo de quanheng duliang*, 103–17.

8 Tao, *Bencao jing jizhu*, 1.53. One *fen* in Tao's time was equivalent to about 3.5 grams. See Guo, *San zhi shisi shiji Zhongguo de quanheng duliang*, 115.

9 Tao, *Bencao jing jizhu*, 5.374. Other examples in this category include "hemp seed" (*mafen*, cannabis) and "cloud fruit" (*yunshi*, Mysore thorn). See 3.247–48 and 7.499–500 in the same book. On hallucinogenic drugs in classical Chinese pharmacy, see Ishida, "Genkiyaku kō," 38–57.

10 Tao, *Bencao jing jizhu*, 6.450–52; 7.471–72; 7.515–16.

11 Tao, *Bencao jing jizhu*, 1.80–88.

12 *Shennong bencao jing jiaozhu*, 1.3–4.

13 Chin, *Zhongguo gudai de yixue, yishi yu zhengzhi*.

14 Lloyd and Sivin, *Way and the Word*, 188–238.

15 *Huangdi neijing suwen jiaozhu*, 8.128–30.

16 *Shennong bencao jing jiaozhu*, 1.4–5.

17 Puett, "Ethics of Responding Properly," 37–68.

18 Tao, *Bencao jing jizhu*, 1.93–125. Besides *The Divine Farmer's Classic*, Tao also consulted a treatise dedicated to drug combinations titled *Drug Correspondences* (Yaodui) to compile this list.

19 Tao, *Bencao jing jizhu*, 1.113.

20 Tao, *Bencao jing jizhu*, 1.11.

21 Tao, *Bencao jing jizhu*, 1.11.

22 On the discussion of dragon's bone, which probably refers to fossilized animal bones, see Nappi, *Monkey and the Inkpot*, 50–68.

23 "Barbarian powder" likely refers to white lead. See Sivin, *Chinese Alchemy*, 278.

24 Tao, *Bencao jing jizhu*, 1.94.

25 Tao, *Bencao jing jizhu*, 1.11.

26 Tao, *Bencao jing jizhu*, 1.80–88.

27 *Shennong bencao jing jiaozhu*, 1.6–7.

28 Tao, *Bencao jing jizhu*, 1.90–93.

29 Being deficient (*xu*) and replete (*shi*) are two opposing states of the body conceived of in Chinese medicine. See Kuriyama, *Expressiveness of the Body and the Divergence of Greek and Chinese Medicine*, 217–31.

30 Tao, *Bencao jing jizhu*, 1.20–21.

31 A different term with the same pronunciation, *paozhi* (roast to restrain), is commonly found in modern pharmaceutical writings in China. This term only started to appear in twelfth-century texts, then gradually became the dominant phrase to designate drug processing. See Zheng Jinsheng, *Yaolin waishi*, 174.

32 Xu Shen, *Shuowen jiezi*, 10a.208, 10b.212.

33 *Maoshi zhengyi*, 15.1095–99.

34 *Maoshi zhengyi*, 15.1098–99. There is a third character in the poem, *fan*, which refers to the roasting of dry meat.

35 *Liji zhengyi*, 28.997.

36 On culinary culture in early China, see Sterckx, *Food, Sacrifice, and Sagehood in Early China*, 49–82; on the intimate relationship between food and medicine in premodern China, see Lo, "Pleasure, Prohibition, and Pain: Food and Medicine in Traditional China," 163–85.

37 *Shennong bencao jing jiaozhu*, 1.5–6.

38 Tao, *Bencao jing jizhu*, 1.39–54.

39 The word *jin*, for example, could refer to a variety of plants not restricted to aconite. See Obringer, *L'aconit et l'orpiment*, 94–99.

40 Obringer, *L'aconit et l'orpiment*, 119–30. On the cultural history of aconite in pre-modern China, see Wei Bing, "Cong *Zhangming xian fuzi ji* kan Songdai shidafu dui fuzi de renshi," 310–22; and Yu Xin, *Zhonggu yixiang*, 189–216.

41 Obringer, *L'aconit et l'orpiment*, 105–6, 139–43.

42 Bisset, "Arrow Poisons in China. Part II," 247–336.

43 Harper, *Early Chinese Medical Literature*, 105. *Wuhui*, which literally means "black beak," refers to the main tubers of aconite with a split, resembling a bird's bill. See Tao, *Bencao jing jizhu*, 5.343.

44 Harper, *Early Chinese Medical Literature*, 352–53. The use of aconite for speedy travel is also recorded in *Ten Thousand Things* (Wanwu), excavated from Shuang-gudui (ca. 165 BCE), in which it is claimed that the ingestion of the plant enables both humans and horses to run fast. See Fuyang Hanjian Zhengli Zu, "Fuyang han-jian *Wanwu*," 38, 39.

45 "Cold damage" (*shanghan*), a disease category originating during the Eastern Han period, refers to a set of acute, severe, and often infectious conditions character-ized by fever. See Mitchell, Ye, and Wiseman, *Shang Han Lun*, 9–19.

46 Yang and Brown, "Wuwei Medical Manuscripts," 241–301. On the formulas includ-ing aconite, see 258, 259, 260, 265, 274, 279, 280, 283–84, 286, 288, 291–92, 293–94, 296–97, 298, and 299.

47 Shi You, *Jijiu pian*, 4.276–77.

48 This estimation is based on a list of commodities with their prices from the Juyan manuscripts (Yu Xin, *Zhonggu yixiang*, 201). Silk was affordable during the Han period, as it was used as a common writing material (Tsien, *Written on Bamboo and Silk*, 130).

49 *Shennong bencao jing jiaozhu*, 1.8. The cold and hot maladies refer to those pathological conditions with typical symptoms of chilling and heating sensa-tions, respectively. This principle of opposites, of course, is not unique to Chinese medicine; a wide variety of healing traditions around the world rely on it to treat illnesses. See Anderson, "'Heating' and 'Cooling' Foods in Hong Kong and Tai-wan," 237–68; and Messer, "Hot/Cold Classifications and Balancing Actions in Mesoamerican Diet and Health," 149–67.

50 *Shennong bencao jing jiaozhu*, 4.205–6. Several other warming drugs, including cinnamon, Sichuan pepper, and ginger, also appear frequently in Han medical formulas. See Yang and Brown, "Wuwei Medical Manuscripts," 241–301.

51 I will explore this issue further in chapter 7.

52 For an excellent study of this murder, see Li Jianmin, *Lüxingzhe de shixue*, 285–324.

53 For example, see Harper, *Early Chinese Medical Literature*, 226, 237, 274, 288, and 297; and Yang and Brown, "Wuwei Medical Manuscripts," 258, 265, and 280. On pharmaceutical techniques during the Han period, see Zheng Jinsheng, *Yaolin waishi*, 178–85.

54 Shang, "*Leigong paozhi lun* youguan wenxian yanjiu," 139–43.

55 Zheng et al., eds., *Dictionary of the Ben Cao Gang Mu*, vol. 3, 254, 256.

56 Although refined arsenic (arsenic trioxide) was one of the most frequently used poisons in late imperial China, it appeared in materia medica writings starting in the tenth century. See Obringer, "Song Innovation in Pharmacotherapy," 197.

57 The original *Treatise on Drug Processing* has long been lost, but sections of it have been preserved in the eleventh-century pharmacological work *Zhenglei bencao*, allowing for reconstruction.

58 "The southern ground of *wu*" (*wudi*) could be a reference to "evading stems" (*dunjia*), a divination system based on the spatial-temporal correspondence between the trigrams from *The Classic of Changes* and the sexagenary cycle. In this system, *wu* corresponds to the direction of due south, so the ground of *wu* could refer to the southern section of the ground in a house. On *dunjia*, see DeWoskin, *Doctors, Diviners, and Magicians of Ancient China*, 25.

59 *Leigong paozhi lun*, 2.58–59.

60 Fan Ye, *Hou Hanshu*, 94.3110–11.

61 Pregadio, *Great Clarity*, 95–96, 99.

62 Fan Ye, *Hou Hanshu*, 83.2770–71.

63 Fan Ye, *Hou Hanshu*, 83.2770, 2777.

64 Fan Ye, *Hou Hanshu*, 82.2745–46.

65 Fan Ye, *Hou Hanshu*, 82.2719.

66 Fan Ye, *Hou Hanshu*, 82.2743–45.

67 The meaning of *fangshi* is subject to multiple interpretations. The term has been variously translated as "masters of methods," "recipe gentlemen," and "technicians," among others. In the eyes of Han literati, they sometimes appeared to be "quacks," especially when they tried to use their occult arts to gain imperial favor and posed a threat to established orders. But this is not always the case, as Han texts also portray them, especially those with no political ambitions, as talented masters with extraordinary faculties. Due to the historical complexity of the term, I leave it untranslated in this book. On the issue of *fangshi*, see DeWoskin, *Doctors, Diviners, and Magicians*; Sivin, "Taoism and Science," ch. VII, 27–30; Harper, *Early Chinese Medical Literature*, 50–54; and Csikszentmihalyi, "Fangshi," 406–9.

68 DeWoskin, *Doctors, Diviners, and Magicians*, 17–22.

69 Shangdang is a region in the northwest (in present-day Shanxi). Tao considered ginseng grown in that area to be of the highest quality, better than that produced from the two Korean kingdoms of Baekje and Goguryeo. Yet people during his time erroneously valued the latter two types more. See Tao, *Bencao jing jizhu*, 3.207–8.

70 Huayin is a region in the northwest (in present-day Shaanxi). Tao considered asarum produced from that area to be one of the best kinds for medicine. See Tao, *Bencao jing jizhu*, 3.220.

71 Tao, *Bencao jing jizhu*, 1.32–35.

72 *Leigong paozhi lun*, 3.101–2.

73 Tao, *Bencao jing jizhu*, 1.33.

74 Mantis eggshells found on the branches of mulberry trees were considered the best, as they could absorb *qi* of the sap from the trees. Tao, *Bencao jing jizhu*, 6.430.

75 Centipedes with red heads and legs were considered the best for medicine. Tao, *Bencao jing jizhu*, 6.442.

76 Tao, *Bencao jing jizhu*, 2.132; 3.253; 4.311; 5.358, 359; 6.443.

77 Tao, *Bencao jing jizhu*, 3.197, 198, 202, 242, 254; 4.292, 320; 5.372; 6.430, 449.

78 Hibino, "Tō Kōkei no *Honzō shūchū* ni kansuru itsu kōsatsu," 1–20; Chen Yuanpeng, "*Bencao jing jizhu* suozai 'Taozhu' zhong de zhishi leixing," 184–212.

79 Tao, *Bencao jing jizhu*, 1.30.

80 For the studies of Xu Zhicai and the influential Xu medical clan, see Fan Ka-wai, *Zhonggu shiqi de yizhe yu bingzhe*, 70–91; Iwamoto, *Tōdai no iyakusho to Tonkō bunken*, 51–77; and Chen Hao, *Shenfen xushi yu zhishi biaoshu zhijian de yizhe zhi yi*, 87–130.

81 Xu Zhicai, *Leigong yaodui*, 1.1.

82 Weatherall, "Drug Therapies," 915–38.

83 Deleuze and Guattari, *Thousand Plateaus*, 282–86. For an excellent study of the concept of "drug assemblage" and its implications in contemporary drug culture, see Fuenzalida, "Pharmakontologies."

CHAPTER 3: FIGHTING POISON WITH POISON

Epigraphs: Soushen houji, 6.47; Wei Zheng et al., *Suishu*, 79.1791.

1 *Soushen houji*, 6.42–43.

2 *Shennong bencao jing jiaozhu*, 1.8.

3 Poo, "The Concept of Ghost in Ancient Chinese Religion," 173–91.

4 Xu Shen, *Shuowen jiezi*, 11a.233.

5 Liu Xi, *Shiming*, 4.885b.

6 Li Jianmin, "Contagion and Its Consequences," 201–22.

7 Ge, *Buji zhouhou fang*, 1.24–26. Earlier scholars have tried to draw a correspondence between demonic infestation and a disease in modern biomedicine, for example, by identifying it as tuberculosis (Yu Yan, *Gudai jibing minghou shuyi*, 223; Fan Xinzhun, *Zhongguo bingshi xinyi*, 96–99). More recently, scholars have shifted to examining demonic influence as part of the cultural fabric of premodern China without flattening the illness to fit it into a modern disease category (Sivin, *Chinese Alchemy*, 297; Li Jianmin, "They Shall Expel Demons," 1132–47). I adopt the approach of the latter group in exploring the rich and changing meanings of demonic infestation in its own cultural milieu. For an exemplary historical study of the disease foot *qi* in Chinese medicine's own framework, see Hilary Smith, *Forgotten Disease*.

8 Harper, "Chinese Demonography of the Third Century B.C.," 459–98.

9 On detailed studies of *zhu* in the grave-quelling writs, see Chen Hao, *Ji zhi cheng shang*, 181–220; and Chen Liang, "Donghan zhenmu wen suojian daowu guanxi de zai sikao," 44–71.

10 Strickmann, *Chinese Magical Medicine*, 58–88; Mollier, "Visions of Evil," 74–100; Lin, *Zhongguo zhonggu shiqi de zongjiao yu yiliao*, 29–84.

11 Yoshikawa, "Seishitsu kō," 125–62; Kleeman, *Celestial Masters*, 222–28.

12 Nickerson, "Great Petition for Sepulchral Plaints," 230–74.

13 This is *The Scripture of Divine Incantations of the Abyssal Caverns* (Taishang dongyuan shenzhou jing), HY 335. On the studies of this Daoist text, see Mollier, *Une apocalypse taoïste du Ve siècle*; Lee Fong-mao, "*Daozang* suoshou zaoqi daoshu de wenyi guan," 417–54.

14 HY 335, 9.1a.

15 HY 335, 8.2b; 11.9a. Another telling example is *nüqing*, a potent herb of the *Paederia* genus that, based on the materia medica literature, could kill demons and avert epidemics. It also appears in the title of a fourth-century Daoist text of demonology, *Demon Statutes of Nüqing* (Nüqing guilü, HY 790), revealing a strong link between poisons and demons. See Strickmann, *Chinese Magical Medicine*, 80–88.

16 Tao Hongjing briefly discussed this etiological model in his *Collected Annotations*. See Tao, *Bencao jing jizhu*, 15–18; and Li Jianmin, "They Shall Expel Demons," 1146–47.

17 Li Linfu et al., *Tang liudian*, 14.410.

18 Despeux, "Gymnastics," 223–61; Kohn, *Chinese Healing Exercises*; Ding, *Zhubing yuanhou lun yangsheng fang daoyin fa yanjiu*.

19 Dolly Yang, "Prescribing 'Guiding and Pulling.'"

20 Chao et al., *Zhubing yuanhou lun jiaozhu*, 24.696–97.

21 This interpretation is based on the fact that the character *zhu* 注 (to pour) is a homonym of the character *zhu* 住 (to reside).

22 Chao et al., *Zhubing yuanhou lun jiaozhu*, 23.669–70.

23 Unschuld, *Huang Di nei jing su wen*, 149–67.

24 Dolly Yang, "Prescribing 'Guiding and Pulling,'" 301–14.

25 Sun, *Beiji qianjin yaofang jiaoshi*, 17.612–20.

26 Sun, *Beiji qianjin yaofang jiaoshi*, 17.615. The Great One (Taiyi) is the name of a deity in the Daoist pantheon. See Andersen, "Taiyi," 956–59.

27 Sun, *Beiji qianjin yaofang jiaoshi*, 17.614–15. Golden teeth (*jinya*) refers to a mineral drug that has a golden color and is about the size of chess pieces (Tao, *Bencao jing jizhu*, 2.179). It is the first of the forty-five ingredients listed in the formula.

28 Kuriyama, "Epidemics, Weather, and Contagion," 3–22; Zhang Zhibin, *Zhongguo gudai yibing liuxing nianbiao*.

29 Lin, *Zhongguo zhonggu shiqi de zongjiao yu yiliao*, 29–85.

30 Sun, *Beiji qianjin yaofang jiaoshi*, 9.340.

31 Barrett, "Climate Change and Religious Response," 139–56.

32 Mollier, *Une apocalypse taoïste du Ve siècle*.

33 Li Linfu et al., *Tang liudian*, 14.334–35.

34 Besides demonic infestation, which is the focus of my analysis, other major types of contagious disorders include "epidemic pestilence" (*yili*), "seasonal *qi*" (*shiqi*), "warm illness" (*wenbing*), and "cold damage" (*shanghan*). For an extensive analysis of these disorders in Chao's work, see (Chang Chia-Feng), "'Jiyi' yu 'xiangran,'" 157–99.

35 On the discussion of epidemics in Chinese medicine in late imperial China, see Hanson, *Speaking of Epidemics in Chinese Medicine*.

36 Shirakawa, "Biko kankei jisetsu," 458–76; Obringer, *L'aconit et l'orpiment*, 226–28.

37 *Chunqiu zuozhuan zhengyi*, 41.1343–44. For a detailed study of this story, see Brown, *Art of Medicine in Early China*, 21–40.

38 *Chunqiu zuozhuan zhengyi*, 41.1340–43.

39 *Zhouyi zhengyi*, 3.108–11; Xing, "Hexagram *Gu*," 20–21.

40 The link between *gu* and female seduction in early China is also visible in a fourth-century BCE divination text. See Cook, "Fatal Case of *Gu* 蠱 Poisoning in Fourth-Century BC China?," 123–49. We should note that the passage in *Zuo Commentary* is He's interpretation of *gu*, not what *The Classic of Changes* says. On the contrary, the divination text reads the sign of *gu* as a favorable condition in which it is suitable to cross a great river.

41 Wind and worms are etymologically related—the character for wind (*feng*) contains the basic element of the character for worms (*chong*). In a first-century dictionary, the entry for wind explains that "once wind moves, vermin come into being." Xu Shen, *Shuowen jiezi*, 13b.284.

42 Xu Shen, *Shuowen jiezi*, 13b.284.

43 Fèvre, "Drôles de bestioles," 57–65; Liu Pao-line, "Yi chong wei xiang."

44 Gan Bao, *Xinjiao soushen ji*, 12.95–96.

45 *Soushen houji*, 2.12–13.

46 For a brief summary, see Fan Ka-wai, "Han-Tang jian zhi gudu," 1–23.

47 Chao et al., *Zhubing yuanhou lun jiaozhu*, 25.716–17.

48 Chao et al., *Zhubing yuanhou lun jiaozhu*, 25.717–18.

49 Zhang Zhuo, *Chaoye qianzai*, 6.158.

50 Sun, *Sun zhenren qianjin fang*, 25.420–25.

51 Sun, *Sun zhenren qianjin fang*, 26.451.

52 On the connection between poison and the heating power of yang, see Obringer, *L'aconit et l'orpiment*, 244; and Li Jianmin, "They Shall Expel Demons," 1120–22.

53 Unschuld, *Medicine in China*, 50–52.

54 Chen Cangqi, *Bencao shiyi jishi*, 6.242–43.

55 The pioneering studies of this aspect of *gu* are de Groot, *Religious System of China*, 826–69; and Feng and Shryock, "Black Magic in China Known as *Ku*," 1–30.

56 Ban, *Hanshu*, 63.2742–45.

57 Loewe, "Case of Witchcraft in 91 B.C.," 159–96; Poo, "Wugu zhi huo de zhengzhi yiyi," 511–38; Cai, *Witchcraft and the Rise of the First Confucian Empire*.

58 "The sinister way" (*zuodao*) is an umbrella term that designates various types of black magic. See von Glahn, *Sinister Way*.

59 Wei Zheng et al., *Suishu*, 79.1790–91. A similar account can be found in Li Yanshou, *Beishi*, 61.2172–73. For previous studies of this episode, see Lu Xiangqian, "Wu Zetian 'weimao shuo' yu Suishi 'maogui zhi yu,'" 81–94; Li Ronghua, "Suidai 'wugu zhi shu' xintan," 78–81; and Doran, "Cat Demon, Gender, and Religious Practice," 689–707.

60 On the identification of *li* as a type of wild cat, see Barrett, *Religious Affiliations of the Chinese Cat*, 16–17, 25–27.

61 Chao et al., *Zhubing yuanhou lun jiaozhu*, 25.724.

62 Ito, *Chūgoku no shinjū, akkitachi*; Sterckx, *Animal and the Daemon in Early China*.

63 Barrett, *Religious Affiliations of the Chinese Cat*, 1–40; Barrett and Strange, "Walking by Itself," 84–98.

64 Liu Xu et al., *Jiu Tangshu*, 51.2170. For detailed studies of this episode, see Lu Xiangqian, "Wu Zetian 'weimao shuo' yu Suishi 'maogui zhi yu,'" 81–94; and Fu, "Wu Zetian 'weimao shuo' zaitan," 96–109.

65 Wei Zheng et al., *Suishu*, 79.1789–90; Lu Xiangqian, "Wu Zetian 'weimao shuo' yu Suishi 'maogui zhi yu,'" 87–88; Doran, "Cat Demon, Gender, and Religious Practice," 692–93.

66 Wei Zheng et al., *Suishu*, 48.1287–88.

67 Wei Zheng et al., *Suishu*, 2.43. Besides the cat demon, the edict also expelled families who were accused of practicing three other types of black magic: *gu* poison (*gudu*), sorcery (*yanmei*), and wild path (*yedao*). For detailed studies of them, see von Glahn, *Sinister Way*; Mollier, *Buddhism and Taoism Face to Face*, 55–99; and Li Jianmin, *Lüxingzhe de shixue*, 251–84.

68 Yang Xiu was a younger brother of the crown prince Yang Guang. I mentioned earlier that his implication in the witchcraft was the outcome of Yang Su's false accusation.

69 Zhang Zhuo, *Chaoye qianzai*, 1.26.

70 Zhangsun et al., *Tanglü shuyi qianjie*, 18.1299–1300; Chen Dengwu, *Cong renjianshi dao youmingjie*, 196–214.

71 Schafer, *Vermilion Bird*.

72 Wei Zheng et al., *Suishu*, 31.886–87.

73 On *gu*'s association with the south, see Fan Ka-wai, *Liuchao Sui-Tang yixue zhi chuancheng yu zhenghe*, 148–53; and Yu Gengzhe, *Tangdai jibing, yiliaoshi chutan*, 180–93.

74 This insight is from Barrett and Strange, "Walking by Itself," 87.

75 The literature on shamans in Chinese history is profuse. For representative studies, see Harper, *Early Chinese Medical Literature*, 173–83; Lin, "Image and Status of Shamans in Ancient China," 397–458; Sivin, *Health Care in Eleventh-Century China*, 93–128; and Hinrichs, *Shamans, Witchcraft, and Quarantine*.

76 The phrase first appeared in *The Record of Clouds and Mist Passing before One's Eyes* (Yunyan guoyan lu) by the Song scholar Zhou Mi (1232–1298). The text describes a foreign material called "Khottal rhino horn" (*guduo xi*), which the author identified as actually the horn of a snake. The substance was extremely poisonous but could also counteract poisons. The logic, the author reasoned, was to "use poison to attack poison." See Weitz, *Zhou Mi's "Record of Clouds and Mist Passing before One's Eyes,"* 82, 312. I am indebted to Fan Ka-wai for bringing this reference to my attention. On the development of this idea in the Buddhist context, see Chen Ming, *Zhonggu yiliao yu wailai wenhua*, 440.

77 Comparatively, we find a similar logic in homeopathy. Developed by the German physician Samuel Hahnemann (1755–1843), the therapy, based on the "principle of similars," uses the pathogenic agent diluted to infinitesimal amounts to cure the disease it causes. Although the rationale of homeopathy resembles that of the medical use of poisons in China, they are also substantially different: the latter

never involves ultrahigh dilutions of medicines, and the former is not about purging the body. See Jonas, Kaptchuk, and Linde, "Critical Overview of Homeopathy," 393–99.

78 Temkin, "Scientific Approach to Disease," 629–47; Rosenberg, *Explaining Epidemics and Other Studies in the History of Medicine*, 293–304.

79 Unschuld, "Traditional Chinese Medicine," 1023–29; Hinrichs, "Catchy Epidemic," 19–62.

80 The two models are not categorically distinct but often work in a linked and dynamic manner in Chinese medical traditions. For example, Chao Yuanfang, in his *On the Origins and Symptoms*, fuses the concept of demons with *qi*; that is, he uses demonic *qi* to explain a variety of maladies. This approach allows him to tie the ontological etiology to the physiology of the body as expounded by the ancient classics. For detailed analysis of the entanglement of the two models, see Yan Liu, "Words, Demons, and Illness," 1–29.

81 Diamond, "Miao and Poison," 1–25; Yu Gengzhe, *Tangdai jibing, yiliaoshi chutan*, 105–19; Hinrichs, *Shamans, Witchcraft, and Quarantine*.

82 Deng, *Zhongguo wugu kaocha*; Wang Ming-ke, "Nüren, bujie yu cunzhai rentong," 699–738.

CHAPTER 4: MEDICINES IN CIRCULATION

Epigraph: Su et al., *Xinxiu bencao*, 1.

1 Wang Pu, *Tang huiyao*, 82.1522–23.

2 The decline of the Tang regime was ushered in by the An Lushan Rebellion. Instigated from the north by the Tang general An Lushan in 755, it triggered a seven-year war that devastated the Tang empire. Although the revolt was eventually suppressed in 763, Tang power was subsequently weakened and decentralized. See Hansen, *Open Empire*, 201–34.

3 Fan Ye, *Hou Hanshu*, 116.3592; Brown, "'Medicine' in Early China," 459–72.

4 Chen Hao, *Shenfen xushi yu zhishi biaoshu zhijian de yizhe zhi yi*, 87–130.

5 Li Linfu et al., *Tang liudian*, 14.409; Miyashita, "Zui-Tō jidai no iryō," 259–88; Ren, "Tangdai de yiliao zuzhi yu yixue jiaoyu," 449–73; Needham, *Science and Civilisation in China*, vol. 6, pt. 6, *Medicine*, 98–105.

6 Iwamoto, *Tōdai no iyakusho to Tonkō bunken*, 60–69.

7 The Tang emperors often bestowed creams on their officials, who used them to protect their skin and enhance their complexion. See Fan Ka-wai, *Dayi jingcheng*, 125–29.

8 Li Linfu et al., *Tang liudian*, 11.324–25.

9 Li Linfu et al., *Tang liudian*, 26.667. The Tang princes lived in the Eastern Palace, a different site from the emperors' residence, and hence they were served by a separate medical office.

10 Li Linfu et al., *Tang liudian*, 11.324–25.

11 The document is preserved in the Pavilion of Heavenly One (Tianyi Ge) in Ningbo, a private library established in the sixteenth century. Previously thought

to be a Ming (1368–1644) text, it was rediscovered in 1998 to be part of a long-lost legal document titled *Ordinances of the Tiansheng Era* (Tiansheng ling) completed in 1029. Significantly, the document contains almost five hundred Tang ordinances dating to the eighth century, many of which are not seen in other extant sources. See Dai, "Tianyi Ge cang Ming chaoben *Guanpin ling* kao," 71–86.

12 Cheng, "Tang Yiji ling fuyuan yanjiu," 552–80.

13 Cheng, "Tang Yiji ling fuyuan yanjiu," 146, 579.

14 I interpret *huanfang* as an abbreviation for *gongren huanfang* (ward for the sick palace maids). The ward, established in the two capitals (Chang'an and Luoyang), offered medical services to the palace maids who were seriously ill. It had its own drug depot, as well as personnel dispatched by the Imperial Medical Office. See Ouyang Xiu, *Xin Tangshu*, 48.1244–45; and Ishino, "Tōdai ryōkyō no miyabito kanbō," 25–35. A different type of organization called "the ward of compassion field and recuperation" (*beitian yangbing fang*) or simply "the ward of recuperation" (*bingfang*) was established at the beginning of the eighth century. Based in Buddhist monasteries, they were state-organized charity sites that provided housing, food, and basic care for the elderly, invalids, and the poor. See Wang Pu, *Tang huiyao*, 49.862–63; and Liu Shu-fen, *Cibei qingjing*, 41–54.

15 The Gates Office (Mensi) was part of the palace guard system that inspected articles that either entered or exited the palace. See Li Linfu et al., *Tang liudian*, 25.640.

16 Zhangsun et al., *Tanglü shuyi qianjie*, 9.740–44.

17 Zhangsun et al., *Tanglü shuyi qianjie*, 26.1795–98.

18 Huo, "'Du' yu zhonggu shehui," 127–49.

19 Zhangsun et al., *Tanglü shuyi qianjie*, 18.1304–11.

20 Zhangsun et al., *Tanglü shuyi qianjie*, 18.1304.

21 Cheng, "Tang Yiji ling fuyuan yanjiu," 139, 573. Due to the lack of corroboration from other sources during the Tang period, the dating of this ordinance is not conclusive. Aconite was not on this list probably because it was frequently used as a medicine, much more so than the other two poisons (see chapter 2).

22 Li Linfu et al., *Tang liudian*, 14.392, 409–10.

23 The two capitals refer to the main capital of Chang'an in the west and the second capital of Luoyang in the east.

24 Cheng, "Tang Yiji ling fuyuan yanjiu," 145–46, 579.

25 *Shangshu zhengyi*, 6.158–205.

26 Cheng, "Tang Yiji ling fuyuan yanjiu," 145–46, 579; Ouyang Xiu, *Xin Tangshu*, 48.1244–45. For a comprehensive list of drugs with their locations in the early Tang period, see Sun, *Qianjin yifang*, 1.5–6; and Yu Gengzhe, *Tangdai jibing, yiliaoshi chutan*, 92–104.

27 Li Linfu et al., *Tang liudian*, 3.79.

28 Du, *Tongdian*, 6.112.

29 Huang Zhengjian, "Shilun Tangdai qianqi huangdi xiaofei de mouxie cemian," 173–211.

30 On a survey of these sources, see Wang Yongxing, "Tangdai tugong ziliao xinian," 60–65, 59. Early scholarship focuses on the symbolic function of these

tribute items (Hibino, "*Shin tōjo* chirishi no tokō nitsuite," 83–99) while more recent studies point out their practical uses (Yu Xin, *Zhonggu yixiang*, 267–93).

31 Du, *Tongdian*, 6.112–31. According to one modern scholar's research, these tribute items were collected between 742 and 755. See Wang Yongxing, "Tangdai tugong ziliao xinian," 62-63.

32 Huang Zhengjian, "Shilun Tangdai qianqi huangdi xiaofei de mouxie cemian," 176–88. The counting is slightly different from Huang's, based on my own analysis. The grouping of medicines and foods is by no means definitive, as it is often hard to distinguish them in premodern China.

33 Yan Qiyan, "Cong Tangdai gongpin yaocai kan Sichuan didao yaocai," 76–81.

34 Su et al., *Xinxiu bencao*, 15.363–65.

35 Su et al., *Xinxiu bencao*, 6.160–63, 8.203; Zhou Zuofeng, "*Tang liudian* jizai de tugong yaocai fenxi," 13–18.

36 Su et al., *Xinxiu bencao*, 5.142.

37 Su et al., *Xinxiu bencao*, 16.424–25.

38 Schafer, *Golden Peaches of Samarkand*, 192–93. Bovine bezoar was another costly product on the list that prompted many counterfeits on the market. See Su et al., *Xinxiu bencao*, 15.362–63.

39 Cheng, "Tang Yiji ling fuyuan yanjiu," 137–38, 578.

40 The work is often touted as the first pharmacopoeia in the world, which appeared eight centuries earlier than *The Nuremberg Pharmacopoeia* in Europe (1542). Yet it is important to note that the Tang text did not in and of itself impose legal regulation of drug prescription, as was evident in the European work. Rather, it functioned as a guidebook for the imperial collection and use of drugs. See Unschuld, *Medicine in China*, 47.

41 Fan Ka-wai, *Dayi jingcheng*, 81. During the Tang period, foot *qi* was a condition whose symptoms were swelling of the feet or the lower legs, perceived of as the result of a plump body. See Hilary Smith, *Forgotten Disease*, 43–65.

42 Su et al., *Xinxiu bencao* (Japan edition), 15.216–20. For a detailed study of these authors, see Wang, Zhang, and Yin, "*Xinxiu bencao* zuanxiu renyuan kao," 200–204; Fan Ka-wai, *Dayi jingcheng*, 78–85; and Chen Hao, *Shenfen xushi yu zhishi biaoshu zhijian de yizhe zhi yi*, 219–43.

43 Liu Xu et al., *Jiu Tangshu*, 47.2048.

44 Su et al., *Xinxiu bencao*, 1–10.

45 Dunhuang manuscript Kyōu 040R.

46 Similar to other early pharmacological texts in China, *Newly Revised Materia Medica* has long been lost to us, but its drug entries, together with a modified preface, have been preserved in Song materia medica texts thanks to the commentary tradition, allowing for the recovery of the Tang treatise. That being said, there are several manuscript fragments dating to the Tang period that contain sections of *Newly Revised Materia Medica*, among which the newly released one from the Kyōu Shōku Collection preserves a preface that is markedly different from the Song editions.

47	The term *jiaoli* 澆醨, in Fan Ka-wai's view, should be read as *yaoli* 堯離, which refers to the rule of Sage Yao in high antiquity, corresponding to the phase of Fire (*li*) in the dynastic cycle. Some Han scholars claimed that their dynasty matched the same propitious phase. Hence, I translate the term as "propitious fortune." See Chang Shu-hao, "Xihan 'yao hou huo de' shuo de chengli," 1–27. I thank Fan Ka-wai for suggesting this interpretation.

48	Zhou here refers to the dynasty of the Northern Zhou (557–581) that the Sui dynasty superseded. Certain Tang scholars, regarding the regimes of the Era of Division as unorthodox, traced the lineage of the Tang directly back to the orthodox rule of the Han dynasty. See Rao, *Zhongguo shixue shang zhi zhengtong lun*, 25–27.

49	Dunhuang manuscript Kyōu 040R, reprinted in *Tonkō hikyū*, vol. 1. The passage is incomplete, and in this reading, a gap is filled by the historian Iwamoto Atsushi based on a thirteenth-century Japanese medical work. See Iwamoto, *Tōdai no iyakusho to Tonkō bunken*, 102–15.

50	Tao, *Bencao jing jizhu*, 5.335–36.

51	*Taishang lingbao wufu xu* (HY 388), 2.19a. The practice of consuming *huangjing* to prolong life was popular among Daoist adepts and social elites from the Era of Division to the Tang period. See Fan Ka-wai, *Zhonggu shiqi de yizhe yu bingzhe*, 304–9; and Arthur, *Early Daoist Dietary Practices*, 115–16.

52	Su et al., *Xinxiu bencao*, 6.153–54, 10.253–55.

53	Su et al., *Xinxiu bencao*, 10.256–58.

54	Su et al., *Xinxiu bencao*, 10.260–61.

55	Su et al., *Xinxiu bencao*, 10.258–59.

56	Dunhuang manuscript Kyōu 040R.

57	Su et al., *Xinxiu bencao*, 8.219, 10.256.

58	Su et al., *Xinxiu bencao*, 11.291.

59	Barrett, *Woman Who Discovered Printing*, 84–98.

60	Wang Pu, *Tang huiyao*, 82.1805; Li Fang et al., *Taiping yulan*, 724.3338a. On a modern reconstruction of some of the formulas in *Guangji fang*, see Feng, *Gu fangshu jiyi*, 26–92.

61	We also see such practice in the Buddhist context. For example, a collection of formulas was carved on one of the Buddhist grottos in Longmen (in present-day Henan) in the mid-seventh century, likely for the same reason of making useful medical knowledge available to the public. See Zhang, Wang, and Stanley-Baker, "Earliest Stone Medical Inscription," 373–88; and Chen Hao, *Shenfen xushi yu zhishi biaoshu zhijian de yizhe zhi yi*, 269–300.

62	Wang Pu, *Tang huiyao*, 82.1522; Du, *Tongdian*, 33.915.

63	Dunhuang manuscript P. 3714. On the dating of this manuscript, see Lu Xiangqian, "Boxihe sanqiyisi hao beimian chuanmafang wenshu yanjiu," 671–74.

64	Su et al., *Xinxiu bencao* (Japan edition), 15.220. This copy is incomplete, containing ten scrolls only.

65	For a general introduction to the Dunhuang manuscripts, see Rong, *Eighteen Lectures on Dunhuang*.

66 *Dunhuang yiyao wenxian jijiao*; Lo and Cullen, eds., *Medieval Chinese Medicine*;
    Despeux, ed., *Médecine, religion et société dans la Chine médiévale*.
67 Dunhuang manuscript Kyōu 040R.
68 Dunhuang manuscript P. 3714.
69 Dunhuang manuscripts S. 4534 and S. 9434.
70 *Dunhuang yiyao wenxian jijiao*, 653–58; Despeux, *Médecine, religion et société
    dans la Chine médiévale*, 211–13.
71 Baums, "Inventing the *Pothi*," 343–62.
72 Iwamoto, *Tōdai no iyakusho to Tonkō bunken*, 169–74.
73 It is possible that these non-native plants were transplanted in Dunhuang for local
    consumption, but direct evidence is lacking.
74 The plant is simply called *su* (betony) in the standard edition of *Newly Revised Mate-
    ria Medica*. See Su et al., *Xinxiu bencao*, 18.469.
75 Substitution was particularly common with the use of potent drugs in Dunhuang.
    For example, gelsemium (*yege*), a highly potent herb that was forbidden by the
    Tang court to circulate among the population, was replaced by phytolacca
    (*danglu*), an herb with similar medical uses but locally available. See P. 3731.
76 Zheng and Dang, "Tangdai Dunhuang sengyi kao," 31–46; Zheng and Gao, "Cong
    Dunhuang wenshu kan Tang-Wudai Dunhuang diqu de yishi zhuangkuang,"
    68–73; Chen Ming, *Dunhuang de yiliao yu shehui*, 59–73.
77 Iwamoto, *Tōdai no iyakusho to Tonkō bunken*, 181–86; Engelhardt, "Dietetics in Tang
    China and the First Extant Works of *Materia Dietetica*," 173–91.
78 The five pungent vegetables are large garlic (*dasuan*), Chinese onion (*caocong*), scal-
    lion (*cicong*), small garlic (*lancong*), and asafetida (*xingqu*). See P. 3777 and P. 3244.
79 On alcohol consumption in Buddhist monasteries, see Liu Shu-fen, *Zhonggu de
    fojiao yu shehui*, 398–435.
80 Fujieda, "Tunhuang Manuscripts: A General Description (Part I)," 1–32; Fujieda,
    "Tunhuang Manuscripts: A General Description (Part II)," 17–39.
81 On a close study of a Dunhuang manuscript in motion, see van Schaik and Galam-
    bos, *Manuscripts and Travellers*.
82 Li Linfu et al., *Tang liudian*, 11.324–25, 14.408–9.
83 Hinrichs, "Governance through Medical Texts and the Role of Print," 217–38; Hin-
    richs, *Shamans, Witchcraft, and Quarantine*.
84 This phenomenon, of course, is not limited to medical manuscripts. For studies of
    manuscript culture in Chinese literature, see Tian, *Tao Yuanming & Manuscript
    Culture*; and Nugent, *Manifest in Words, Written on Paper*.

CHAPTER 5: MEDICINES IN PRACTICE

Epigraph: Sun, *Sun Zhenren qianjin fang*, 12.202.
1 Sun, *Sun Zhenren qianjin fang*, 12.199–202.
2 Farquhar, *Knowing Practice*; Sivin, "Text and Experience in Classical Chinese Medi-
    cine," 195–98; Li Jianmin, *Lüxingzhe de shixue*, 67–91.

3   Lei, "How Did Chinese Medicine Become Experiential?," 334. In this sense, the term carries a meaning similar to *experientia*, the Latin root of the English word "experience." *Experientia* refers to "a trial, proof, experiment; knowledge gained by repeated trials." Information extracted from Online Etymology Dictionary (www.etymonline.com).

4   Prior to the Song dynasty, the term appears in a collection of miracle tales (fifth or sixth century) and denotes the efficacy of divination techniques. See *Soushen houji*, 2.15–16.

5   Wei Zheng et al., *Suishu*, 34.1042–46; Liu Xu et al., *Jiu Tangshu*, 47.2049–50; Ouyang Xiu, *Xin Tangshu*, 59.1567–73.

6   This genre initially appeared in governmental archives during the Han dynasty, fell out of fashion in the medieval period except a brief revival in the twelfth century, and started to proliferate from the sixteenth century on. See Cullen, "*Yi'an* 醫案 (Case Statements)," 297–323; Grant, *Chinese Physician*; Furth, "Producing Medical Knowledge through Cases," 125–51; and Goldschmidt, "Reasoning with Cases," 19–51.

7   Ban, *Hanshu*, 30.1777–78.

8   Harper, *Early Chinese Medical Literature*, 221–304.

9   Yang and Brown, "Wuwei Medical Manuscripts," 241–301.

10 Fan Ka-wai, *Liuchao suitang yixue zhi chuancheng yu zhenghe*.

11 Wei Zheng et al., *Suishu*, 34.1040–50.

12 Fan Ka-wai, *Zhonggu shiqi de yizhe yu bingzhe*, 70–91.

13 Wei Zheng et al., *Suishu*, 34.1050; Liu Xu et al., *Jiu Tangshu*, 47.2049.

14 Cheng, "Tang Yiji ling fuyuan yanjiu," 137, 578; Fan Ka-wai, *Zhonggu shiqi de yizhe yu bingzhe*, 190–93.

15 Wei Zheng et al., *Suishu*, 34.1041, 1042, 1045. On the elevation of Zhang during the Northern Song period, see Goldschmidt, *Evolution of Chinese Medicine*, 69–102; and Brown, *Art of Medicine in Early China*, 110–29.

16 Chen Yanzhi, *Xiaopin fang*; Ishida, "*Shōbon hō* no igaku shisō," 254–76.

17 Linghu, *Zhoushu*, 47.839–44; Li Yanshou, *Beishi*, 90.2977–79; Yao Sengyuan, *Jiyan fang*. It is also possible that the name refers to a different text since we find several medical works with such a title in the Sui and Tang bibliographical records.

18 Gan Zuwang, *Sun Simiao pingzhuan*.

19 Chen Hao, "Zai xieben yu yinben zhijian de fangshu," 69–85; Zheng Jinsheng, *Yaolin waishi*, 306–18.

20 The exact year of Sun's birth is still debatable given the contradictory accounts in different sources. A new piece of evidence, the epitaph of Sun Xing, one of Sun's sons, indicates that the physician's time of birth might have been the late sixth century. Since Sun died in 682, he was a centenarian, which is possible given the emphasis in his works on the cultivation of longevity. See Hu Mingzhao, "Cong xinchu Sun Xing muzhi tanxi yaowang shengzunian," 406–10.

21 *Da Tang xishi bowuguan cang muzhi*, 326–27.

22 Sun, *Sun Zhenren qianjin fang*, 1.1–2; Liu Xu et al., *Jiu Tangshu*, 191.5094–97; Ouyang Xiu, *Xin Tangshu*, 196.5596–98; Sivin, *Chinese Alchemy*, 81–144.

23 Wang Pu, *Tang huiyao*, 82.1523–24.

24 *Da Tang xishi bowuguan cang muzhi*, 326–27. On Sun's ties to the court, see Chen Hao, *Shenfen xushi yu zhishi biaoshu zhijian de yizhe zhi yi*, 162–93.

25 Ingesting water (*fushui*) refers to a fasting practice that involved the ritual imbibing of water. Both Daoist and Buddhist adepts during the Tang period adopted the technique to cultivate longevity and obtain transcendence. See Fan Ka-wai, *Zhonggu shiqi de yizhe yu bingzhe*, 113–33.

26 On Sun's connection to Daoism and Buddhism, see Sakade, *Chūgoku shisō kenkyū*, 246–82; on Sun's alchemy, see Sivin, *Chinese Alchemy*.

27 Sun, *Qianjin yifang*.

28 Sun, *Qianjin yifang*, 2–4.14–58.

29 The Tang editions of *Essential Formulas* have long been lost. The earliest complete copy of the text is the Song edition produced in the eleventh century. A different edition of the text (*Sun Zhenren qianjin fang*), which contains twenty scrolls, was discovered in the late eighteenth century and is considered to bear fewer traces of Song editorial changes and to preserve more features of the Tang text. My study relies on this edition for the extant scrolls (*juan* 1–5, 11–15, 21–30) and the Song edition for the rest of the scrolls (*juan* 6–10, 16–20). Moreover, I also consulted a Japanese edition (*Zhenben qianjin fang*) dated to the fourteenth century, with only the first scroll extant that preserves certain Tang traits of the book. See Okanishi, *Sō izen iki kō*, 795–835.

30 The preface is based on the Japanese edition *Zhenben qianjin fang*. See Sun, *Sun Zhenren qianjin fang*, 1.613.

31 Sun, *Sun Zhenren qianjin fang*, 1.613–14.

32 Fan Ka-wai, *Dayi jingcheng*, 167.

33 For an explanation of these schemes, see Sivin, *Traditional Medicine in Contemporary China*, 43–80.

34 On Bian Que in the history of Chinese medicine, see Brown, *Art of Medicine in Early China*, 41–62.

35 Sun, *Sun Zhenren qianjin fang*, 5.122, 15.286, 21.298, 22.332–38, 23.350, 23.369. Sun valued the works of these ancient figures, making it clear in the preface that he believed these eminent physicians possessed true medical knowledge originating in the distant past.

36 Sun, *Sun Zhenren qianjin fang*, 1.9–10.

37 This is most evident in *juan* 26, which includes more than four hundred formulas. Most of them use only one ingredient to treat emergencies such as sudden death, snake poisoning, injuries caused by beatings, and burns. Tellingly, Sun offers no theoretical discussion at all in this section.

38 Sun, *Sun Zhenren qianjin fang*, 1.614.

39 Li Jianmin, *Lüxingzhe de shixue*, 39–54.

40 Sun, *Sun Zhenren qianjin fang*, 3.83, 3.86, 11.164, 13.223.

41 Liu Xu et al., *Jiu Tangshu*, 191.5096; Ouyang Xiu, *Xin Tangshu*, 9.1571.

42 Sun, *Sun Zhenren qianjin fang*, 12.199–211, 23.345–77.

43 The specific mention of eighteen years of no pregnancies in this formula indicates that such information was derived from a particular medical case.

44 During the Tang period, one *liang* was equivalent to about forty grams; one *fen*, a quarter of a *liang*, was equivalent to about ten grams. See Guo, *San zhi shisi shiji Zhongguo de quanheng duliang*, 169, 191.

45 Sun, *Sun Zhenren qianjin fang*, 2.28.

46 Although this formula doesn't specify what these effects are, other medical texts point out that aconite could induce the sensations of numbness and dizziness. See *Jingui yaolüe*, 2.70.

47 Sun attributes another formula in his book to the magistrate of the Northern Land, who, as Sun specifies, is a figure in the Eastern Han dynasty. See Sun, *Sun Zhenren qianjin fang*, 25.422.

48 Sun, *Sun Zhenren qianjin fang*, 5.116.

49 Sun, *Sun Zhenren qianjin fang*, 15.280.

50 For some examples of these phrases, see Sun, *Sun Zhenren qianjin fang*, 2.46, 3.74, 3.88, 4.107, 11.169, 11.185, 21.318, 24.391, 26.459.

51 The term "efficacy phrases" was coined by the historian of medicine Claire Jones. In her study of medieval English medical manuscripts, she identified these phrases at the end of many formulas and argued that they reveal the authoritative or popular voice rather than empirical knowledge. See Jones, "Formula and Formulation," 199–209.

52 For example, see Chen Yanzhi, *Xiaopin fang*; and Yao Sengyuan, *Jiyan fang*.

53 For a translation and brief analysis of some of these cases, see Sivin, "Seventh-Century Chinese Medical Case History," 267–73.

54 Sun, *Sun Zhenren qianjin fang*, 11.180.

55 "The dragon illness" involved the formation of a coagulation in the abdomen upon eating celery. See Chao, *Zhubing yuanhou lun jiaozhu*, 19.585.

56 Sun, *Beiji qianjin yaofang jiaoshi*, 7.280, 20.711; Sun, *Sun Zhenren qianjin fang*, 21.313.

57 Sun, *Beiji qianjin yaofang jiaoshi*, 7.271; Sun, *Sun Zhenren qianjin fang*, 21.297–98. Later medical cases during the early modern period give patients a stronger voice to negotiate therapeutic options with physicians. See Tu, *Jiuming*; and Bian, "Documenting Medications," 103–23. A similar phenomenon also arose in early modern Europe. See Pomata, *Contracting a Cure*.

58 Sun, *Sun Zhenren qianjin fang*, 24.401–2. "Great wind" refers to a severe, wind-induced condition, the symptoms of which resemble leprosy. See Leung, *Leprosy in China*, 17–59.

59 Sun, *Beiji qianjin yaofang jiaoshi*, 7.280; Sun, *Sun Zhenren qianjin fang*, 12.211, 23.365.

60 Sun, *Sun Zhenren qianjin fang*, 23.365.

61 Su et al., *Xinxiu bencao*, 8.222–23.

62 Gan Zizhen could be the name of a court physician who appears in another medical case of Sun (see my discussion later in this section).

63 Sun, *Sun Zhenren qianjin fang*, 23.349.

64 Sun included the formula from Granny Rong of Qizhou elsewhere in the same section of his book (Sun, *Sun Zhenren qianjin fang*, 23.347). It merits our attention that both this formula and the one from Gan Zizhen are linked to elderly women, indicating their role in medicinal preparation that likely took place in domestic spaces. See Lee Jen-der, *Nüren de Zhongguo yiliao shi*, 305–48.

65 Sun, *Sun Zhenren qianjin fang*, 15.284, 25.422.

66 Sun, *Sun Zhenren qianjin fang*, 12.211. For further discussion of the detoxification of potent minerals in Chinese alchemy, see chapter 7.

67 Sun, *Beiji qianjin yaofang jiaoshi*, 20.706–8; Chao, *Zhubing yuanhou lun jiaozhu*, 22.648–51.

68 Sun, *Beiji qianjin yaofang jiaoshi*, 20.711.

69 Chen Hao, *Shenfen xushi yu zhishi biaoshu zhijian de yizhe zhi yi*, 131–40.

70 Sun, *Sun Zhenren qianjin fang*, 24.388, 25.420, 25.423.

71 On the concept of phlegm (*tan*) in Chinese medicine and its Indian connection, see Köhle, "Confluence of Humors," 465–93.

72 On the identification of this monk, see Fan Ka-wai, *Zhonggu shiqi de yizhe yu bing-zhe*, 127–28.

73 Sun, *Sun Zhenren qianjin fang*, 12.202.

74 This worldview, that the highest principle, or Dao, is utterly inscrutable and unpredictable, can be traced back to the ancient philosophical works *Laozi* and *Zhuangzi*. See Sivin, "On the Limits of Empirical Knowledge," 165–89.

75 Sun, *Sun Zhenren qianjin fang*, 26.447.

76 Sun, *Sun Zhenren qianjin fang*, 1.3.

77 Classical Chinese medicine considers the Spleen and the Stomach to be closely related. The *qi* of the Spleen fosters the digestion of grains in the Stomach. To treat diarrhea, therefore, one needs to tackle the root of the problem, namely, the malfunction of the Spleen. See Chao, *Zhubing yuanhou lun jiaozhu*, 17.522.

78 In a separate passage, Sun remarks that drugs such as ginger, cinnamon, and ginseng were expensive and hard to obtain during his time. See Sun, *Beiji qianjin yaofang jiaoshi*, 10.365.

79 Sun, *Sun Zhenren qianjin fang*, 15.287–88.

80 Sun, *Sun Zhenren qianjin fang*, 23.357–58.

81 On the use of feces in Chinese medicine, see Despeux, "Chinese Medicinal Excrement," 139–69.

82 Pomata, "Medical Case Narrative," 1–23; Pomata, "Medical Case Narrative in Pre-Modern Europe and China," 15–46.

83 McVaugh, "*Experimenta* of Arnold of Villanova," 107–18.

84 This epistemic orientation became more pronounced during the Song period, when scholar-officials integrated personal experience of healing and empirical knowledge in general into their writings. See Chen Yun-ju, "Accounts of Treating *Zhang* ("miasma") Disorders," 205–54; and Zuo, *Shen Gua's Empiricism*.

85 Wang Tao, *Waitai miyao fang*, 1.3–6; Fan Ka-wai, *Zhonggu shiqi de yizhe yu bingzhe*, 153–85.

CHAPTER 6: ALLURING STIMULANT

Epigraph: Chen Yanzhi, *Xiaopin fang*, 9.164.

1   Li Yanshou, *Nanshi*, 32.839–40. The physician Xu Sibo in this story came from the prestigious Xu family, practitioners of medicine for eight generations. See Fan Ka-wai, *Zhonggu shiqi de yizhe yu bingzhe*, 78–80.

2   Yu Jiaxi, "Hanshi San kao," 181–226; Wagner, "Lebensstil und Drogen im Chinesischen Mittelalter," 79–178.

3   Liu Yiqing, *Shishuo xinyu jianshu*, 2.74; Mather, *Shih-shuo Hsin-yü*, 37.

4   A similar origin story can be found in later physicians' works. See Chao, *Zhubing yuanhou lun jiaozhu*, 6.177; and Sun, *Sun Zhenren qianjin fang*, 25.413.

5   Chen Shou, *Sanguo zhi*, 9.292; Chao, *Zhubing yuanhou lun jiaozhu*, 6.177.

6   Tang, *Wei-Jin xuanxue lungao*; Wagner, *Language, Ontology, and Political Philosophy in China*.

7   He Yan was executed in 249 because the general whom he served, Cao Shuang, was eliminated in a power struggle at the court of Wei. See Chen Shou, *Sanguo zhi*, 9.282–88.

8   Liu Yiqing, *Shishuo xinyu jianshu*, 23.726–65; Mather, *Shih-shuo Hsin-yü*, 399–422; Yü, "Individualism and the Neo-Taoist Movement in Wei-Chin China," 121–56.

9   Lu Xun, "Wei-Jin fengdu ji wenzhang yu yao ji jiu zhi guanxi," 486–507. Also see Wagner, "Lebensstil und Drogen im Chinesischen Mittelalter," 118–35.

10 Chao, *Zhubing yuanhou lun jiaozhu*, 6.177; Sun, *Sun Zhenren qianjin fang*, 25.413.

11 Ouyang Xun, *Yiwen leiju*, 75.1292.

12 Yan Kejun, *Quan Jin wen*, 22–26.1580–1611; Yu Jiaxi, "Hanshi San kao," 194–98; Richter and Chace, "Trouble with Wang Xizhi," 86–88.

13 Satō, "Ō Gishi to Goseki San," 1–13.

14 Tamba, *Yixin fang/Ishimpō*, 19.394. The former aspiration intimates the alchemical practice of ingesting elixirs to achieve the transcendence of the body. These two goals, namely, the enhancement of life and the transformation of the body, entailed related but distinct practices. Sharing Qin's view, Tao Hongjing also placed Five-Stone Powder in the category of "worldly formulas" rather than "transcendent formulas." See Tao, *Bencao jing jizhu*, 1.11.

15 Tamba, *Yixin fang/Ishimpō*, 19.395.

16 Besides Huiyi, we also find the eminent monk Huiyuan (334–416), who took the powder at an old age, as well as the monks Zhibin and Daohong, who both produced medical writings on the powder. See Huijiao, *Gaoseng zhuan*, 6.221–22; and Wei Zheng et al., *Suishu*, 34.1041.

17 Chao, *Zhubing yuanhou lun jiaozhu*, 6.177.

18 Wei Shou, *Weishu*, 2.44. An important detail of the story is that the emperor only started to suffer from the powder after the Prefect of Grand Physicians, who might have been involved in prescribing the powder for the monarch, died, suggesting that medical guidance was central to the proper use of the drug.

19 Shen Ruiwen, *An Lushan fusan kao*, 133–75.

20 Chao, *Zhubing yuanhou lun jiaozhu*, 6.177–207; Epler, "Concept of Disease," 255–62. In the history of Chinese medicine, Huangfu Mi has been primarily remembered as a medical scholar who capably compiled and edited ancient medical classics. Yet prior to the Song period, he figured prominently in heated discussions of Five-Stone Powder. On the changing image of Huangfu Mi in Chinese medical history, see Brown, *Art of Medicine in Early China*, 130–50.

21 Yu Jiaxi, "Hanshi San kao," 186–87.

22 Fang et al., *Jinshu*, 51.1409–18; DeClercq, *Writing against the State*, 159–205.

23 Fang et al., *Jinshu*, 68.1825–26; Akahori, "Kanshoku San to yōjō," 117–21.

24 Liu Yiqing, *Shishuo xinyu jianshu*, 23.731.

25 Wagner, "Lebensstil und Drogen im Chinesischen Mittelalter," 115–16; Akahori, "Kanshoku San to yōjō," 132–36.

26 Ge, *Baopuzi waipian jiaojian*, 26.16–18.

27 *Shennong bencao jing jiaozhu*, 2.26–27.

28 Sivin, *Traditional Medicine in Contemporary China*, 70–80. Specifically, the green-blue clay (phase Wood) nourishes the Liver, the red clay (phase Fire) nourishes the Heart, the yellow clay (phase Earth) nourishes the Spleen, the white clay (phase Metal) nourishes the Lungs, and the black clay (phase Water) nourishes the Kidneys.

29 *Zhouli zhushu*, 5.137.

30 Sima, *Shiji*, 105.2810–11. For a translation of the full case, see Hsu, *Pulse Diagnosis in Early Chinese Medicine*, 87–88; on the historical context of Chunyu Yi's cases, see Brown, *Art of Medicine in Early China*, 63–86.

31 Sima, *Shiji*, 105.2796.

32 Guangzhou Shi Wenwu Guanli Weiyuanhui, *Xihan Nanyue wang mu*, vol. 1, 141. The kingdom of Nanyue, with its capital in Panyu (present-day Guangzhou), was established by a Qin general during the chaotic period of the Qin-Han transition, and later annexed to the Han empire in 111 BCE. See Twitchett and Loewe, eds., *Cambridge History of China*, vol. 1, 451–53.

33 Li Ling, "Wushi kao," 345–46.

34 *Jingui yaolüe*, 23.631; Jing and Xiao, "Zhonggu fusan de chengyin ji chuancheng," 342–47.

35 *Jingui yaolüe*, 5.134.

36 Chao, *Zhubing yuanhou lun jiaozhu*, 6.177.

37 Yu Jiaxi, "Hanshi San kao," 208.

38 Many of these formulas are preserved in Sun Simiao's *Qianjin yifang, juan* 22. See also the summary of these formulas in Obringer, *L'aconit et l'orpiment*, 153–61.

39 Li Fang et al., *Taiping yulan*, 722.3331a. Little is known about Jin Shao. Sun Simiao placed him among a group of eminent physicians during the Era of Division and included two formulas from Jin in his medical work. See Sun, *Sun Zhenren qianjin fang*, 1.3; and Sun, *Qianjin yifang*, 15.170a, 22.266a.

40 Wang Tao, *Waitai miyao fang*, 15.276.

41 Tao, *Bencao jing jizhu*, 2.168–69. Modern chemical analysis has shown that heat-
    ing can reduce the toxicity of arsenolite. See Wang Kuike et al., "Shen de lishi zai
    Zhongguo," 14–38.

42 This hypothesis was proposed by the historian of chemistry Wang Kuike. See
    Wang Kuike, "'Wushi San' xinkao," 87.

43 Obringer, *L'aconit et l'orpiment*, 173–75, 188.

44 Needham et al., *Science and Civilisation in China*, vol. 5, pt. II, 282–94.

45 Chao, *Zhubing yuanhou lun jiaozhu*, 5.164–65.

46 Chao, *Zhubing yuanhou lun jiaozhu*, 6.199.

47 Tao, *Bencao jing jizhu*, 2.138, 141, 142, 143, 144, 152, 154, 168. The exceptions are limo-
    nite (plain) and kalinite (cooling). Given kalinite is the only cooling agent on the list,
    it is possible that arsenolite, rather than kalinite, was actually used in the powder.

48 Tao, *Bencao jing jizhu*, 2.168. Arsenic poisoning causes the inflammation of
    the stomach, vomiting, and diarrhea, leading to extreme thirst and dehydration.
    These symptoms are consistent with the warming nature of the mineral as
    defined in Chinese materia medica texts. See Whorton, *Arsenic Century*, 7–16.

49 The text has long been lost, but sections of it have been preserved in later medical
    works. The discussion on Five-Stone Powder is preserved in *Yixin fang/Ishimpō*,
    juan 19. A similar passage is also in *Zhubing yuanhou lun*, *juan* 6.

50 Tamba, *Yixin fang/Ishimpō*, 19.395.

51 Chao, *Zhubing yuanhou lun jiaozhu*, 6.174.

52 Xu Shen, *Shuowen jiezi*, 12b.270.

53 Sun, *Sun Zhenren qianjin fang*, 23.360–67; 25.412–20.

54 Wei Zheng et al., *Suishu*, 34.1040–50; Liu Xu et al., *Jiu Tangshu*, 47.2047–51; Ouyang
    Xiu, *Xin Tangshu*, 59.1566–73.

55 Tamba, *Yixin fang/Ishimpō*, 19.394.

56 Tamba, *Yixin fang/Ishimpō*, 19.395.

57 Chao, *Zhubing yuanhou lun jiaozhu*, 6.180–85.

58 Tamba, *Yixin fang/Ishimpō*, 19.396–97.

59 Tamba, *Yixin fang/Ishimpō*, 19.394–95. The former was espoused by the monk
    Huiyi, the latter by Qin Chengzu.

60 Tao's comment is cited in *Formulas of the Lesser Grade* (fifth century), which is
    preserved in *Arcane Essentials from the Imperial Library* (eighth century). See
    Wang Tao, *Waitai miyao fang*, 37.752. "Waiting at the stump" is a reference to a
    story in the ancient philosophical text *Hanfeizi*. In the story, a farmer had the
    good fortune of obtaining a rabbit who had accidentally run into a stump and
    died. After that, he waited at the stump, expecting more such fortunes, but to no
    avail. See *Hanfeizi jijie*, 49.442–43.

61 Chao, *Zhubing yuanhou lun jiaozhu*, 6.168–73; Sun, *Sun Zhenren qianjin fang*,
    25.413–17. Little is known about Daohong, and only excerpts of his text are pre-
    served in Sui and Tang medical sources. According to *On the Origins and Symp-
    toms of All Illnesses*, he lived in the south during the Era of Division and excelled
    at treating the disorders caused by Five-Stone Powder. See Chao, *Zhubing yuan-
    hou lun jiaozhu*, 6.168.

62 Chao, *Zhubing yuanhou lun jiaozhu*, 6.174–77.

63 Wang Kuike, "'Wushi San' xinkao," 80–87.

64 Tao, *Bencao jing jizhu*, 2.154–56. The most famous case is that of the Tang scholar Han Yu (768–824), who allegedly suffered from sulfur poisoning. See Hu and Hu, "Han Yu 'zuruo buneng bu' yu 'tuizhi fu liuhuang' kaobian," 193–212; and Davis, "Lechery, Substance Abuse, and . . . Han Yu?," 89–91.

65 Sun, *Qianjin yifang*, 22.261a. The five exhaustions and seven injuries refer to severe conditions of viscera depletion, especially the depletion of the Kidneys that leads to sexual malfunction. See Chao, *Zhubing yuanhou lun jiaozhu*, 3.86–89.

66 Sun, *Qianjin yifang*, 15.167a.

67 Sun Simiao was not the first physician to propose the highly restrictive use of the powder. The sixth-century physician Yao Sengyuan held a similar view. In a medical case described in *The History of the Zhou*, he encountered a patient who contracted a *qi* disorder that led to panting and fluster. The family of the patient was tempted to treat him with Five-Stone Powder, probably intrigued by its panacea reputation. Yao rejected the idea and prescribed a specific formula that cured the patient. See Linghu, *Zhoushu*, 47.841–42.

68 Sun, *Sun Zhenren qianjin fang*, 25.413.

69 Sun, *Sun Zhenren qianjin fang*, 25.412.

70 Sun, *Sun Zhenren qianjin fang*, 25.413.

71 For a detailed study of the culture of ingesting stalactite during the Tang period, see Sakade, "Zui-Tō jidai niokeru shōnyūseki fukuyō no ryūkō nitsuite," 615–44.

72 On the *zhen* bird, see chapter 1.

73 Sun, *Sun Zhenren qianjin fang*, 25.412–13.

74 Lu Xun, "Wei-Jin fengdu ji wenzhang yu yao ji jiu zhi guanxi," 494; Yu Jiaxi, "Han-shi San kao," 181–82; Li Ling, "Yaodu yijia," 35–38. The similarity between Five-Stone Powder and opium was first proposed by the Qing scholar Yu Zhengxie (1775–1840). See Yu Zhengxie, "Hanshi San," 7.212–13 (cited by Yu Jiaxi above).

75 Wagner, "Lebensstil und Drogen im Chinesischen Mittelalter," 174–77.

76 Zheng, *Social Life of Opium in China*.

77 For example, see Wagner, "Lebensstil und Drogen im Chinesischen Mittelalter," 135–49.

78 Tomes, *Remaking the American Patient*, 234–40.

79 Etkin, "'Side Effects,'" 99–113; Etkin, "Negotiation of 'Side' Effects," 17–32.

CHAPTER 7: DYING TO LIVE

Epigraph: Chuze, *Taiqing shibi ji* (HY 881), 3.11a.

1 On *fangshi*, see chapter 2.

2 Lard (*zhufang*) was mainly used for making ointments in Chinese medicine. Occasionally it was ingested to treat emergencies. See Ge, *Buji zhouhou fang*, 1.22. I have not yet been able to identify what "grain lacquer" (*guqi*) is.

3 Liu Xu et al., *Jiu Tangshu*, 132.3649.

4   Zhao Yi, *Ershier shi zhaji*, 398–99.

5   In comparison to outer alchemy, inner alchemy (*neidan*) focused on various techniques of meditation to achieve transcendence without ingesting potent substances. In this chapter, for simplicity, I use the word "alchemy" to refer only to the practices of outer alchemy.

6   Needham et al., *Science and Civilisation in China*, vol. 5, pt. II, pt. III, and pt. IV; Ho, *Explorations in Daoism*.

7   Sivin, "Chinese Alchemy and the Manipulation of Time," 512–26; Pregadio, *Great Clarity*.

8   Ho and Needham, "Elixir Poisoning in Medieval China," 221–51.

9   Strickmann, "On the Alchemy of T'ao Hung-ching," 123–92.

10 Needham et al., *Science and Civilisation in China*, vol. 5, pt. IV, 472–91.

11 This sense of upward movement is evident in the affinity of the early writing of *xian* to *qian*, which means "ascend" or "transfer." See Miura, "*Xianren*," 1092–94.

12 Gruman, *History of Ideas about the Prolongation of Life*.

13 My understanding of *xian* is informed by Yü, "Life and Immortality in the Mind of Han China," 80–122; Needham et al., *Science and Civilisation in China*, vol. 5, pt. II, 71–127; Bokenkamp, *Early Daoist Scriptures*, 21–23; Campany, *To Live as Long as Heaven and Earth*, 4–5; Stanley-Baker, "Cultivating Body, Cultivating Self," 34–40; and Pregadio, "Which Is the Daoist Immortal Body?," 385–407.

14 Sima, *Shiji*, 6.247; Schafer, "Transcendent Vitamin," 27–38.

15 Sima, *Shiji*, 28.1385.

16 On alchemy in Chinese antiquity, see Li Ling, "Liandanshu de qiyuan he fushi zhuyou," 301–40. An important text in the Daoist canon, *Token for the Agreement of the Three According to the Book of Changes* (Zhouyi cantong qi), was traditionally treated as a Han alchemical work, but more recent studies have shown that the text was originally a work of prognostication and only became associated with alchemy during the Era of Division. See Pregadio, "Early History of the *Zhouyi cantong qi*," 149–76.

17 Fang et al., *Jinshu*, 72.1910–13; Campany, *To Live as Long as Heaven and Earth*, 13–17.

18 Ge lamented that, though in possession of instructional books given by Zheng Yin for more than twenty years, he still couldn't practice alchemy, due to the lack of resources. See Ge, *Baopuzi neipian jiaoshi*, 4.71.

19 Ge, *Baopuzi neipian jiaoshi*, 4.72.

20 Ge, *Baopuzi neipian jiaoshi*, 4.71–72.

21 Ge, *Baopuzi neipian jiaoshi*, 4.82–83.

22 Pregadio, "Seeking Immortality in Ge Hong's *Baopuzi Neipian*," 437–39.

23 Ge, *Baopuzi neipian jiaoshi*, 4.72.

24 *Huangdi neijing suwen jiaozhu*, 43.565; Unschuld, *Huang Di nei jing su wen*, vol. 2, 163–67.

25 Ge, *Baopuzi neipian jiaoshi*, 15.272; Fan Ka-wai, "*Ge xianweng Zhouhou beijifang*," 88–94; Stanley-Baker, "*Ge xianweng zhouhou beiji fang*," forthcoming.

26 Ge, *Baopuzi neipian jiaoshi*, 4.77, 9.172.

27   Ge, *Baopuzi neipian jiaoshi*, 13.240.

28   Ge, *Baopuzi neipian jiaoshi*, 3.53–54.

29   To be sure, certain alchemical texts in medieval China concern only the imagination and cosmic contemplation of elixir-making rather than putting alchemy into practice (Sivin, "Chinese Alchemy and the Manipulation of Time," 512–26; Bokenkamp, *Early Daoist Scriptures*, 289–95), but we also have abundant textual and material evidence for the actual making and ingesting of elixirs, as I will demonstrate shortly.

30   Fang et al., *Jinshu*, 8.208–9.

31   Wei Shou, *Weishu*, 114.3049.

32   Li Yanshou, *Beishi*, 89.2931.

33   Alchemists during the Era of Division consisted of mainly two groups: *fangshi*, who were technical adepts versed in various magical arts, and Daoist practitioners, especially in the sect of the Great Clarity (Taiqing). See Pregadio, *Great Clarity*.

34   Yao Silian, *Liangshu*, 51.742; Jia, *Huayang Tao yinju neizhuan* (HY 300), 2.13b.

35   Li Yanshou, *Nanshi*, 76.1899. Not surprisingly, Tao's intimate relationship with the court helped him promote the Daoist sect that he established in Maoshan. See Zhong, *Tao Hongjing pingzhuan*, 125–35; and Pettit, "Learning from Maoshan."

36   Li Yanshou, *Nanshi*, 76.1899.

37   My study of Tao's alchemy is primarily based on *Inner Biography of the Hermit Tao from Huayang* (Huayang Tao yinju neizhuan), compiled by Jia Song during the Tang dynasty. Although this is a much later text, it preserves information that matches up well with Tao's own writings that are preserved only in fragments, allowing me to reconstruct Tao's alchemical practice with certain confidence. See Jia, *Huayang Tao yinju neizhuan* (HY 300); Strickmann, "On the Alchemy of T'ao Hung-ching," 123–92; Sakade, *Chūgoku shisō kenkyū*, 113–46; and Zhong, *Tao Hongjing pingzhuan*, 135–62.

38   The procedure is described in an alchemical text dated to the early Era of Division, *Essential Instructions on the Scripture of the Reverted Elixir in Nine Cycles of the Perfected of the Great Ultimate*. See *Taiji zhenren jiuzhuan huandan jing yaojue* (HY 889), 1b–4a; Strickmann, "On the Alchemy of T'ao Hung-ching," 143–46; and Pregadio, *Great Clarity*, 193–200. Fabrizio Pregadio offered a full translation of the text, on which my summary is based.

39   Jia, *Huayang Tao yinju neizhuan* (HY 300), 2.8b–11b. We can trace this idea of choosing a sacred site for alchemy back to Ge Hong's writings. See Ge, *Baopuzi neipian*, 4.84–85.

40   Wei Zheng et al., *Suishu*, 35.1093.

41   Jia, *Huayang Tao yinju neizhuan* (HY 300), 2.5b.

42   Tao, *Bencao jing jizhu*, 1.33, 2.148–49.

43   Chen Yuanpeng, "*Bencao jing jizhu* suozai 'Taozhu' zhong de zhishi leixing," 184–212.

44   Jia, *Huayang Tao yinju neizhuan* (HY 300), 2.12a–12b.

45   Jia, *Huayang Tao yinju neizhuan* (HY 300), 2.13a–13b. *Instructions on Elixirs* is likely the abbreviated title of a lost alchemical text.

46 Jia, *Huayang Tao yinju neizhuan* (HY 300), 2.14a. The same source narrates that in 524, Tao made another attempt at compounding the elixir, finally succeeding when the product radiated the variegated colors of a rainbow. But we don't know what Tao did with the elixir. Another source reveals that Tao presented a certain Sublimated Elixir to Emperor Wu sometime before 519. Both the emperor and Tao ingested it and felt their bodies become light (Li Yanshou, *Nanshi*, 76.1899). Michel Strickmann has argued that what they ingested was not a deadly drug but a "tonic iatro-alchemical compound" (Strickmann, "On the Alchemy of T'ao Hung-ching," 162–63). In any case, both the emperor and Tao lived long lives—the emperor died at 86 and Tao at 81—suggesting that they never took a lethal elixir.

47 One such daring alchemist is Tao's disciple Zhou Ziliang (497–516), who died of elixir poisoning at the age of twenty. See Zhou Ziliang, *Zhoushi mingtong ji* (HY 302), 1.3a–4a, 4.19a–20b; and Bokenkamp, "Answering a Summons," 188–202.

48 Sakade, *Chūgoku shisō kenkyū*, 138–40.

49 On the early history of the Shangqing movement, see Strickmann, "Mao Shan Revelations," 1–64; and Robinet, *Taoism*, 114–48.

50 Pregadio, *Great Clarity*, 43–47; Chang Chaojan, "You xian er zhen," 260–326; Stanley-Baker, "Daoists and Doctors."

51 *Huangdi jiuding shendan jingjue* (HY 885), 14.2a.

52 *Yin zhenjun jinshi wu xianglei* (HY 906), 33a.

53 *Jinshi bu wujiu shu jue* (HY 907), 7a.

54 Schafer, *Golden Peaches of Samarkand*, 215–21; Liao Jui-yui, *Tangdai fushi yangsheng yanjiu*, 73–95; Chen Ming, *Zhonggu yiliao yu wailai wenhua*, 278–96.

55 Bokenkamp, "Li Bai, Huangshan, and Alchemy," 29–55.

56 Shaanxi Sheng Bowuguan Geweihui Xiezuo Xiaozu, "Xi'an nanjiao Hejiacun faxian Tangdai jiaocang wenwu," 30–42; Geng, "Xi'an nanjiao Tangdai jiaocang li de yiyao wenwu," 56–60; Qi and Shen, *Huawu da Tang chun*, 150–55.

57 Even without detailed explanation, the effort required to manage the potency of alchemical ingredients is already visible during the Era of Division. For instance, a text titled *Oral Instructions of the Heavenly Master on the Classics of the Great Clarity* briefly describes the methods of detoxifying gold and silver. See *Taiqing jing tianshi koujue* (HY 883), 5b–8b.

58 Pregadio, *Great Clarity*, 241–54.

59 *Huangdi jiuding shendan jingjue* (HY 885), 6.4a. On *zhen*-laced alcohol, see chapter 1.

60 Ge, *Baopuzi neipian jiaoshi*, 4.72; Zhao Kuanghua, "Woguo gudai 'chousha liangong' de yanjin jiqi huaxue chengjiu," 128–53.

61 Tao, *Bencao jing jizhu*, 2.129–30.

62 *Huangdi jiuding shendan jingjue* (HY 885), 13.1b.

63 In Tang materia medica, mercury was relegated to the middle group of drugs, suggesting its lowered value. See Su et al., *Xinxiu bencao*, 4.107.

64 *Huangdi jiuding shendan jingjue* (HY 885), 11.1a–11b. On the history of mercury in Chinese medicine and alchemy, see Liu and Kuriyama, "Fluid Being."

65 Pregadio, *Great Clarity*, 169; Chen Guofu, *Chen Guofu daozang yanjiu lunwen ji*, 320–24.

66 *Huangdi jiuding shendan jingjue* (HY 885), 11.9a–9b.

67 Tao, *Bencao jing jizhu*, 6.397–98, 7.510, 7.514.

68 The other two yang drugs are sal ammoniac and flakes of gold and silver.

69 Pregadio, "Elixirs and Alchemy," 179–80.

70 *Huangdi jiuding shendan jingjue* (HY 885), 10.4b, 11.5a–6a.

71 *Huangdi jiuding shendan jingjue* (HY 885), 20.17a. One tip of the jade-knife (*daogui*) is a size unit in classical Chinese pharmacy. It is four times the size of a small bean, which is eight times the size of a millet grain. Hence, from the dose of one tip of the jade-knife to that of half a millet grain, we see a difference of sixty-four times. See Tao, *Bencao jing jizhu*, 1.38–39.

72 *Shennong bencao jing jiaozhu*, 1.8. Also see chapter 2.

73 Fang et al., *Jinshu*, 72.1913.

74 On the studies of *shijie*, see Robinet, "Metamorphosis and Deliverance," 37–70; Cedzich, "Corpse Deliverance," 1–68; Campany, *To Live as Long as Heaven and Earth*, 52–60; and Pregadio, "Which Is the Daoist Immortal Body?," 389–92.

75 Ge, *Baopuzi neipian jiaoshi*, 2.20.

76 Ge, *Baopuzi neipian jiaoshi*, 3.52–53.

77 Shen Yue, *Songshu*, 45.1377–78.

78 *Hu* is a unit of volume measurement. During the Era of Division, one *hu* was equivalent to about 0.2 liters. See Qiu, *Zhongguo lidai duliangheng kao*, 254–55.

79 Tao, *Zhen'gao* (HY 1016), 10.5a.

80 Tao, *Zhen'gao* (HY 1016), 5.8a–8b. A similar but more famous story is that of Wei Boyang. Wei, a Daoist master, brought three disciples to a mountain to compound an elixir. After the elixir was made, he pronounced that it was an elixir with *du*. He then fed it to a dog, who died instantly. Despite this, Wei, together with one trusting disciple, ingested the elixir and died too. Terrified, the other two disciples fled, only to realize later that Wei and his unflinching follower had become transcendents. See Campany, *To Live as Long as Heaven and Earth*, 379–80, 543–44.

81 Chen Guofu, *Daozang yuanliu kao*, 314–15.

82 Chuze, *Taiqing shibi ji* (HY 881), 2.7a.

83 Chuze, *Taiqing shibi ji* (HY 881), 3.11a. The original quote is from the ancient text *The Book of Documents* (Shangshu). See *Shangshu zhengyi*, 10.294–95.

84 The triple *jiao* (*sanjiao*) is one of the six palace-viscera in classical Chinese medicine, with no counterpart in modern biomedicine. Functionally, it controls the opening of water channels in the body and regulates digestion and excretion. See *Huangdi neijing suwen jiaozhu*, 8.129, 9.150; and Sivin, *Traditional Medicine in Contemporary China*, 125.

85 Chuze, *Taiqing shibi ji* (HY 881), 3.10b–11a. Unlike certain early medical texts that deem pain to be a symptom of abnormal circulation of *qi* inside the body, this alchemical text regards pain and other strong bodily sensations as therapeutic manifestations of powerful *qi* from the elixir. See Lo, "Tracking the Pain," 191–211.

86   In particular, worms figured prominently in the Daoist imagination of sickness as innate, destructive creatures residing in one's body that pose a perpetual menace to life. See Toshiaki Yamada, "Longevity Techniques," 99–124; Huang Shih-shan Susan, "Daoist Imagery of Body and Cosmos, Part 2," 33–64; and Yan Liu, "Words, Demons, and Illness," 19–23.

87   Chuze, *Taiqing shibi ji* (HY 881), 3.11b–12a.

88   Skar and Pregadio, "Inner Alchemy (*Neidan*)," 464–97; Yokote, "Daoist Internal Alchemy," 1053–1110.

89   Besides two formula books (see chapter 5), Sun Simiao also compiled an alchemical text titled *Essential Instructions from the Classics of Elixirs of the Great Clarity* (Taiqing danjing yaojue), which, with regard to the therapeutic use of elixirs, resembles *The Record from the Stone Wall*. See Sivin, *Chinese Alchemy*.

CONCLUSION

Epigraph: Gu Yanwu, *Rizhi lu jishi*, 6.279–80. The passage is quoted in Yu Yan, "Duyao bian," 4.

1   Fan Ka-wai, "Liu Yuxi yu *Chuanxin fang*," 111–44.

2   Liu Yuxi, *Liu Yuxi ji*, 6.77.

3   Liu Zongyuan, "Yu Cui lianzhou lun shi zhongru shu," 515–18.

4   Davis, "Lechery, Substance Abuse, and . . . Han Yu?," 89–91; Fan Ka-wai, *Zhonggu shiqi de yizhe yu bingzhe*, 200–222.

5   Han, "Gu taixue boshi Lijun muzhiming," 2655–57.

6   Chen Yuanpeng, *Liang Song de "shangyi shiren" yu "ruyi."*

7   Bian, *Know Your Remedies*.

8   Li Shizhen, *Bencao gangmu*, 17.1113–29.

9   Gu Yanwu, *Rizhi lu jishi*, 6.280.

10   Lei, *Neither Donkey nor Horse*; Andrews, *Making of Modern Chinese Medicine*.

11   On the globalization of Chinese medicine and its consequences, see Barnes, "World of Chinese Medicine and Healing," 284–378.

12   Hanson, "Is the 2015 Nobel Prize a Turning Point for Traditional Chinese Medicine?"

13   Rao, Li, and Zhang, "Drug from Poison," 495–502. Arsenic trioxide, a refined product from arsenic ores, entered Chinese pharmacy during the Song dynasty. Called *pishuang*, it was considered an effective drug to treat intermittent fevers. See Obringer, "Song Innovation in Pharmacotherapy," 192–213.

14   Lord et al., "Urothelial Malignant Disease and Chinese Herbal Nephropathy," 1515–16; Hao, "Cong lishi jiaodu kexue lixing renshi zhongyao de dufu zuoyong," 57. In the latest development in this controversy, the newest edition of the government-issued *Pharmacopoeia of China* (Zhongguo yaodian), released in 2020, has eliminated aristolochia from its drug list (www.sohu.com/a/402929732 _233656, accessed August 1, 2020).

15   Throughout this book, I have used "drug" and "medicine" interchangeably to translate *yao* so as to underscore the fluid meaning of the word over the course of Chinese history. On the changed meaning of the word "drug" from medicine to an

object of substance abuse in early twentieth-century America, see Parascandola, "Drug Habit," 156–67.

16 Martin Lee, *Smoke Signals*; Dufton, *Grass Roots*.

17 Pollan, *How to Change Your Mind*, 331–96.

18 Herzberg, *Happy Pills in America*; Greene and Watkins, eds., *Prescribed*.

19 Centers for Disease Control and Prevention (www.cdc.gov/nchs/fastats/drug -use-therapeutic.htm, accessed August 1, 2020). The data are based on the period 2013–16.

20 Information from the National Institute on Drug Abuse (www.drugabuse.gov /drugs-abuse/opioids/opioid-overdose-crisis#one, accessed August 1, 2020).

21 On an excellent new study of the history of licit drug abuse in twentieth-century America, see Herzberg, *White Market Drugs*.

BIBLIOGRAPHY

ABBREVIATION

HY — Location of a text in the *Zhengtong daozang* 正統道藏, edited in 1445

MANUSCRIPTS

Dunhuang Manuscripts

BIBLIOTHÈQUE NATIONALE DE FRANCE, PARIS

P. 3714 (fragment of *Newly Revised Materia Medica*, 669 or later)
P. 3822 (fragment of *Newly Revised Materia Medica*)

BRITISH LIBRARY, LONDON

S. 4534 (fragment of *Newly Revised Materia Medica*)
S. 9434 (fragment of *Newly Revised Materia Medica*)

KYŌU SHŌKU COLLECTION 杏雨書屋, TAKEDE SCIENCE FOUNDATION, OSAKA

Kyōu 040R in *Tonkō hikyū* 敦煌秘笈. Osaka: Takeda Kagaku Shinkō Zaidan, 2009.
(fragment of *Newly Revised Materia Medica*, late ninth century)

OMIYA LIBRARY OF RYUKOKU UNIVERSITY, KYOTO

Preface to *Collected Annotations on the Classic of Materia Medica*, eighth century

Turfan Manuscript

STAATSBIBLIOTHEK ZU BERLIN, BERLIN

Ch. 1036 (fragment of *Collected Annotations on the Classic of Materia Medica*, seventh century)

OTHER PRIMARY SOURCES

Ban Gu 班固 (32–92). *Hanshu* 漢書. Taipei: Dingwen Shuju, 1986.

Chao Yuanfang 巢元方 et al. *Zhubing yuanhou lun jiaozhu* 諸病源候論校注. 610. Edited by Ding Guangdi 丁光迪. Beijing: Renmin Weisheng Chubanshe, 1991.

Chen Cangqi 陳藏器 (ca. 687–757). *Bencao shiyi jishi* 本草拾遺輯釋. 739. Edited by Shang Zhijun 尚志鈞. Hefei: Anhui Kexue Jishu Chubanshe, 2003.

Chen Shou 陳壽 (233–297). *Sanguo zhi* 三國志. Taipei: Dingwen Shuju, 1980.

Chen Yanzhi 陳延之. *Xiaopin fang* 小品方. Fifth century. Edited by Gao Wenzhu 高文鑄. Beijing: Zhongguo Zhongyiyao Chubanshe, 1995.

Chunqiu zuozhuan zhengyi 春秋左傳正義. Ca. fourth century BCE. Beijing: Beijing Daxue Chubanshe, 2000.

Chuze xiansheng 楚澤先生. *Taiqing shibi ji* 太清石壁記. 758 or 759. HY 881.

Da Tang xishi bowuguan cang muzhi 大唐西市博物館藏墓誌. Edited by Hu Ji 胡戟 and Rong Xinjiang 榮新江. Beijing: Beijing Daxue Chubanshe, 2012.

Du You 杜佑 (735–812). *Tongdian* 通典. 801. Edited by Wang Wenjin 王文錦 et al. Beijing: Zhonghua Shuju, 1988.

Dunhuang yiyao wenxian jijiao 敦煌醫藥文獻輯校. Edited by Ma Jixing 馬繼興 et al. Nanjing: Jiangsu Guji Chubanshe, 1998.

Fan Ye 范曄 (398–445). *Hou Hanshu* 後漢書. Taipei: Dingwen Shuju, 1981.

Fang Xuanling 房玄齡 (579–648) et al. *Jinshu* 晉書. Taipei: Dingwen Shuju, 1980.

Gan Bao 干寶 (fourth century). *Xinjiao soushen ji* 新校搜神記. Edited by Hu Huaichen 胡懷琛. Shanghai: Shangwu Yinshuguan, 1957.

Ge Hong 葛洪 (283–343). *Baopuzi neipian jiaoshi* 抱朴子內篇校釋. Edited by Wang Ming 王明. Beijing: Zhonghua Shuju, 1985.

———. *Baopuzi waipian jiaojian* 抱朴子外篇校箋. Edited by Yang Mingzhao 楊明照. Beijing: Zhonghua Shuju, 1991.

———. *Buji zhouhou fang* 補輯肘後方. Edited by Shang Zhijun. Hefei: Anhui Kexue Jishu Chubanshe, 1996.

Gu Yanwu 顧炎武 (1613–1682). *Rizhi lu jishi* 日知錄集釋. 1695. Edited by Huang Rucheng 黃汝成. Shanghai: Shanghai Guji Chubanshe, 2006.

Gu Yewang 顧野王 (519–581). *Songben yupian* 宋本玉篇. Beijing: Zhongguo Shudian, 1983.

Han Yu 韓愈 (768–824). "Gu taixue boshi Lijun muzhiming" 故太學博士李君墓誌銘. In *Hanyu wenji huijiao jianzhu* 韓愈文集彙校箋注, edited by Liu Zhenlun 劉真倫 and Yue Zhen 岳珍, 2655–57. Beijing: Zhonghua Shuju, 2010.

Hanfeizi jijie 韓非子集解. Edited by Wang Xianshen 王先慎. Beijing: Zhonghua Shuju, 1998.

Huangdi jiuding shendan jingjue 黃帝九鼎神丹經訣. Seventh century. HY 885.

Huangdi neijing suwen jiaozhu 黃帝內經素問校注. Han period. Edited by Guo Aichun 郭靄春. Beijing: Renmin Weisheng Chubanshe, 1992.

Huijiao 慧皎 (497–554). *Gaoseng zhuan* 高僧傳. Edited by Tang Yongtong 湯用彤. Beijing: Zhonghua Shuju, 1992.

Jia Song 賈嵩. *Huayang Tao yinju neizhuan* 華陽陶隱居內傳. Tang period. HY 300.

Jingui yaolüe 金匱要略. Attributed to Zhang Zhongjing 張仲景 (150–219). Taipei: Zhiyin Chubanshe, 2002.

Jinshi bu wujiu shu jue 金石簿五九數訣. Tang period. HY 907.

Laozi jiaoshi 老子校釋. Edited by Zhu Qianzhi 朱謙之. Beijing: Zhonghua Shuju, 1984.

Leigong paozhi lun 雷公炮炙論. Attributed to Lei Xiao 雷斅 (fifth century). Edited by Shang Zhijun. Hefei: Anhui Kexue Jishu Chubanshe, 1991.

Li Fang 李昉 et al. *Taiping yulan* 太平御覽. 984. Taipei: Shangwu Yinshuguan, 1975.

Li Linfu 李林甫 et al. *Tang liudian* 唐六典. 739. Edited by Chen Zhongfu 陳仲夫. Beijing: Zhonghua Shuju, 1992.

Li Shizhen 李時珍 (1518–1593). *Bencao gangmu* 本草綱目. Beijing: Renmin Weisheng Chubanshe, 1975.

Li Yanshou 李延壽 (seventh century). *Beishi* 北史. Taipei: Dingwen Shuju, 1980.

———. *Nanshi* 南史. Taipei: Dingwen Shuju, 1981.

Liji zhengyi 禮記正義. Beijing: Beijing Daxue Chubanshe, 2000.

Linghu Defen 令狐德棻 (583–666) et al. *Zhoushu* 周書. Taipei: Dingwen Shuju, 1980.

Liu An 劉安 et al. *Huainanzi* 淮南子. Second century BCE. Edited by Liu Wendian 劉文典. Beijing: Zhonghua Shuju, 1989.

Liu Xi 劉熙. *Shiming* 釋名. Third century. In *Han Wei congshu* 漢魏叢書, collected by Wang Mo 王謨. Taipei: Dahua Shuju, 1983.

Liu Xu 劉昫 et al. *Jiu Tangshu* 舊唐書. Tenth century. Taipei: Dingwen Shuju, 1981.

Liu Yiqing 劉義慶 (403–444). *Shishuo xinyu jianshu* 世說新語箋疏. Edited by Yu Jiaxi 余嘉錫. Taipei: Huazheng Shuju, 1984.

Liu Yuxi 劉禹錫 (772–842). *Liu Yuxi ji* 劉禹錫集. Beijing: Zhonghua Shuju, 1990.

Liu Zongyuan 柳宗元 (773–819). "Yu Cui lianzhou lun shi zhongru shu" 與崔連州論石鍾乳書. In *Liu Hedong ji* 柳河東集, 515–18. Shanghai: Shanghai Guji Chubanshe, 2008.

Lü Buwei 呂不韋 (292–235 BCE) et al. *Lüshi chunqiu jishi* 呂氏春秋集釋. Edited by Xu Weiyu 許維遹. Beijing: Zhonghua Shuju, 2009.

Maoshi zhengyi 毛詩正義. Beijing: Beijing Daxue Chubanshe, 2000.

Nüqing guilü 女青鬼律. Fourth century. HY 790.

Ouyang Xiu 歐陽修 (1007–1072). *Xin Tangshu* 新唐書. Taipei: Dingwen Shuju, 1981.

Ouyang Xun 歐陽詢 (557–641). *Yiwen leiju* 藝文類聚. Edited by Wang Shaoying 汪紹楹. Shanghai: Shanghai Guji Chubanshe, 1999.

Shangshu zhengyi 尚書正義. Beijing: Beijing Daxue Chubanshe, 2000.

Shen Yue 沈約 (441–513). *Songshu* 宋書. Taipei: Dingwen Shuju, 1980.

Shennong bencao jing jiaozhu 神農本草經校注. Han period. Edited by Shang Zhijun. Beijing: Xueyuan Chubanshe, 2008.

Shennong bencao jing jizhu 神農本草經輯注. Edited by Ma Jixing et al. Beijing: Renmin Wensheng Chubanshe, 1995.

Shi You 史游 (first century BCE). *Jijiu pian* 急就篇. Changsha: Yuelu Shushe, 1989.

Sima Qian 司馬遷 (145–ca. 86 BCE). *Shiji* 史記. Taipei: Dingwen Shuju, 1981.

Soushen houji 搜神後記. Fifth or sixth century. Edited by Wang Shaoying. Beijing: Zhonghua Shuju, 1981.

Su Jing 蘇敬 et al. *Xinxiu bencao* 新修本草. 659. Edited by Shang Zhijun. Hefei: Anhui Kexue Jishu Chubanshe, 1981.

———. *Xinxiu bencao* 新修本草. Facsimile of 10 *juan* preserved in Japan. 731. Shanghai: Shanghai Guji Chubanshe, 1985.

Sun Simiao 孫思邈 (581?–682). *Qianjin yifang* 千金翼方. 680s. Taipei: Zhongguo Yiyao Yanjiusuo, 1974.

———. *Sun Zhenren qianjin fang (fu zhenben qianjin fang)* 孫真人千金方（附真本千金方）. 650s. Edited by Li Jingrong 李景榮 et al. Beijing: Renmin Weisheng Chubanshe, 1996.

———. *Beiji qianjin yaofang jiaoshi* 備急千金要方校釋. 650s. Edited by Li Jingrong et al. Beijing: Renmin Weisheng Chubanshe, 1997.

Taiji zhenren jiuzhuan huandan jing yaojue 太極真人九轉還丹經要訣. Early Era of Division. HY 889.

Taiqing jing tianshi koujue 太清經天師口訣. Era of Division. HY 883.

Taishang dongyuan shenzhou jing 太上洞淵神咒經. Fifth century. HY 335.

Taishang lingbao wufu xu 太上靈寶五符序. Late third century. HY 388.

Tamba Yasuyori 丹波康賴 (912–995). *Yixin fang/Ishimpō* 醫心方. 984. Edited by Gao Wenzhu et al. Beijing: Huaxia Chubanshe, 1996.

Tao Hongjing 陶弘景 (456–536). *Bencao jing jizhu* 本草經集注. Ca. 500. Edited by Shang Zhijun and Shang Yuansheng 尚元勝. Beijing: Renmin Weisheng Chubanshe, 1994.

———. *Zhen'gao* 真誥. 499. HY 1016.

Tianyi Ge cang Ming chaoben Tiansheng ling jiaozheng 天一閣藏明鈔本天聖令校證. 1032. Edited by Tianyi Ge Bowuguan 天一閣博物館 and Zhongguo Shehui Kexueyuan Lishi Yanjiusuo Tiansheng Ling Zhengli Ketizu 中國社會科學院歷史研究所天聖令整理課題組. Beijing: Zhonghua Shuju, 2006.

Wang Chong 王充 (27–97). *Lunheng jiaoshi* 論衡校釋. Edited by Huang Hui 黃暉. Beijing: Zhonghua Shuju, 1990.

Wang Pu 王溥 (922–982). *Tang huiyao* 唐會要. Beijing: Zhonghua Shuju, 1955.

Wang Tao 王燾. *Waitai miyao fang* 外臺秘要方. 752. Edited by Gao Wenzhu. Beijing: Huaxia Chubanshe, 1993.

Wei Shou 魏收 (507–572). *Weishu* 魏書. Taipei: Dingwen Shuju, 1980.

Wei Zheng 魏徵 et al. *Suishu* 隋書. 636. Taipei: Dingwen Shuju, 1980.

Wu Pu 吳普. *Wu Pu bencao* 吳普本草. Third century. Edited by Shang Zhijun. Beijing: Renmin Weisheng Chubanshe, 1987.

Xu Shen 許慎 (ca. 55–ca. 149). *Shuowen jiezi* 說文解字. 100. Beijing: Zhonghua Shuju, 1963.

Xu Zhicai 徐之才 (492–572). *Leigong yaodui* 雷公藥對. Edited by Shang Zhijun and Shang Yuansheng. Hefei: Anhui Kexue Jishu Chubanshe, 1994.

Yan Kejun 嚴可均 (1762–1843). *Quan Jin wen* 全晉文. In *Quan shanggu Sandai Qin-Han Sanguo Liuchao wen* 全上古三代秦漢三國六朝文. Beijing: Zhonghua Shuju, 1991.

Yao Sengyuan 姚僧垣 (499–583). *Jiyan fang* 集驗方. Edited by Fan Xingzhun 范行準. Beijing: Zhongyi Guji Chubanshe, 2019.

Yao Silian 姚思廉 (557–637). *Liangshu* 梁書. Taipei: Dingwen Shuju, 1980.

Yin zhenjun jinshi wu xianglei 陰真君金石五相類. Tang period. HY 906.

Yu Zhengxie 俞正燮 (1775–1840). "Hanshi San" 寒食散. In *Guisi cungao* 癸巳存稿, 212–13. Shenyang: Liaoning Jiaoyu Chubanshe, 2003.

Zhang Hua 張華 (third century). *Bowu zhi jiaozheng* 博物志校證. Edited by Fan Ning 范寧. Beijing: Zhonghua Shuju, 1980.

Zhang Zhuo 張鷟 (660?–740). *Chaoye qianzai* 朝野僉載. Beijing: Zhonghua Shuju, 2005.

Zhangsun Wuji 長孫無忌 et al. *Tanglü shuyi qianjie* 唐律疏議籤解. 653. Edited by Liu Junwen 劉俊文. Beijing: Zhonghua Shuju, 1996.

Zhao Yi 趙翼 (1727–1814). *Ershier shi zhaji* 二十二史劄記. 1795. Beijing: Zhonghua Shuju, 1963.

Zhou Mi 周密 (1232–1298). *Yunyan guoyan lu* 雲煙過眼錄. Edited by Deng Zimian 鄧子勉. Beijing: Zhonghua Shuju, 2018.

Zhou Ziliang 周子良 (497–516). *Zhoushi mingtong ji* 周氏冥通記. Edited by Tao Hongjing. 517. HY 302.

Zhouli zhushu 周禮注疏. Beijing: Beijing Daxue Chubanshe, 1999.

Zhouyi zhengyi 周易正義. Beijing: Beijing Daxue Chubanshe, 1999.

SECONDARY SOURCES

Akahori, Akira 赤堀昭. "Drug Taking and Immortality." In *Taoist Meditation and Longevity Techniques*, edited by Livia Kohn in cooperation with Yoshinobu Sakade, 73–98. Ann Arbor: Center for Chinese Studies, University of Michigan, 1989.

Akahori Akira. "Kanshoku San to yōjō" 寒食散と養生. In *Chūgoku kodai yōjō shisō no sōgōteki kenkyū* 中国古代養生思想の総合的研究, edited by Sakade Yoshinobu 坂出祥伸, 116–43. Tokyo: Hirakawa Shuppansha, 1988.

Andersen, Poul. "Taiyi." In *The Encyclopedia of Taoism*, edited by Fabrizio Pregadio, 956–59. London: Routledge, 2008.

Anderson, Eugene N. "'Heating' and 'Cooling' Foods in Hong Kong and Taiwan." *Social Science Information* 19.2 (1980): 237–68.

Andrews, Bridie. *The Making of Modern Chinese Medicine, 1850–1960*. Vancouver: University of British Columbia Press, 2014.

Appadurai, Arjun, ed. *The Social Life of Things: Commodities in Cultural Perspective*. Cambridge: Cambridge University Press, 1986.

Arnold, David. *Colonizing the Body: State Medicine and Epidemic Disease in Nineteenth-Century India*. Berkeley: University of California Press, 1993.

———. *Toxic Histories: Poison and Pollution in Modern India*. Cambridge: Cambridge University Press, 2016.

Arthur, Shawn. *Early Daoist Dietary Practices: Examining Ways to Health and Longevity*. Lanham, MD: Lexington Books, 2013.

Barnes, Linda L. "A World of Chinese Medicine and Healing: Part One and Two." In *Chinese Medicine and Healing: An Illustrated History*, edited by TJ Hinrichs and

Linda L. Barnes, 284–378. Cambridge, MA: Belknap Press of Harvard University Press, 2013.

Barrett, T. H. *The Religious Affiliations of the Chinese Cat: An Essay Towards an Anthropozoological Approach to Comparative Religion*. The Louis Jordan Occasional Papers in Comparative Religion 2. London: School of Oriental and Asian Studies, 1998.

———. "Climate Change and Religious Response: The Case of Early Medieval China." *Journal of the Royal Asiatic Society* 17.2 (2007): 139–56.

———. *The Woman Who Discovered Printing*. New Haven, CT: Yale University Press, 2008.

Barrett, T. H., and Mark Strange. "Walking by Itself: The Singular History of the Chinese Cat." In *Animals Through Chinese History: Earliest Times to 1911*, edited by Roel Sterckx, Martina Siebert, and Dagmar Schäfer, 84–98. Cambridge: Cambridge University Press, 2019.

Baums, Stefan. "Inventing the *Pothi*: The Adoption and Spread of a New Manuscript Format in Indian Buddhism." In *Body and Cosmos: Studies in Early Indian Medical and Astral Sciences in Honor of Kenneth G. Zysk*, edited by Toke Lindegaard Knudsen, Jacob Schmidt-Madsen, and Sara Speyer, 343–62. Leiden, Netherlands: Brill, 2020.

Beck, Lily, trans. *De materia medica*, by Pedanius Dioscorides of Anazarbus. Hildesheim, Germany: Olms-Weidmann, 2017.

Bian, He. "Documenting Medications: Patients' Demand, Physicians' Virtuosity, and Genre-Mixing of Prescription-Cases (*Fang'an*) in Seventeenth-Century China." *Early Science and Medicine* 22.1 (2017): 103–23.

———. *Know Your Remedies: Pharmacy and Culture in Early Modern China*. Princeton, NJ: Princeton University Press, 2020.

Biller, Peter, and Joseph Ziegler, eds. *Religion and Medicine in the Middle Ages*. York Studies in Medieval Theology III. York, UK: York Medieval Press, 2001

Bisset, N. G. "Arrow Poisons in China. Part I." *Journal of Ethnopharmacology* 1.4 (1979): 325–84.

———. "Arrow Poisons in China. Part II. *Aconitum*–Botany, Chemistry, and Pharmacology." *Journal of Ethnopharmacology* 4.3 (1981): 247–336.

Bokenkamp, Stephen R. "Answering a Summons." In *Religions of China in Practice*, edited by Donald S. Lopez Jr., 188–202. Princeton, NJ: Princeton University Press, 1996.

———. *Early Daoist Scriptures*. Berkeley: University of California Press, 1997.

———. "Li Bai, Huangshan, and Alchemy." *T'ang Studies* 25 (2007): 29–55.

Bol, Peter K. *Neo-Confucianism in History*. Cambridge, MA: Harvard University Asia Center, 2008.

Boltz, William. *The Origin and Early Development of the Chinese Writing System*. New Haven, CT: American Oriental Society, 1994.

Brook, Timothy. "Medievality and the Chinese Sense of History." *The Medieval History Journal* 1.1 (1998): 145–64.

Brown, Miranda. *The Art of Medicine in Early China: The Ancient and Medieval Origins of a Modern Archive*. New York: Cambridge University Press, 2015.

———. "'Medicine' in Early China." In *Routledge Handbook of Early Chinese History*, edited by Paul R. Goldin, 459–72. Abingdon, UK: Routledge, 2018.

Bynum, Caroline. "Material Continuity, Personal Survival, and the Resurrection of the Body: A Scholastic Discussion in Its Medieval and Modern Contexts." *History of Religions* 30.1 (1990): 51–85.

———. "Why All the Fuss about the Body? A Medievalist's Perspective." *Critical Inquiry* 22.1 (1995): 1–33.

Cai, Liang. *Witchcraft and the Rise of the First Confucian Empire*. Albany: State University of New York Press, 2014.

Campany, Robert Ford. *To Live as Long as Heaven and Earth: A Translation and Study of Ge Hong's Traditions of Divine Transcendents*. Berkeley: University of California Press, 2002.

Cedzich, Ursula-Angelika. "Corpse Deliverance, Substitute Bodies, Name Change, and Feigned Death: Aspects of Metamorphosis and Immortality in Early Medieval China." *Journal of Chinese Religions* 29.1 (2001): 1–68.

Chang Chaojan 張超然. "You xian er zhen: *Ziyang zhenren neizhuan* suo biaoshi de xin xiudao lujing" 由仙而真：《紫陽真人內傳》所標示的新修道路徑. *Dandao yanjiu* 丹道研究 1 (2006): 260–326.

Chang Shu-hao 張書豪. "Xihan 'yao hou huo de' shuo de chengli" 西漢「堯後火德」說的成立. *Hanxue yanjiu* 漢學研究 29.3 (2011): 1–27.

Chen Dengwu 陳登武. *Cong renjianshi dao youmingjie—Tangdai de fazhi, shehui yu guojia* 從人間世到幽冥界—唐代的法制、社會與國家. Beijing: Beijing Daxue Chubanshe, 2007.

Chen Guofu 陳國符. *Daozang yuanliu kao* 道藏源流攷. Beijing: Zhonghua Shuju, 1963.

———. *Chen Guofu daozang yanjiu lunwen ji* 陳國符道藏研究論文集. Shanghai: Shanghai Guji Chubanshe, 2004.

Chen Hao 陳昊. "Zai xieben yu yinben zhijian de fangshu—Songdai *Qianjin fang* de shuji shi" 在寫本與印本之間的方書—宋代《千金方》的書籍史. *Zhongyiyao zazhi* 中醫藥雜誌 24.S1 (2013): 69–85.

———. *Shenfen xushi yu zhishi biaoshu zhijian de yizhe zhi yi—6-8 shiji Zhongguo de shuji zhixu, weiyi zhi ti yu yixue shenfen de fuxian* 身分敘事與知識表述之間的醫者之意—6-8世紀中國的書籍秩序、為醫之體與醫學身分的浮現. Shanghai: Shanghai Guji Chubanshe, 2019.

———. *Ji zhi cheng shang—Qin-Song zhijian de jibing mingyi yu lishi xushi zhong de cunzai* 疾之成殤—秦宋之間的疾病名義與歷史敘事中的存在. Shanghai: Shanghai Guji Chubanshe, 2020.

Chen Liang 陳亮. "Donghan zhenmu wen suojian daowu guanxi de zai sikao" 東漢鎮墓文所見道巫關係的再思考. *Xingxiang shixue* 形象史學 9.1 (2019): 44–71.

Chen Ming 陳明. *Shufang yiyao—Chutu wenshu yu xiyu yixue* 殊方異藥—出土文書與西域醫學. Beijing: Beijing Daxue Chubanshe, 2005.

———. *Zhonggu yiliao yu wailai wenhua* 中古醫療與外來文化. Beijing: Beijing Daxue Chubanshe, 2013.

———. *Dunhuang de yiliao yu shehui* 敦煌的醫療與社會. Beijing: Zhongguo Dabaike Quanshu Chubanshe, 2018.

Chen Yuanpeng 陳元朋. *Liang Song de "shangyi shiren" yu "ruyi"—jianlun qi zai Jin-Yuan de liubian* 兩宋的「尚醫士人」與「儒醫」—兼論其在金元的流變. Taipei: Guoli Taiwan Daxue Chuban Weiyuanhui, 1997.

———. "*Bencao jing jizhu* suozai 'Taozhu' zhong de zhishi leixing, yaochan fenbu yu beifang yaowu de shuru" 《本草經集注》所載「陶注」中的知識類型、藥產分布與北方藥物的輸入. *Zhongguo shehui lishi pinglun* 中國社會歷史評論 12 (2011): 184–212.

Chen Yun-ju. "Accounts of Treating *Zhang* ("miasma") Disorders in Song Dynasty Lingnan: Remarks on Changing Literary Forms of Writing Experience." *Hanxue yanjiu* 漢學研究 34.3 (2016): 205–54.

Cheng Jin 程錦. "Tang Yiji ling fuyuan yanjiu" 唐醫疾令復原研究. In *Tianyi Ge cang Ming chaoben Tiansheng ling jiaozheng* 天一閣藏明鈔本天聖令校證, 552–80. Beijing: Zhonghua Shuju, 2006.

Chin Shih-chi 金仕起. *Zhongguo gudai de yixue, yishi yu zhengzhi* 中國古代的醫學、醫史與政治. Taipei: Zhengda Chubanshe, 2010.

Collard, Franck. *The Crime of Poison in the Middle Ages*. Translated by Deborah Nelson-Campbell. Westport, CT: Praeger, 2008.

Collard, Franck, and Évelyne Samama, eds. *Le corps à l'épreuve: Poisons, remèdes et chirurgie: aspects des practiques médicales dans l'Antiquité et au Moyen-Âge*. Langres, France: D. Guéniot, 2002.

Cook, Constance A. "A Fatal Case of *Gu* 蠱 Poisoning in Fourth-Century BC China." *East Asian Science, Technology, and Medicine* 44 (2016): 123–49.

———. "Exorcism and the Spirit Turtle." In *Thinking about Early China: Essays in Honor of Sarah Allan*, edited by Constance Cook, Susan Blader, and Christopher Foster, forthcoming.

Copp, Paul. *The Body Incantatory: Spells and the Ritual Imagination in Medieval Chinese Buddhism*. New York: Columbia University Press, 2014.

Csikszentmihalyi, Mark. "*Fangshi*." In *The Encyclopedia of Taoism*, edited by Fabrizio Pregadio, 406–9. London: Routledge, 2008.

Cullen, Christopher. "*Yi'an* 醫案 (Case Statements): The Origins of a Genre of Chinese Medical Literature." In *Innovation in Chinese Medicine*, edited by Elisabeth Hsu, 297–323. Cambridge: Cambridge University Press, 2001.

Dai Jianguo 戴建國. "Tianyi Ge cang Ming chaoben *Guanpin ling* kao" 天一閣藏明抄本《官品令》考. *Lishi yanjiu* 歷史研究 3 (1999): 71–86.

Daston, Lorraine, ed. *Things That Talk: Object Lessons from Art and Science*. New York: Zone Books, 2004.

Davis, Timothy M. "Lechery, Substance Abuse, and . . . Han Yu?" *Journal of the American Oriental Society* 135.1 (2015): 71–92.

de Groot, J. J. M. *The Religious System of China: Its Ancient Forms, Evolution, History and Present Aspect, Manners, Customs and Social Institutions Connected Therewith*.

Vol. 5, book II. Reprint of Leiden, Netherlands: E. J. Brill, 1892–1910; Taipei: Ch'eng Wen Publishing Company, 1972.

DeClercq, Dominik. *Writing against the State: Political Rhetorics in Third and Fourth Century China.* Leiden, Netherlands: Brill, 1998.

Deleuze, Gilles, and Félix Guattari. *A Thousand Plateaus: Capitalism and Schizophrenia.* Translated by Brian Massumi. Minneapolis: University of Minnesota Press, 1987.

Deng Qiyao 鄧啟耀. *Zhongguo wugu kaocha* 中國巫蠱考察. Shanghai: Shanghai Wenyi Chubanshe, 1999.

d'Errico, Francesco et al. "Early Evidence of San Material Culture Represented by Organic Artifacts from Border Cave, South Africa." *Proceedings of the National Academy of Sciences* 109.33 (2012): 13214–19.

Derrida, Jacques. "Plato's Pharmacy." In *Dissemination*, translated by Barbara Johnson, 61–171. Chicago: University of Chicago Press, 1981.

Despeux, Catherine. "Gymnastics: The Ancient Tradition." In *Taoist Meditation and Longevity Techniques*, edited by Livia Kohn in cooperation with Yoshinobu Sakade, 223–61. Ann Arbor: Center for Chinese Studies, University of Michigan, 1989.

———. "The System of the Five Circulatory Phases and the Six Seasonal Influences (*wuyun liuqi*), a Source of Innovation in Medicine under the Song (960–1279)." In *Innovation in Chinese Medicine*, edited by Elisabeth Hsu, 121–65. Cambridge: Cambridge University Press, 2001.

———, ed. *Médecine, religion et société dans la Chine médiévale: étude de manuscrits chinois de Dunhuang et de Turfan.* Paris: Collège de France, Institut des Hautes Études Chinoises, 2010.

———. "Chinese Medicinal Excrement: Is There a Buddhist Influence on the Use of Animal Excrement-Based Recipes in Medieval China?" *Asian Medicine* 12.1–2 (2017): 139–69.

DeWoskin, Kenneth. *Doctors, Diviners, and Magicians of Ancient China: Biographies of Fang-shih.* New York: Columbia University Press, 1983.

Diamond, Norma. "The Miao and Poison: Interactions on China's Southwest Frontier." *Ethnology* 27.1 (1988): 1–25.

Dien, Albert E., and Keith N. Knapp, eds. *The Cambridge History of China.* Vol. 2, *The Six Dynasties, 220–589.* Cambridge: Cambridge University Press, 2019.

Ding Guangdi 丁光迪. *Zhubing yuanhou lun yangsheng fang daoyin fa yanjiu* 諸病源候論養生方導引法研究. Beijing: Renmin Weisheng Chubanshe, 2010.

Doran, Rebecca. "The Cat Demon, Gender, and Religious Practice: Towards Reconstructing a Medieval Chinese Cultural Pattern." *Journal of the American Oriental Society* 135.4 (2015): 689–707.

Duden, Barbara. *The Woman beneath the Skin: A Doctor's Patients in Eighteenth-Century Germany.* Translated by Thomas Dunlap. Cambridge, MA: Harvard University Press, 1991.

Dufton, Emily. *Grass Roots: The Rise and Fall and Rise of Marijuana in America.* New York: Basic Books, 2017.

Dumbacher, John et al. "Homobatrachotoxin in the Genus *Pitohui*: Chemical Defense in Birds?" *Science* 258.5083 (1992): 799–801.

Engelhardt, Ute. "Dietetics in Tang China and the First Extant Works of *Materia Dietetica*." In *Innovation in Chinese Medicine*, edited by Elisabeth Hsu, 173–91. Cambridge: Cambridge University Press, 2001.

Epler, Deane C., Jr. "The Concept of Disease in Two Third Century Chinese Medical Texts." PhD diss., University of Washington, 1977.

Etkin, Nina L. "'Side Effects': Cultural Constructions and Reinterpretations of Western Pharmaceuticals." *Medical Anthropology Quarterly* 6.2 (1992): 99–113.

———. "The Negotiation of 'Side' Effects in Hausa (Northern Nigeria) Therapeutics." In *Medicines: Meanings and Contexts*, edited by Nina L. Etkin and Michael L. Tan, 17–32. Quezon City, Philippines: Health Action Information Network in coordination with the Medical Anthropology Unit, University of Amsterdam, 1994.

Fan Ka-wai 范家偉. "Han-Tang jian zhi gudu" 漢唐間之蠱毒. In *Dushi cungao* 讀史存稿, edited by Li Hanji 黎漢基, 1–23. Hong Kong: Xuefeng Wenhua Shiye Gongsi, 1998.

———. *Liuchao Sui-Tang yixue zhi chuancheng yu zhenghe* 六朝隋唐醫學之傳承與整合. Hong Kong: Zhongwen Daxue Chubanshe, 2004.

———. *Dayi jingcheng—Tangdai guojia, xinyang yu yixue* 大醫精誠—唐代國家、信仰與醫學. Taipei: Dongda Tushu Gongsi, 2007.

———. "Liu Yuxi yu *Chuanxin fang*—yi Tangdai nanfang xingxiang, bianguan he yanfang wei zhongxin de kaocha" 劉禹錫與《傳信方》—以唐代南方形象、貶官和驗方為中心的考察. In *Cong yiliao kan zhongguo shi* 從醫療看中國史, edited by Li Jianmin 李建民, 111–44. Taipei: Lianjing Chuban Shiye Gufen Youxian Gongsi, 2008.

———. *Zhonggu shiqi de yizhe yu bingzhe* 中古時期的醫者與病者. Shanghai: Fudan Daxue Chubanshe, 2010.

———. "The Period of Division and the Tang Period." In *Chinese Medicine and Healing: An Illustrated History*, edited by TJ Hinrichs and Linda L. Barnes, 65–96. Cambridge, MA: Belknap Press of Harvard University Press, 2013.

———. *Beisong jiaozheng yishuju xintan—yi guojia yu yixue wei zhongxin* 北宋校正醫書局新探—以國家與醫學為中心. Hong Kong: Zhonghua Shuju, 2014.

———. "Ge xianweng Zhouhou beijifang." In *Early Medieval Chinese Texts: A Bibliographical Guide*, edited by Cynthia L. Chennault, Keith N. Knapp, Alan J. Berkowitz, and Albert E. Dien, 88–94. Berkeley, CA: Institute of East Asian Studies, 2015.

Fan Xingzhun 范行準. *Zhongguo yixue shilüe* 中國醫學史略. Beijing: Zhongyi Guji Chubanshe, 1986.

———. *Zhongguo bingshi xinyi* 中國病史新義. Beijing: Zhongyi Guji Chubanshe, 1989.

Farquhar, Judith. *Knowing Practice: The Clinical Encounter of Chinese Medicine*. Boulder, CO: Westview Press, 1994.

Feng Hanyong 馮漢鏞. *Gu fangshu jiyi* 古方書輯佚. Beijing: Renmin Weisheng Chubanshe, 1993.

Feng, H. Y., and J. K. Shryock. "The Black Magic in China Known as *Ku*." *Journal of the American Oriental Society* 55 (1935): 1–30.

Fèvre, Francine. "Drôles de bestioles: qu'est-ce qu'un *chong*?" *Anthropozoologica* 18 (1993): 57–65.

Findlen, Paula, ed. *Early Modern Things: Objects and Their Histories, 1500–1800.* New York: Routledge, 2013.

Fu Ting 付婷. "Wu Zetian 'weimao shuo' zaitan—jianlun Tangdai 'mao' de xingxiang" 武則天 "畏貓說" 再探—兼論唐代 "貓" 的形象. *Tangshi luncong* 唐史論叢 15 (2012): 96–109.

Fuenzalida, Ariel. "Pharmakontologies: Philosophy and the Question of Drugs." PhD diss., University of Western Ontario, 2009.

Fujieda, Akira. "The Tunhuang Manuscripts: A General Description (Part I)." *Zinbun: Memoirs of the Research Institute for Humanistic Studies, Kyoto University* 9 (1966): 1–32.

———. "The Tunhuang Manuscripts: A General Description (Part II)." *Zinbun: Memoirs of the Research Institute for Humanistic Studies, Kyoto University* 10 (1967): 17–39.

Furth, Charlotte. "Producing Medical Knowledge through Cases: History, Evidence, and Action." In *Thinking with Cases: Specialist Knowledge in Chinese Cultural History*, edited by Charlotte Furth, Judith T. Zeitlin, and Ping-chen Hsiung, 125–51. Honolulu: University of Hawai'i Press, 2007.

Fuyang Hanjian Zhengli Zu 阜陽漢簡整理組. "Fuyang hanjian *Wanwu*" 阜陽漢簡 《萬物》. *Wenwu* 文物 4 (1988): 36–47.

Gan Zuwang 干祖望. *Sun Simiao pingzhuan* 孫思邈評傳. Nanjing: Nanjing Daxue Chubanshe, 1995.

Gao Wenzhu 高文鑄. *Waitai miyao fang congkao* 外臺秘要方叢考. In *Waitai miyao fang* 外臺秘要方, edited by Gao Wenzhu, 839–978. Beijing: Huaxia Chubanshe, 1993.

Geng Jianting 耿鑒庭. "Xi'an nanjiao Tangdai jiaocang li de yiyao wenwu" 西安南郊唐代窖藏裏的醫藥文物. *Wenwu* 文物 1 (1972): 56–60.

Gibbs, Frederick W. *Poison, Medicine, and Disease in Late Medieval and Early Modern Europe.* London: Routledge, 2019.

Goldschmidt, Asaf. *The Evolution of Chinese Medicine: Song Dynasty, 960–1200.* London: Routledge, 2009.

———. "Reasoning with Cases: The Transmission of Clinical Medical Knowledge in Twelfth-Century Song China." In *Antiquarianism, Language, and Medical Philology: From Early Modern to Modern Sino-Japanese Medical Discourses*, edited by Benjamin Elman, 19–51. Leiden, Netherlands: Brill, 2015.

Grant, Joanna. *A Chinese Physician: Wang Ji and the "Stone Mountain Medical Case Histories."* London: RoutledgeCurzon, 2003.

Greene, Jeremy, and Elizabeth Watkins, eds. *Prescribed: Writing, Filling, Using, and Abusing the Prescription in Modern America.* Baltimore: Johns Hopkins University Press, 2012.

Grell, Ole Peter, Andrew Cunningham, and Jon Arrizabalaga, eds. *"It All Depends on the Dose": Poisons and Medicines in European History.* London: Routledge, 2018.

Gruman, Gerald. *A History of Ideas about the Prolongation of Life: The Evolution of Prolongevity Hypotheses to 1800*. Philadelphia: American Philosophical Society, 1966.

Guangzhou Shi Wenwu Guanli Weiyuanhui 廣州市文物管理委員會. *Xihan Nanyue wang mu* 西漢南越王墓. Beijing: Wenwu Chubanshe, 1991.

Guo Zhengzhong 郭正忠. *San zhi shisi shiji Zhongguo de quanheng duliang* 三至十四世紀中國的權衡度量. Beijing: Zhongguo Shehui Kexue Chubanshe, 1993.

Hansen, Valerie. *The Open Empire: A History of China to 1800*. New York: W. W. Norton & Company, 2015.

Hanson, Marta. *Speaking of Epidemics in Chinese Medicine: Disease and the Geographic Imagination in Late Imperial China*. London: Routledge, 2011.

———. "Is the 2015 Nobel Prize a Turning Point for Traditional Chinese Medicine?" *The Conversation*, October 5, 2015.

Hao Baohua 郝保華. "Cong lishi jiaodu kexue lixing renshi zhongyao de dufu zuoyong" 從歷史角度科學理性認識中藥的毒副作用. *Dulixue shi yanjiu wenji* 毒理學史研究文集 2 (2003): 57.

Harper, Donald. "A Chinese Demonography of the Third Century B.C." *Harvard Journal of Asiatic Studies* 45.2 (1985): 459–98.

———. *Early Chinese Medical Literature: The Mawangdui Medical Manuscripts*. New York: Kegan Paul International, 1998.

———. "Physicians and Diviners: The Relation of Divination to the Medicine of the *Huangdi neijing* (Inner canon of the Yellow Thearch)." *Extrême-Orient, Extrême-Occident* 21 (1999): 91–110.

Herzberg, David. *Happy Pills in America: From Miltown to Prozac*. Baltimore: Johns Hopkins University Press, 2009.

———. *White Market Drugs: Big Pharma and the Hidden History of Addiction in America*. Chicago: University of Chicago Press, 2020.

Hibino Takeo 日比野丈夫. "*Shin Tōjo* chirishi no tokō nitsuite" 新唐書地理志の土貢について. *Tōhō gakuhō* 東方学報 17 (1949): 83–99.

———. "Tō Kōkei no *Honzō shūchū* ni kansuru itsu kōsatsu—tokuni sanchi no hensen nitsuite" 陶弘景の本草集注に関する一考察—とくに産地の変遷について. *Kyōu* 杏雨 1 (1998): 1–20.

Hinrichs, TJ. "Governance through Medical Texts and the Role of Print." In *Knowledge and Text Production in an Age of Print: China, 900–1400*, edited by Lucille Chia and Hilde De Weerdt, 217–38. Leiden, Netherlands: Brill, 2011.

———. "The Catchy Epidemic: Theorization and its Limits in Han to Song Period Medicine." *East Asian Science, Technology, and Medicine* 41 (2015): 19–62.

———. *Shamans, Witchcraft, and Quarantine: The Medical Transformation of Governance and Southern Customs in Mid-Imperial China*. Cambridge, MA: Harvard University Asia Center, forthcoming.

Ho Peng Yoke. *Explorations in Daoism: Medicine and Alchemy in Literature*. London: Routledge, 2007.

Ho Ping-Yü, and Joseph Needham. "Elixir Poisoning in Medieval China." *Janus* 48 (1959): 221–51.

Holcombe, Charles. "Was Medieval China Medieval? (Post-Han to Mid-Tang)." In *A Companion to Chinese History*, edited by Michael Szonyi, 106–17. Hoboken, NJ: Wiley Blackwell, 2017.

Horden, Peregrine. "What's Wrong with Early Medieval Medicine?" *Social History of Medicine* 24.1 (2011): 5–25.

Hsu, Elisabeth. *Pulse Diagnosis in Early Chinese Medicine: The Telling Touch*. Cambridge: Cambridge University Press, 2010.

Hu Axiang 胡阿祥 and Hu Haitong 胡海桐. "Han Yu 'zuruo buneng bu' yu 'tuizhi fu liuhuang' kaobian" 韓愈 "足弱不能步" 與 "退之服硫黃" 考辨. *Zhonghua wenshi luncong* 中華文史論叢 98.2 (2010): 193–212.

Hu Mingzhao 胡明曌. "Cong xinchu Sun Xing muzhi tanxi yaowang shengzunian" 從新出孫行墓誌探析藥王生卒年. In *Chutu wenxian yanjiu* 出土文獻研究, vol. 10, 406–10. Beijing: Zhonghua Shuju, 2011.

Hu Pingsheng 胡平生 and Han Ziqiang 韓自強. "*Wanwu* lüeshuo"《萬物》略說. *Wenwu* 文物 4 (1988): 48–54.

Hu, Shiu-ying. *An Enumeration of Chinese Materia Medica*. Hong Kong: Chinese University Press, 1980.

Huang, Shih-shan Susan. "Daoist Imagery of Body and Cosmos. Part 2: Body Worms and Internal Alchemy." *Journal of Daoist Studies* 4 (2011): 33–64.

Huang Zhengjian 黃正建. "Shilun Tangdai qianqi huangdi xiaofei de mouxie cemian—yi *Tongdian* juanliu suoji changgong wei zhongxin" 試論唐代前期皇帝消費的某些側面—以《通典》卷六所記常貢為中心. *Tang yanjiu* 唐研究 6 (2000): 173–211.

Hulsewé, A. F. P. *Remnants of Ch'in Law: An Annotated Translation of the Ch'in Legal and Administrative Rules of the 3rd Century B.C. Discovered in Yün-meng Prefecture, Hu-pei Province, in 1975*. Leiden, Netherlands: Brill, 1985.

Huo Bin 霍斌. "'Du' yu zhonggu shehui" "毒" 與中古社會. Master's thesis, Shaanxi Normal University, 2012.

Ishida Hidemi 石田秀実. "*Shōbon hō* no igaku shisō"「小品方」の医学思想. In his *Kokoro to karada: Chūgoku kodai niokeru shintai no shisō* こころとからだ: 中国古代における身体の思想, 254–76. Fukuoka: Chūgoku Shoten, 1995.

———. "Genkiyaku kō" 見鬼藥考. *Tōhō shūkyō* 東方宗教 96 (2000): 38–57.

Ishino Tomohiro 石野智大. "Tōdai ryōkyō no miyabito kanbō" 唐代両京の宮人患坊. *Hōshigaku kenkyūkai kaihō* 法史学研究会会報 13 (2008): 25–35.

Ito Kiyoshi 伊藤清司. *Chūgoku no shinjū, akkitachi: Sengaikyō no sekai* 中国の神獣・悪鬼たち: 山海経の世界. Tokyo: Tōhō Shoten, 1986.

Iwamoto Atsushi 岩本篤志. *Tōdai no iyakusho to Tonkō bunken* 唐代の医薬書と敦煌文献. Tokyo: Kadokawa Gakugei Shuppan, 2015.

Jing Shuhui 景蜀慧 and Xiao Rong 肖榮. "Zhonggu fusan de chengyin ji chuancheng: cong Huangfu Mi dao Sun Simiao" 中古服散的成因及傳承: 從皇甫謐到孫思邈. *Tang yanjiu* 唐研究 13 (2007): 337–68.

Jonas, Wayne B., Ted J. Kaptchuk, and Klaus Linde. "A Critical Overview of Homeopathy." *Annals of Internal Medicine* 138 (2003): 393–99.

Jones, Claire. "Formula and Formulation: 'Efficacy Phrases' in Medieval English Medical Manuscripts." *Neuphilologische Mitteilungen* 99 (1998): 199–209.

Kaptchuk, Ted J. *The Web That Has No Weaver: Understanding Chinese Medicine.* New York: McGraw-Hill, 2000.

Kawahara Hideki 川原秀城. *Dokuyaku wa kuchi ni nigashi—Chūgoku no bunjin to furō fushi* 毒薬は口に苦し—中国の文人と不老不死. Tokyo: Taishūkan Shoten, 2001.

Kieschnick, John. *The Impact of Buddhism on Chinese Material Culture.* Princeton, NJ: Princeton University Press, 2003.

Kleeman, Terry. *Celestial Masters: History and Ritual in Early Daoist Communities.* Cambridge, MA: Harvard University Asia Center, 2016.

Knapp, Keith. "Did the Middle Kingdom Have a Middle Period? The Problem of 'Medieval' in China's History." *Education about Asia* 12.2 (2007): 8–13.

Köhle, Natalie. "A Confluence of Humors: Āyurvedic Conceptions of Digestion and the History of Chinese 'Phlegm' (*tan* 痰)." *Journal of the American Oriental Society* 136.3 (2016): 465–93.

Kohn, Livia, ed., in cooperation with Yoshinobu Sakade. *Taoist Meditation and Longevity Techniques.* Ann Arbor: Center for Chinese Studies, University of Michigan, 1989.

———. *Chinese Healing Exercises: The Tradition of Daoyin.* Honolulu: University of Hawai'i Press, 2008.

Kuo Ho-Hsiang 郭賀翔. "Sui-Tang yiji zhong guanyu du de xin renshi—yi sanda yiji wei zhongxin de tantao" 隋唐醫籍中關於毒的新認識—以三大醫籍為中心的探討. Master's thesis, National Tsing Hua University, 2006.

Kuriyama, Shigehisa. *The Expressiveness of the Body and the Divergence of Greek and Chinese Medicine.* New York: Zone Books, 1999.

———. "Epidemics, Weather, and Contagion in Traditional Chinese Medicine." In *Contagion: Perspectives from Pre-Modern Societies*, edited by Lawrence I. Conrad and Dominik Wujastyk, 3–22. Aldershot, UK: Ashgate, 2000.

Latour, Bruno. *We Have Never Been Modern.* Translated by Catherine Porter. Cambridge, MA: Harvard University Press, 1993.

Lau Nap Yin 柳立言. "Hewei 'Tang-Song biange'?" 何謂「唐宋變革」? *Zhonghua wenshi luncong* 中華文史論叢 81 (2006): 125–71.

Lee Fong-mao 李豐楙. "*Daozang* suoshou zaoqi daoshu de wenyi guan—yi *Nüqing guilü* ji *Dongyuan shenzhou jing* weizhu"《道藏》所收早期道書的瘟疫觀—以《女青鬼律》及《洞淵神咒經》為主. *Zhongguo wenzhe yanjiu jikan* 中國文哲研究集刊 3 (1993): 417–54.

Lee Jen-der 李貞德. *Nüren de Zhongguo yiliao shi—Han-Tang zhijian de jiankang zhaogu yu xingbie* 女人的中國醫療史—漢唐之間的健康照顧與性別. Taipei: Sanmin Shuju, 2008.

Lee, Martin A. *Smoke Signals: A Social History of Marijuana—Medical, Recreational, and Scientific.* New York: Scribner, 2012.

Lei, Sean Hsiang-lin. "How Did Chinese Medicine Become Experiential? The Political Epistemology of *Jingyan*." *Positions* 10.2 (2002): 333–64.

———. *Neither Donkey nor Horse: Medicine in the Struggle over China's Modernity.* Chicago: University of Chicago Press, 2014.

Leung, Angela Ki Che. *Leprosy in China: A History*. New York: Columbia University Press, 2009.

Li, Hui-lin. "The Origin and Use of Cannabis in Eastern Asia: Their Linguistic-Cultural Implications." In *Cannabis and Culture*, edited by Vera Rubin, 51–62. Berlin: De Gruyter Mouton, 1975.

Li Jianmin 李建民. "Contagion and Its Consequences: The Problem of Death Pollution in Ancient China." In *Medicine and the History of the Body: Preeceedings of the 20th, 21st and 22nd International Symposium on the Comparative History of Medicine—East and West*, edited by Yasuo Otsuka, Shizu Sakai, and Shigehisa Kuriyama, 201–22. Tokyo: Ishiyaku EuroAmerica, 1999.

———. *Sisheng zhiyu—Zhou-Qin-Han maixue zhi yuanliu* 死生之域—周秦漢脈學之源流. Taipei: Zhongyang Yanjiuyuan Lishi Yuyan Yanjiusuo, 2000.

———. "They Shall Expel Demons: Etiology, the Medical Canon and the Transformation of Medical Techniques before the Tang," translated by Sabine Wilms. In *Early Chinese Religion, Part One: Shang through Han (1250 BC–220 AD)*, edited by John Lagerwey and Marc Kalinowski, vol. 2, 1103–50. Leiden, Netherlands: Brill, 2008.

———. *Huatuo yincang de shoushu* 華佗隱藏的手術. Taipei: Dongda Tushu Gufen Youxian Gongsi, 2011.

———. *Lüxingzhe de shixue* 旅行者的史學. Taipei: Yunchen Wenhua Shiye Gufen Youxian Gongsi, 2011.

Li Ling 李零. "Wushi kao" 五石考. In his *Zhongguo fangshu xukao* 中國方術續考, 341–49. Beijing: Dongfang Chubanshe, 2000.

———. "Yaodu yijia" 藥毒一家. In his *Zhongguo fangshu xukao*, 28–38. Beijing: Dongfang Chubanshe, 2000.

———. "Liandanshu de qiyuan he fushi zhuyou" 煉丹術的起源和服食祝由. In his *Zhongguo fangshu kao (xiuding ben)* 中國方術考（修訂本）, 301–40. Beijing: Dongfang Chubanshe, 2001.

Li Ronghua 李榮華. "Suidai 'wugu zhi shu' xintan" 隋代 "巫蠱之術" 新探. *Wuyi daxue xuebao* 五邑大學學報 12.3 (2010): 78–81.

Liao Jui-yui 廖芮茵. *Tangdai fushi yangsheng yanjiu* 唐代服食養生研究. Taipei: Xuesheng Shuju, 2004.

Liao Yuqun 廖育群. *Qi Huang yidao* 歧黃醫道. Shenyang: Liaoning Jiaoyu Chubanshe, 1991.

———. "Kaoding *Mingyi bielu* jiqi yu Tao Hongjing zhushu de guanxi" 考訂《名醫別錄》及其與陶弘景著述的關係. *Ziran kexueshi yanjiu* 自然科學史研究 11.3 (1992): 261–69.

———. "Yindu gudai yaowu fenlei fa jiqi keneng dui Zhongguo yixue chansheng de yingxiang" 印度古代藥物分類法及其可能對中國醫學產生的影響. *Ziran bianzhengfa tongxun* 自然辯證法通訊 17.2 (1995): 56–63.

———. *Renshi Yindu chuantong yixue* 認識印度傳統醫學. Taipei: Dongda Tushu Gongsi, 2003.

———. "Zhongguo chuantong yixue de 'chuantong' yu 'geming'" 中國傳統醫學的「傳統」與「革命」. In his *Yizhe yi ye—Renshi Zhongguo chuantong yixue* 醫者意也—認識中國傳統醫學, 209–25. Taipei: Dongda Tushu Gongsi, 2003.

Lin, Fu-shih 林富士. "The Image and Status of Shamans in Ancient China." In *Early Chinese Religion, Part One: Shang through Han (1250 BC–220 AD)*, edited by John Lagerwey and Marc Kalinowski, vol. 1, 397–458. Leiden, Netherlands: Brill, 2008.

Lin Fu-shih. *Zhongguo zhonggu shiqi de zongjiao yu yiliao* 中國中古時期的宗教與醫療. Taipei: Lianjing Chuban Shiye Gufen Youxian Gongsi, 2008.

Liu Pao-line 劉寶玲. "Yi chong wei xiang—Han-Tang shiqi yiji zhong de chong" 以蟲為象—漢唐時期醫籍中的蟲. Master's thesis, National Tsing Hua University, 2004.

Liu Shu-fen 劉淑芬. *Zhonggu de fojiao yu shehui* 中古的佛教與社會. Shanghai: Shanghai Guji Chubanshe, 2008.

———. *Cibei qingjing: Fojiao yu zhonggu shehui shenghuo* 慈悲清淨：佛教與中古社會生活. Beijing: Shangwu Yinshuguan, 2017.

Liu, Yan. "Poisonous Medicine in Ancient China." In *History of Toxicology and Environmental Health Series: Toxicology in Antiquity*, edited by Philip Wexler, 431–39. London: Elsevier, 2019.

———. "Words, Demons, and Illness: Incantatory Healing in Medieval China." *Asian Medicine* 14 (2019): 1–29.

Liu, Yan, and Shigehisa Kuriyama. "Fluid Being: Mercury in Chinese Medicine and Alchemy." In *Fluid Matter(s): Flow and Transformation in the History of the Body*, edited by Natalie Köhle and Shigehisa Kuriyama. Canberra: Australian National University Press, 2020.

Lloyd, Geoffrey, and Nathan Sivin. *The Way and the Word: Science and Medicine in Early China and Greece*. New Haven, CT: Yale University Press, 2002.

Lo, Vivienne. "Tracking the Pain: *Jue* and the Formation of a Theory of Circulating *Qi* through the Channels." *Sudhoffs Archiv* 83.2 (1999): 191–211.

———. "The Influence of Nurturing Life Culture on the Development of Western Han Acumoxa Therapy." In *Innovation in Chinese Medicine*, edited by Elisabeth Hsu, 19–51. Cambridge: Cambridge University Press, 2001.

———. "Pleasure, Prohibition, and Pain: Food and Medicine in Traditional China." In *Of Tripod and Palate: Food, Politics, and Religion in Traditional China*, edited by Roel Sterckx, 163–85. New York: Palgrave Macmillan, 2004.

———. *Potent Flavours: A History of Nutrition in China*. London: Reaktion Books, forthcoming.

Lo, Vivienne, and Christopher Cullen, eds. *Medieval Chinese Medicine: The Dunhuang Medical Manuscripts*. London: RoutledgeCurzon, 2005.

Loewe, Michael. "The Case of Witchcraft in 91 B.C.: Its Historical Setting and Effect on Han Dynastic History." *Asia Major* 15.2 (1970): 159–96.

Lord, Graham et al. "Urothelial Malignant Disease and Chinese Herbal Nephropathy." *Lancet* 358.9292 (2001): 1515–16.

Lu, Gwei-Djen, and Joseph Needham. *Celestial Lancets: A History and Rationale of Acupuncture and Moxa*. Cambridge: Cambridge University Press, 1980.

Lu Xiangqian 盧向前. "Boxihe sanqiyisi hao beimian chuanmafang wenshu yanjiu" 伯希和三七一四號背面傳馬坊文書研究. In *Dunhuang Tulufan wenxian yanjiu lunji* 敦煌吐魯番文獻研究論集, 671–74. Beijing: Zhonghua Shuju, 1982.

———. "Wu Zetian 'weimao shuo' yu Suishi 'maogui zhi yu'" 武則天 "畏貓說" 與 隋室 "貓鬼之獄." *Zhongguo shi yanjiu* 中國史研究 1 (2006): 81–94.

Lu Xun 魯迅. "Wei-Jin fengdu ji wenzhang yu yao ji jiu zhi guanxi" 魏晉風度及文章 與藥及酒之關係 (1927). In *Lu Xun quanji* 魯迅全集, vol. 3, 486–507. Shanghai: Renmin Wenxue Chubanshe, 1973.

Marcon, Federico. *The Knowledge of Nature and the Nature of Knowledge in Early Modern Japan.* Chicago: University of Chicago Press, 2015.

Mather, Richard B., trans. *Shih-shuo Hsin-yü: A New Account of Tales of the World.* Ann Arbor: Center for Chinese Studies, University of Michigan, 2002.

Mayanagi Makoto 真柳誠. "Chintori—Jitsuzai kara densetsu e" 鳩鳥—実在から伝 説へ. In *Mono no imēji: Honzō to hakubutsugaku e no shōtai* 物のイメージ・本草 と博物学への招待, edited by Yamada Keiji 山田慶兒, 151–85. Tokyo: Asahi Shin- bunsha, 1994.

———. "The Three *Juan* Edition of *Bencao jizhu* and Excavated Sources," translated by Sumiyo Umekawa. In *Medieval Chinese Medicine: The Dunhuang Medical Manuscripts*, edited by Vivienne Lo and Christopher Cullen, 306–21. London: RoutledgeCurzon, 2005.

McVaugh, Michael. "The *Experimenta* of Arnald of Villanova." *Journal of Medieval and Renaissance Studies* 1.1 (1971): 107–18.

Messer, Ellen. "Hot/Cold Classifications and Balancing Actions in Mesoamerican Diet and Health." In *The Body in Balance: Humoral Medicines in Practice*, edited by Peregrine Horden and Elisabeth Hsu, 149–67. New York: Berghahn Books, 2013.

Miller, Daniel, ed. *Materiality.* Durham, NC: Duke University Press, 2005.

Mitchell, Craig, Feng Ye, and Nigel Wiseman, trans. *Shang Han Lun: On Cold Dam- age.* Brookline, MA: Paradigm Publications, 1999.

Miura Kunio. "*Xianren.*" In *The Encyclopedia of Taoism*, edited by Fabrizio Pregadio, 1092–94. London: Routledge, 2008.

Miyakawa, Hisayuki. "An Outline of the Naitō Hypothesis and Its Effects on Japa- nese Studies of China." *Far Eastern Quarterly* 14.4 (1955): 533–52.

Miyashita Saburō 宮下三郎. "Zui-Tō jidai no iryō" 隋唐時代の医療. In *Chūgoku chūsei kagaku gijutsushi no kenkyū* 中国中世科学技術史の研究, edited by Yabuuchi Kiyoshi 藪内清, 259–88. Tokyo: Kadokawa Shoten, 1963.

Mollier, Christine. *Une apocalypse taoïste du Vᵉ siècle: le Livre des incantations divines des grottes abyssales.* Paris: Collège de France, Institut des Hautes Études Chi- noises, 1990.

———. "Visions of Evil: Demonology and Orthodoxy in Early Daoism." In *Daoism in History: Essays in Honour of Liu Ts'un-yan*, edited by Benjamin Penny, 74–100. London: Routledge, 2006.

———. *Buddhism and Taoism Face to Face: Scripture, Ritual, and Iconographic Exchange in Medieval China.* Honolulu: University of Hawai'i Press, 2008.

Mou Runsun 牟潤孫. "Duyao kukou" 毒藥苦口. In his *Haiyi zazhu* 海遺雜著, 437– 38. Hong Kong: Zhongwen Daxue Chubanshe, 1990.

Nappi, Carla. *The Monkey and the Inkpot: Natural History and Its Transformations in Early Modern China.* Cambridge, MA: Harvard University Press, 2009.

Needham, Joseph et al. *Science and Civilisation in China.* Vol. 5, *Chemistry and Chemical Technology.* Cambridge: Cambridge University Press, 1974 (pt. II), 1976 (pt. III), and 1980 (pt. IV).

Needham, Joseph, with the collaboration of Lu Gwei-Djen and edited by Nathan Sivin. *Science and Civilisation in China.* Vol. 6, pt. VI, *Medicine.* Cambridge: Cambridge University Press, 2000.

Nickerson, Peter. "The Great Petition for Sepulchral Plaints." In *Early Daoist Scriptures,* by Stephen Bokenkamp, 230–74. Berkeley: University of California Press, 1997.

Nugent, Christopher. *Manifest in Words, Written on Paper: Producing and Circulating Poetry in Tang Dynasty China.* Cambridge, MA: Harvard University Asia Center, 2010.

Nylan, Michael. *The Five "Confucian" Classics.* New Haven, CT: Yale University Press, 2001.

Obringer, Frédéric. *L'aconit et l'orpiment: Drogues et poisons en Chine ancienne et médiévale.* Paris: Fayard, 1997.

———. "A Song Innovation in Pharmacotherapy: Some Remarks on the Use of White Arsenic and Flowers of Arsenic." In *Innovation in Chinese Medicine,* edited by Elisabeth Hsu, 192–213. Cambridge: Cambridge University Press, 2001.

Okanishi Tameto 岡西為人. *Sō izen iki kō* 宋以前醫籍考. Beijing: Renmin Weisheng Chubanshe, 1958.

Parascandola, John. "The Drug Habit: The Association of the Word 'Drug' with Abuse in American History." In *Drugs and Narcotics in History,* edited by Roy Porter and Mikuláš Teich, 156–67. Cambridge: Cambridge University Press, 1995.

———. *King of Poisons: A History of Arsenic.* Washington, DC: Potomac Books, 2012.

Pettit, J. E. E. "Learning from Maoshan: Temple Construction in Early Medieval China." PhD diss., Indiana University, 2013.

Pollan, Michael. *How to Change Your Mind: What the New Science of Psychedelics Teaches Us about Consciousness, Dying, Addiction, Depression, and Transcendence.* New York: Penguin Press, 2018.

Pomata, Gianna. *Contracting a Cure: Patients, Healers, and the Law in Early Modern Bologna.* Baltimore: Johns Hopkins University Press, 1998.

———. "Observation Rising: Birth of an Epistemic Genre, 1500–1650." In *Histories of Scientific Observation,* edited by Lorraine Daston and Elizabeth Lunbeck, 45–80. Chicago: University of Chicago Press, 2011.

———. "The Medical Case Narrative: Distant Reading of an Epistemic Genre." *Literature and Medicine* 32.1 (2014): 1–23.

———. "The Medical Case Narrative in Pre-Modern Europe and China: Comparative History of an Epistemic Genre." In *A Historical Approach to Casuistry: Norms and Exceptions in a Comparative Perspective,* edited by Carlo Ginzburg and Lucio Biasiori, 15–46. London: Bloomsbury Academic, 2019.

Poo, Mu-chou 蒲慕州. "The Concept of Ghost in Ancient Chinese Religion." In *Religion and Chinese Society.* Vol. I: *Ancient and Medieval China,* edited by John Lagerwey, 173–91. Hong Kong: Chinese University Press, 2004.

Poo Mu-chou. "Wugu zhi huo de zhengzhi yiyi" 巫蠱之禍的政治意義. *Zhongyang yanjiuyuan lishi yuyan yanjiusuo jikan* 中央研究院歷史語言研究所集刊 57.3 (1987): 511–38.

Porkert, Manfred. *The Theoretical Foundations of Chinese Medicine: Systems of Correspondence*. Cambridge, MA: MIT Press, 1974.

Pregadio, Fabrizio. "Elixirs and Alchemy." In *Daoism Handbook*, edited by Livia Kohn, 165–95. Leiden, Netherlands: Brill, 2000.

———. "The Early History of the *Zhouyi cantong qi*." *Journal of Chinese Religions* 30 (2002): 149–76.

———. *Great Clarity: Daoism and Alchemy in Early Medieval China*. Stanford, CA: Stanford University Press, 2006.

———. "Which Is the Daoist Immortal Body?" *Micrologus* 26 (2018): 385–407.

———. "Seeking Immortality in Ge Hong's *Baopuzi Neipian*." In *Dao Companion to Xuanxue* 玄學 *(Neo-Daoism)*, edited by David Chai, 427–56. Cham, Switzerland: Springer, 2020.

Puett, Michael. "The Ethics of Responding Properly: The Notion of *Qing* 情 in Early Chinese Thought." In *Love and Emotions in Traditional Chinese Literature*, edited by Halvor Eifring, 37–68. Leiden, Netherlands: Brill, 2004.

Qi Dongfang 齊東方 and Shen Qinyan 申秦雁. *Huawu da Tang chun* 花舞大唐春. Beijing: Wenwu Chubanshe, 2003.

Qiu Guangming 丘光明. *Zhongguo lidai duliangheng kao* 中國歷代度量衡考. Beijing: Kexue Chubanshe, 1992.

Rao, Yi, Runhong Li, and Daqing Zhang. "A Drug from Poison: How the Therapeutic Effect of Arsenic Trioxide on Acute Promyelocytic Leukemia Was Discovered." *Science China: Life Sciences* 56.6 (2013): 495–502.

Rao Zongyi 饒宗頤. *Zhongguo shixue shang zhi zhengtong lun—Zhongguo shixue guannian tantao zhiyi* 中國史學上之正統論—中國史學觀念探討之一. Hong Kong: Longmen Shudian, 1977.

Ren Yucai 任育才. "Tangdai de yiliao zuzhi yu yixue jiaoyu" 唐代的醫療組織與醫學教育. In *Zhongyang yanjiuyuan guoji hanxue huiyi lunwen ji (Lishi kaogu zu)* 中央研究院國際漢學會議論文集（歷史考古組）, 449–73. Taipei: Zhongyang Yanjiu Yuan, 1980.

Richter, Antje, and Charles Chace. "The Trouble with Wang Xizhi: Illness and Healing in a Fourth-Century Chinese Correspondence." *T'oung Pao* 103.1–3 (2017): 33–93.

Riddle, John. *Dioscorides on Pharmacy and Medicine*. Austin: University of Texas Press, 1985.

Rinella, Michael. *Pharmakon: Plato, Drug Culture, and Identity in Ancient Athens*. Lanham, MD: Lexington Books, 2011.

Robinet, Isabelle. "Metamorphosis and Deliverance from the Corpse in Taoism." *History of Religions* 19.1 (1979): 37–70.

———. *Taoism: Growth of a Religion*. Translated by Phyllis Brooks. Stanford, CA: Stanford University Press, 1997.

Rong Xinjiang. *Eighteen Lectures on Dunhuang*. Translated by Imre Galambos. Leiden, Netherlands: Brill, 2013.

Rosenberg, Charles E. *Explaining Epidemics and Other Studies in the History of Medicine*. Cambridge: Cambridge University Press, 1992.

Sakade Yoshinobu 坂出祥伸, ed. *Chūgoku kodai yōjō shisō no sōgōteki kenkyū* 中国古代養生思想の総合的研究. Tokyo: Hirakawa Shuppansha, 1988.

———. "Zui-Tō jidai niokeru shōnyūseki fukuyō no ryūkō nitsuite" 隋唐時代における鐘乳石服用の流行について. In *Chūgoku kodai kagaku shiron* 中國古代科學史論, edited by Yamada Keiji 山田慶兒 and Tanaka Tan 田中淡, 615–44. Kyoto: Kyoto Daigaku Jinbun Kagaku Kenkyūsho, 1989.

———. *Chūgoku shisō kenkyū: Iyaku yōjō, kagaku shisō hen* 中國思想研究: 醫藥養生・科學思想篇. Osaka: Kansai Daigaku Shuhanbu, 1999.

Salguero, C. Pierce. "The Buddhist Medicine King in Literary Context: Reconsidering an Early Medieval Example of Indian Influence on Chinese Medicine and Surgery." *History of Religions* 48.3 (2009): 183–210.

———. *Translating Buddhist Medicine in Medieval China*. Philadelphia: University of Pennsylvania Press, 2014.

Satō Toshiyuki 佐藤利行. "Ō Gishi to Goseki San" 王羲之と五石散. *Hiroshima daigaku daigakuin bungaku kenkyūka ronshū* 広島大学大学院文学研究科論集 65.1 (2005): 1–13.

Schafer, Edward H. *The Golden Peaches of Samarkand: A Study of T'ang Exotics*. Berkeley: University of California Press, 1963.

———. *The Vermilion Bird: T'ang Images of the South*. Berkeley: University of California Press, 1967.

———. "The Transcendent Vitamin: Efflorescence of Lang-kan." *Chinese Science* 3 (1978): 27–38.

Scheid, Volker. *Chinese Medicine in Contemporary China: Plurality and Synthesis*. Durham, NC: Duke University Press, 2002.

Schipper, Kristofer. *The Taoist Body*. Translated by Karen C. Duval. Berkeley: University of California Press, 1994.

Shaanxi Sheng Bowuguan Geweihui Xiezuo Xiaozu 陝西省博物館革委會寫作小組. "Xi'an nanjiao Hejiacun faxian Tangdai jiaocang wenwu" 西安南郊何家村發現唐代窖藏文物. *Wenwu* 文物 1 (1972): 30–42.

Shang Zhijun 尚志鈞. "*Leigong paozhi lun* youguan wenxian yanjiu"《雷公炮炙論》有關文獻研究. In *Leigong paozhi lun* 雷公炮炙論, edited by Shang Zhijun, 139–43. Hefei: Anhui Kexue Jishu Chubanshe, 1991.

Shaughnessy, Edward L., trans. *I Ching: The Classic of Changes*. New York: Ballantine Books, 1996.

Shen Ruiwen 沈睿文. *An Lushan fusan kao* 安祿山服散考. Shanghai: Shanghai Guji Chubanshe, 2015.

Shi Zhicheng 史志誠. "Zhongguo gudai duzi jiqi xiangguan cihui kao" 中國古代毒字及其相關詞彙考. *Dulixue shi yanjiu wenji* 毒理學史研究文集 3 (2004): 1–9.

Shirakawa Shizuka 白川靜. "Biko kankei jisetsu—Chūgoku kodai niokeru jujutsu girei no ichimen" 媚蠱關係字説—中国古代における呪術儀禮の一面. In his *Kōkotsu kinbungaku ronshū* 甲骨金文学論集, 443–503. Kyoto: Hōyū Shoten, 1974.

Siraisi, Nancy. *Medieval and Early Renaissance Medicine: An Introduction to Knowledge and Practice*. Chicago: University of Chicago Press, 1990.

Sivin, Nathan. "A Seventh-Century Chinese Medical Case History." *Bulletin of the History of Medicine* 41.3 (1967): 267–73.

———. *Chinese Alchemy: Preliminary Studies.* Cambridge, MA: Harvard University Press, 1968.

———. "Chinese Alchemy and the Manipulation of Time." *Isis* 67.4 (1976): 512–26.

———. *Traditional Medicine in Contemporary China: A Partial Translation of Revised Outline of Chinese Medicine (1972) with an Introductory Study on Change in Present-Day and Early Medicine.* Ann Arbor: Center for Chinese Studies, University of Michigan, 1987.

———. "On the Limits of Empirical Knowledge in Chinese and Western Science." In *Rationality in Question: On Eastern and Western Views of Rationality*, edited by Shlomo Biderman and Ben-Ami Scharfstein, 165–89. Leiden, Netherlands: Brill, 1989.

———. "On the Word 'Taoist' as a Source of Perplexity. With Special Reference to the Relations of Science and Religion in Traditional China." In *Medicine, Philosophy and Religion in Ancient China: Researches and Reflections*, 303–30. Aldershot, UK: Variorum, 1995.

———. "Taoism and Science." In *Medicine, Philosophy and Religion in Ancient China: Researches and Reflections*, ch. VII, 1–72. Aldershot, UK: Variorum, 1995.

———. "Text and Experience in Classical Chinese Medicine." In *Knowledge and the Scholarly Medical Traditions*, edited by Don Bates, 177–204. Cambridge: Cambridge University Press, 1995.

———. *Health Care in Eleventh-Century China.* New York: Springer, 2015.

Skar, Lowell, and Fabrizio Pregadio. "Inner Alchemy (*Neidan*)." In *Daoism Handbook*, edited by Livia Kohn, 464–97. Leiden, Netherlands: Brill, 2000.

Smith, Hilary. *Forgotten Disease: Illnesses Transformed in Chinese Medicine.* Stanford, CA: Stanford University Press, 2017.

Smith, Paul Jakov, and Richard von Glahn, eds. *The Song-Yuan-Ming Transition in Chinese History.* Cambridge, MA: Harvard University Asia Center, 2003.

Stanley-Baker, Michael. "Cultivating Body, Cultivating Self: A Critical Translation and History of the Tang Dynasty *Yangxing yanming lu* 養性延命錄 (Records of Cultivating Nature and Extending Life)." Master's thesis, Indiana University, 2006.

———. "Daoists and Doctors: The Role of Medicine in Six Dynasties Shangqing Daoism." PhD diss., University College London, 2013.

———. "*Ge xianweng zhouhou beiji fang.*" In *Daozang jiyao Catalogue*, edited by Vincent Goossaert, Elena Valussi, and Lai Chi Tim. Hong Kong: Chinese University of Hong Kong Press, forthcoming.

Steavu, Dominic. "Paratextuality, Materiality, and Corporeality in Medieval Chinese Religions: Talismans (*fu*) and Diagrams (*tu*)." *Journal of Medieval Worlds* 1.4 (2019): 11–40.

Sterckx, Roel. *The Animal and the Daemon in Early China.* Albany: State University of New York Press, 2002.

———. *Food, Sacrifice, and Sagehood in Early China.* Cambridge: Cambridge University Press, 2011.

Stevenson, Lloyd. *The Meaning of Poison*. Lawrence: University of Kansas Press, 1959.

Strickmann, Michel. "The Mao Shan Revelations: Taoism and the Aristocracy." *T'oung Pao* 63.1 (1977): 1–64.

———. "On the Alchemy of T'ao Hung-ching." In *Facets of Taoism: Essays in Chinese Religion*, edited by Holmes Welch and Anna Seidel, 123–92. New Haven, CT: Yale University Press, 1979.

———. *Chinese Magical Medicine*. Edited by Bernard Faure. Stanford, CA: Stanford University Press, 2002.

Tackett, Nicolas. *The Origins of the Chinese Nation: Song China and the Forging of an East Asian World Order*. Cambridge: Cambridge University Press, 2017.

Tambiah, Stanley. *Magic, Science, Religion, and the Scope of Rationality*. Cambridge: Cambridge University Press, 1990.

Tang Yongtong 湯用彤. *Wei-Jin xuanxue lungao* 魏晉玄學論稿. Beijing: Renmin Chubanshe, 1957.

Taylor, Kim. *Chinese Medicine in Early Communist China, 1945–1963: A Medicine of Revolution*. London: RoutledgeCurzon, 2005.

Temkin, Owsei. "The Scientific Approach to Disease: Specific Entity and Individual Sickness." In *Scientific Change: Historical Studies in the Intellectual, Social and Technical Conditions for Scientific Discovery and Technical Innovation, from Antiquity to the Present*, edited by A. C. Crombie, 629–47. New York: Basic Books, 1963.

Tian, Xiaofei. *Tao Yuanming and Manuscript Culture: The Record of a Dusty Table*. Seattle: University of Washington Press, 2005.

Tōdō Akiyasu 藤堂明保. *Kanji gogen jiten* 漢字語源辞典. Tokyo: Gakutōsha, 1965.

Tomes, Nancy. *Remaking the American Patient: How Madison Avenue and Modern Medicine Turned Patients into Consumers*. Chapel Hill: University of North Carolina Press, 2016.

Touwaide, Alain. "Les poisons dans le monde antique et byzantin: introduction à une analyse systémique." *Revue d'histoire de la pharmacie* 290 (1991): 265–81.

Tsien, Tsuen-hsuin. *Written on Bamboo and Silk: The Beginnings of Chinese Books and Inscriptions*. Chicago: University of Chicago Press, 2004.

Tu Feng-en 涂豐恩. *Jiuming—Ming-Qing Zhongguo de yisheng yu bingren* 救命—明清中國的醫生與病人. Taipei: Sanmin Shuju, 2012.

Twitchett, Denis, and Michael Loewe, eds. *The Cambridge History of China*. Vol. 1: *The Ch'in and Han Empires, 221 B.C.–A.D. 220*. Cambridge: Cambridge University Press, 1986.

Unschuld, Paul U. "Zur Bedeutung des Terminus *tu* 毒 in der traditionellen medizinisch-pharmazeutischen Literatur Chinas." *Sudhoffs Archiv* 59.2 (1975): 165–83.

———. "Ma-wang-tui *Materia Medica*: A Comparative Analysis of Early Chinese Pharmaceutical Knowledge." *Zinbun: Memoirs of the Research Institute for Humanistic Studies, Kyoto University* 18 (1982): 11–63.

———. *Medicine in China: A History of Pharmaceutics*. Berkeley: University of California Press, 1986.

———. "Traditional Chinese Medicine: Some Historical and Epistemological Reflections." *Social Science & Medicine* 24.12 (1987): 1023–29.

———. *Huang Di nei jing su wen: Nature, Knowledge, Imagery in an Ancient Chinese Medical Text.* Berkeley: University of California Press, 2003.

van Schaik, Sam, and Imre Galambos. *Manuscripts and Travellers: The Sino-Tibetan Documents of a Tenth-Century Buddhist Pilgrim.* Berlin: De Gruyter, 2012.

Vogel, Hans Ulrich, and Günter Dux, eds. *Concepts of Nature: A Chinese-European Cross-Cultural Perspective.* Leiden, Netherlands: Brill, 2010.

von Glahn, Richard. *The Sinister Way: The Divine and the Demonic in Chinese Religious Culture.* Berkeley: University of California Press, 2004.

———. *The Economic History of China: From Antiquity to the Nineteenth Century.* Cambridge: Cambridge University Press, 2016.

Wagner, Rudolf G. "Lebensstil und Drogen im Chinesischen Mittelalter." *T'oung Pao* 59.1 (1973): 79–178.

———. *Language, Ontology, and Political Philosophy in China: Wang Bi's Scholarly Exploration of the Dark (Xuanxue).* Albany: State University of New York, 2003.

Wang Jiakui 王家葵. *Tao Hongjing congkao* 陶弘景叢考. Jinan: Qilu Shushe, 2003.

Wang Jiakui and Zhang Ruixian 張瑞賢. *"Shennong bencao jing" yanjiu*《神農本草經》研究. Beijing: Beijing Kexue Jishu Chubanshe, 2001.

Wang Jiakui, Zhang Ruixian, and Yin Hai 銀海. *"Xinxiu bencao zuanxiu renyuan kao"*《新修本草》纂修人員考. *Zhonghua yishi zazhi* 中華醫史雜誌 30.4 (2000): 200–204.

Wang Kuike 王奎克. "'Wushi San' xinkao" "五石散" 新考. In *Zhongguo gudai huaxueshi yanjiu* 中國古代化學史研究, edited by Zhao Kuanghua 趙匡華, 80–87. Beijing: Beijing Daxue Chubanshe, 1985.

Wang Kuike et al. "Shen de lishi zai Zhongguo" 砷的歷史在中國. In *Zhongguo gudai huaxueshi yanjiu*, edited by Zhao Kuanghua, 14–38. Beijing: Beijing Daxue Chubanshe, 1985.

Wang Ming-ke 王明珂. "Nüren, bujie yu cunzhai rentong: Minjiang shangyou de duyaomao gushi" 女人、不潔與村寨認同: 岷江上游的毒藥貓故事. *Zhongyang yanjiuyuan lishi yuyan yanjiusuo jikan* 中央研究院歷史語言研究所集刊 70.3 (1999): 699–738.

Wang Yongxing 王永興. "Tangdai tugong ziliao xinian—Tangdai tugong yanjiu zhiyi" 唐代土貢資料系年—唐代土貢研究之一. *Beijing daxue xuebao* 北京大學學報 4 (1982): 60–65, 59.

Weatherall, Miles. "Drug Therapies." In *Companion Encyclopedia of the History of Medicine*, vol. 2, edited by W. F. Bynum and Roy Porter, 915–38. London: Routledge, 1993.

Webster, Charles. *Paracelsus: Medicine, Magic and Mission at the End of Time.* New Haven, CT: Yale University Press, 2008.

Wei Bing 韋兵. "Cong *Zhangming xian fuzi ji* kan Songdai shidafu dui fuzi de renshi" 從《彰明縣附子記》看宋代士大夫對附子的認識. In *Songshi yanjiu lunwen ji* 宋史研究論文集, edited by Deng Xiaonan 鄧小南 et al., 310–22. Zhengzhou: Henan Daxue Chubanshe, 2014.

Weitz, Ankeney. *Zhou Mi's "Record of Clouds and Mist Passing before One's Eyes": An Annotated Translation.* Leiden, Netherlands: Brill, 2002.

Whorton, James. *The Arsenic Century: How Victorian Britain Was Poisoned at Home, Work, and Play*. Oxford: Oxford University Press, 2010.

Whyte, Susan Reynolds, Sjaak van der Geest, and Anita Hardon, eds. *Social Lives of Medicines*. Cambridge: Cambridge University Press, 2002.

Wilms, Sabine. *The Divine Farmer's Classic of Materia Medica: Shen Nong Bencao Jing*. Corbett, OR: Happy Goat Productions, 2016.

Xing, Wen. "The Hexagram *Gu*." In *Chinese Medicine and Healing: An Illustrated History*, edited by TJ Hinrichs and Linda Barnes, 20–21. Cambridge, MA: Belknap Press of Harvard University Press, 2013.

Yamada Keiji 山田慶兒. "The Formation of the *Huang-ti Nei-ching*." *Acta Asiatica* 36 (1979): 67–89.

———. "Hongzō no kigen" 本草の起源. In *Chūgoku kodai kagaku shiron* 中國古代科學史論, edited by Yamada Keiji and Tanaka Tan, 451–567. Kyoto: Kyoto Daigaku Jinbun Kagaku Kenkyūsho, 1989.

———. *Honzō to yume to renkinjutsu to—Busshitsuteki sōzōryoku no genshōgaku* 本草と夢と錬金術と—物質的想像力の現象学. Tokyo: Asahi Shinbunsha, 1997.

Yamada, Toshiaki. "Longevity Techniques and the Compilation of the *Lingbao wufuxu*." In *Taoist Meditation and Longevity Techniques*, edited by Livia Kohn in cooperation with Yoshinobu Sakade, 99–124. Ann Arbor: Center for Chinese Studies, University of Michigan, 1989.

Yan Qiyan 嚴奇岩. "Cong Tangdai gongpin yaocai kan Sichuan didao yaocai" 從唐代貢品藥材看四川地道藥材. *Zhonghua yishi zazhi* 中華醫史雜誌 33.2 (2003): 76–81.

Yang, Dolly. "Prescribing 'Guiding and Pulling': The Institutionalisation of Therapeutic Exercise in Sui China (581–618 CE)." PhD diss., University College London, 2018.

Yang, Yong, and Miranda Brown. "The Wuwei Medical Manuscripts: A Brief Introduction and Translation." *Early China* 40 (2017): 241–301.

Yates, Frances A. *Giordano Bruno and the Hermetic Tradition*. Chicago: University of Chicago Press, 1964.

Yokote Yutaka. "Daoist Internal Alchemy." In *Modern Chinese Religion I: Song-Liao-Jin-Yuan (960–1368 AD)*, vol. 2, edited by John Lagerwey and Pierre Marsone, 1053–1110. Leiden, Netherlands: Brill, 2014.

Yoshikawa Tadao 吉川忠夫. "Seishitsu kō" 靜室考. *Tōhō gakuhō* 東方学報 59 (1987): 125–62.

Yu Gengzhe 于賡哲. *Tangdai jibing, yiliaoshi chutan* 唐代疾病、醫療史初探. Beijing: Zhongguo Shehui Kexue Chubanshe, 2011.

Yu Jiaxi 余嘉錫. "Hanshi San kao" 寒食散考 (1938). In *Yu Jiaxi lunxue zazhu* 余嘉錫論學雜著, 181–226. Beijing: Zhonghua Shuju, 1963.

Yu Shuenn-Der 余舜德, ed. *Tiwu ruwei: Wu yu shentigan de yanjiu* 體物入微：物與身體感的研究. Hsinchu: Guoli Qinghua Daxue Chubanshe, 2008.

Yu Xin 余欣. *Zhonggu yixiang: Xieben shidai de xueshu, xinyang yu shehui* 中古異相：寫本時代的學術、信仰與社會. Shanghai: Shanghai Guji Chubanshe, 2011.

Yu Yan 余巖. *Gudai jibing minghou shuyi* 古代疾病名候疏義. Beijing: Renmin Weisheng Chubanshe, 1953.

———. "Duyao bian" 毒藥辨 (1928). In *Yixue geming lunxuan* 醫學革命論選, 1–4. Taipei: Yiwen Yinshuguan, 1976.

Yü, Ying-shih. "Life and Immortality in the Mind of Han China." *Harvard Journal of Asiatic Studies* 25 (1964–65): 80–122.

———. "Individualism and the Neo-Taoist Movement in Wei-Chin China." In *Individualism and Holism: Studies in Confucian and Taoist Values*, edited by Donald J. Munro, 121–56. Ann Arbor: Center for Chinese Studies, University of Michigan, 1985.

Zhang Guangda 張廣達. "Neiteng Hunan de Tang-Song biange shuo jiqi yingxiang" 內藤湖南的唐宋變革說及其影響. *Tang yanjiu* 唐研究 11 (2005): 5–71.

Zhang Jiafeng 張嘉鳳. "'Jiyi' yu 'xiangran': yi *Zhubing yuanhou lun* wei zhongxin shilun Wei-Jin zhi Sui-Tang zhijian yiji de jibingguan" 「疾疫」與「相染」：以《諸病源候論》為中心試論魏晉至隋唐之間醫籍的疾病觀. In *Jibing de lishi* 疾病的歷史, edited by Lin Fu-shih 林富士, 157–99. Taipei: Lianjing Chuban Shiye Gufen Youxian Gongsi, 2011.

Zhang Ruixian, Wang Jiakui, and Michael Stanley-Baker. "The Earliest Stone Medical Inscription." In *Imagining Chinese Medicine*, edited by Vivienne Lo and Penelope Barrett, 373–88. Leiden, Netherlands: Brill, 2018.

Zhang Zhibin 張志斌. *Zhongguo gudai yibing liuxing nianbiao* 中國古代疫病流行年表. Fuzhou: Fujian Kexue Jishu Chubanshe, 2007.

Zhao Kuanghua 趙匡華. "Woguo gudai 'chousha liangong' de yanjin jiqi huaxue chengjiu" 我國古代 "抽砂煉汞" 的演進及其化學成就. In *Zhongguo gudai huaxueshi yanjiu* 中國古代化學史研究, edited by Zhao Kuanghua, 128–53. Beijing: Beijing Daxue Chubanshe, 1985.

Zheng Binglin 鄭炳林 and Dang Xinling 黨新玲. "Tangdai Dunhuang sengyi kao" 唐代敦煌僧醫考. *Dunhuang xue* 敦煌學 20 (1995): 31–46.

Zheng Binglin and Gao Wei 高偉. "Cong Dunhuang wenshu kan Tang-Wudai Dunhuang diqu de yishi zhuangkuang" 從敦煌文書看唐五代敦煌地區的醫事狀況. *Xibei minzu xueyuan xuebao* 西北民族學院學報 1 (1997): 68–73.

Zheng Jinsheng 鄭金生. *Yaolin waishi* 藥林外史. Taipei: Sanmin Shuju, 2005.

Zheng Jinsheng, Nalini Kirk, Paul D. Buell, and Paul U. Unschuld, eds. *Dictionary of the Ben Cao Gang Mu. Vol. 3: Persons and Literary Sources.* Berkeley: University of California Press, 2018.

Zheng, Yangwen. *The Social Life of Opium in China.* Cambridge: Cambridge University Press, 2005.

Zhong Guofa 鍾國發. *Tao Hongjing pingzhuan* 陶弘景評傳. Nanjing: Nanjing Daxue Chubanshe, 2005.

Zhou Zuofeng 周左鋒. "*Tang liudian* jizai de tugong yaocai fenxi"《唐六典》記載的土貢藥材分析. *Jiangxi zhongyi xueyuan xuebao* 江西中醫學院學報 23.4 (2011): 13–18.

Zuo, Ya. *Shen Gua's Empiricism.* Cambridge, MA: Harvard University Asia Center, 2018.

INDEX

Ingram Content Group UK Ltd.
Milton Keynes UK
UKHW010640220323
418970UK00005B/312